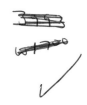
Diagnosis and Management of
Liver Disease

Diagnosis and Management of Liver Disease

Edited by

Ralph Kirsch

Medical Research Council
Liver Research Centre
University of Cape Town, South Africa

Simon Robson

Medical Research Council
Liver Research Centre
University of Cape Town, South Africa

and

Charles Trey

Gastroenterology Associates PC
Massachusetts, USA

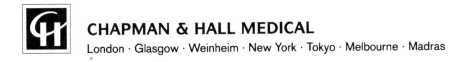

CHAPMAN & HALL MEDICAL
London · Glasgow · Weinheim · New York · Tokyo · Melbourne · Madras

Published by Chapman & Hall, 2–6 Boundary Row, London SE1 8HN, UK

Chapman & Hall, 2–6 Boundary Row, London SE1 8HN, UK

Blackie Academic & Professional, Wester Cleddens Road, Bishopbriggs, Glasgow G64 2NZ, UK

Chapman & Hall GmbH, Pappelallee 3, 69469 Weinheim, Germany

Chapman & Hall USA, One Penn Plaza, 41st Floor, New York NY 10119, USA

Chapman & Hall Japan, Kyowa Building, 3F, 2-2-1 Hirakawacho, Chiyoda-ku, Tokyo 102, Japan

Chapman & Hall Australia, Thomas Nelson Australia, 102 Dodds Street, South Melbourne, Victoria 3205, Australia

Chapman & Hall India, R. Seshadri, 32 Second Main Road, CIT East, Madras 600 035, India

First edition 1995

© 1995 Chapman & Hall

Typeset in 10pt Palatino by Saxon Graphics Ltd, Derby

Printed in Great Britain at the Alden Press, Oxford

ISBN 0 412 57570 1

A catalogue record for this book is available from the British Library

Library of Congress Catalog Card Number: 94-69670

∞ Printed on acid-free text paper, manufactured with ANSI/NISO Z39.48-1992 and ANSI/NISO Z39.48-1984 (Permanence of Paper).

Contents

Colour plates appear between pages 80 and 81

Contents

Contents

Contents

Contents

List of contributors

Dr Susan Adams
MRC/UCT Liver Research Centre, Department of Medicine, University of Cape Town, Observatory 7925, South Africa

Professor Irwin Arias
Department of Physiology, Tufts University, Boston, Massachusetts 02111, USA.

Professor Nathan Bass
Division of Gastroenterology, 1120 Health Sciences West, Box 0538, San Francisco, CA 94143, USA

Dr Steve Beningfield
Department of Radiology, Groote Schuur Hospital, Observatory 7925, South Africa

Professor Lawrence Blendis
Room 223, 9th Floor, Eaton Wing, Toronto General Hospital, Toronto, Canada

Professor Tom Bothwell
Department of Medicine, University of the Witwatersrand, 7 York Road, Parktown 2194, Johannesburg, South Africa

Professor Ian Bouchier
Department of Medicine, Royal Infirmary, Lauriston Place, Edinburgh EH3 9YW, UK

Dr Tom Boyer
Emory University School of Medicine, Division of Digestive Disease, Drawer, AL, Atlanta, GA 30322, USA

Dr Morag Chisholm
Department of Haematology, Southampton General Hospital, Southampton SO9 4XY, UK

Professor Harold Conn
VA Hospital, West Spring Street, West Haven, Connecticut 06516, USA

Ms Collette Cywes
MRC/UCT Liver Research Centre, Department of Medicine, University of Cape Town, Observatory 7925, South Africa

Dr Geoffrey Dusheiko
Department of Medicine, Royal Free Hospital, Hampstead, London NW3 2QG, UK

Professor Mario Ehlers
Department of Biochemistry, Medical School, University of Cape Town, Observatory 7925, South Africa

Professor Jack Franks
Department of Anesthesiology, Vanderbilt University, Nashville, TN 37232, USA

Dr Pauline Hall
Department of Pathology, Flinders Medical Centre, South Australia 5042

Dr Richard Hift
MRC/UCT Liver Research Centre, Department of Medicine, University of Cape Town, Observatory 7925, South Africa

Professor Michael James
Department of Anaesthetics, Groote Schuur Hospital, Observatory 7925, South Africa

Professor Kasimir Jaskiewicz
Department of Anatomical Pathology, Medical School, University of Cape Town, Observatory 7925, South Africa

Professor Delawir Kahn
Renal Unit, Groote Schuur Hospital, Observatory 7925, South Africa

Dr Jay Kambam
Department of Anesthesiology, Vanderbilt University, Nashville, TN 37232, USA

Professor Michael Kew
Department of Medicine, University of the
Witwatersrand, 7 York Road, Parktown 2194,
South Africa

Professor Ralph Kirsch
MRC/UCT Liver Research Centre, Department
of Medicine, University of Cape Town,
Observatory 7925, South Africa

Professor Jake Krige
Department of Surgery, University of Cape
Town, Observatory 7925, South Africa

Dr Didier Lebrec
Liver Research Unit, L'hôpital de Beaujon,
Clichy, Cedex 92118, France

Dr Eric Lemmer
Department of Gastroenterology, Groote
Schuur Hospital, Observatory 7925, South
Africa

Professor Neil McIntyre
Department of Medicine, Royal Free Hospital,
Hampstead, London NW3 2QG, UK

Dr Peter Meissner
MRC/UCT Liver Research Centre, Department
of Medicine, University of Cape Town,
Observatory 7925, South Africa

Dr James Neuberger
The Liver Unit, The Queen Elizabeth Hospital,
Edgbaston, Birmingham B15 2TH, UK

Professor Stephen O'Keefe
Department of Gastroenterology, Groote
Schuur Hospital, Observatory 7925, South
Africa

Professor Lawrie Powell
Department of Medicine, Royal Brisbane
Hospital, Brisbane 4029, Australia

Dr Caroline Riely
University of Tennessee, Rm 555D, Memphis,
TN 38163, USA

Professor Simon Robson
MRC/UCT Liver Research Centre, Department
of Medicine, University of Cape Town,
Observatory 7925, South Africa

Professor Rudi Schmid
School of Medicine, University of California,
San Francisco, CA 94143, USA

Professor David Shafritz
Liver Research Center, Albert Einstein College
of Medicine, 13 Morris Park Avenue, Bronx,
NY 10461, USA

Professor Ahmed Simjee
Department of Medicine, University of Natal,
PO Box 17039, Congella 4013, South Africa

Dr Wendy Spearman
MRC/UCT Liver Research Centre, Department
of Medicine, University of Cape Town,
Observatory 7925, South Africa

Professor Thomas Starzl
Department of Surgery, School of Medicine,
University of Pittsburgh, 3601 Fifth Avenue,
Pittsburgh, PA 15123, USA

Professor John Terblanche
Department of Surgery, University of Cape
Town, Observatory 7925, South Africa

Professor Charles Trey
Department of Gastroenterology, New
England Deaconess Hospital, Harvard Medical
School, Boston, MA 02215, USA

Dr Anton van Wyk
MRC/UCT Liver Research Centre, Department
of Medicine, University of Cape Town,
Observatory 7925, South Africa

Dr Michael Voigt
MRC/UCT Liver Research Centre, Department
of Medicine, University of Cape Town,
Observatory 7925, South Africa

Professor Roger Williams
Liver Unit, King's College Hospital, London
SE5 8RX, UK

Preface

Our aim in producing this book was to provide our readers with an easy to read, relatively short volume containing the information required to manage most patients with liver disease. In doing so we have tried to fill the ever increasing gap between the chapter or two on hepatology in general medical text books, which are usually insufficient, and the detailed texts on liver and biliary diseases which may be too detailed for those practicing or studying internal medicine or gastroenterology. We were further encouraged to produce this book after finding that the four volumes of its predecessor, *Liver Update 1991*, in our university library had had to be replaced because they had literally become worn out.

In order to maintain a relatively constant style and approach we decided that each chapter should, in the first instance, be prepared by a member of the Medical Research Council/ University of Cape Town Liver Research Centre and that these 'first drafts' then be sent to authorities in each field who would add, delete or, where necessary, rewrite the text until they were satisfied with the end result. We were responsible for the final edit. Because many of the recent advances in hepatology require a background knowledge of modern immunology and molecular biology we have included chapters aimed at introducing our readers to these areas. We are indebted to our colleagues, not only for meeting our deadlines, but also for agreeing to donate their royalties to a fund which will allow persons disadvantaged by apartheid to study the liver. We also wish to thank the Medical Research Council of South Africa and the University of Cape Town for their continued support. This book would not have been possible without the constant help and many additional hours of work by Isabel Batho and Lavinia Petersen. Finally, we would like to thank our publisher, Peter Altman, for his commitment to this project and his willingness to help us at all times.

REK
SCR
CT
Cape Town, 1994

Clinical evaluation of liver disease

RALPH KIRSCH, SIMON ROBSON and NATHAN BASS

INTRODUCTION

The evaluation of liver function requires the rational combination of the clinical examination with laboratory tests, radiological imaging and liver histology. In each instance the clinical findings will 'call the tune'. Thus minimal jaundice in a healthy young man may require little more than a blood count, serum bilirubin and liver enzymes to confirm the diagnosis of Gilbert's syndrome, while icterus in an ill, middle-aged person complaining of chills, abdominal pain and itching will require a combination of biochemical and imaging techniques in order to diagnose a stone in the common bile duct.

The clinical evaluation must always seek to identify potentially treatable conditions, such as Wilson's disease and hemochromatosis, even although these are rare, and must exclude infections or iatrogenic factors known to influence the health of patients with deranged liver function. A proper evaluation should lead not only to a diagnosis but also to a reasonably accurate prognosis. The latter has become increasingly important with the advent of organ replacement since it is vital in determining the optimal time for liver transplantation.

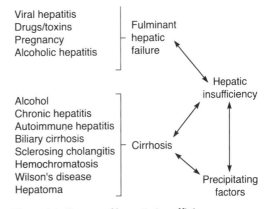

Figure 1.1 Causes of hepatic insufficiency

In this chapter the clinical features of hepatic insufficiency are described. This is followed by chapters on the biochemical, radiological and histological assessment of liver function.

Hepatic insufficiency is the final common pathway down which patients with any form of liver disease may travel (Fig. 1.1). It may arise acutely, as in fulminant viral hepatitis, fatty liver of pregnancy or paracetamol toxicity or may, as in alcoholic cirrhosis or chronic hepatitis, develop over many years.

The progression of the disease may be intermittent because of varying alcohol consumption or modification of its natural history by treatment with corticosteroids. Clinical presentation may occur at any time during this period of progression to cirrhosis, often as a result of a temporary exacerbation of hepatocellular damage or because of an incidental clinical or laboratory finding. Unfortunately the usual presentation is with hepatocellular failure or portal hypertension. In such patients the disease is well advanced. It is obviously important to recognize patients in the latent phase of their disease or before cirrhosis has supervened. Thus liver disease should be actively sought in:

1. Patients presenting with features of alcohol abuse such as depression, malnutrition, vitamin deficiency, gastritis, pancreatitis, peptic ulceration, peripheral neuropathy, anorexia or loss of libido.
2. Patients with autoimmune or connective tissue disorders, inflammatory bowel disease and sarcoidosis.
3. Patients with neurological features of Wilson's disease or the diabetes or endocrinopathy of hemochromatosis. These may occur prior to established, clinically obvious liver disease.
4. Patients with incidental physical findings such as spider nevi, Dupuytren's contracture, gynecomastia, pigmentation or hepatosplenomegaly.
5. Patients with abnormal liver function tests, positive autoantibodies or markers of viral infection.
6. Relatives of patients with familial disorders, such as alpha-1 antitrypsin deficiency, hemochromatosis and Wilson's disease.

Extraneous factors such as infections, surgery, or the injudicious use of sedatives or diuretics may precipitate patients with compensated liver disease into a state of hepatic insufficiency. In these cases the condition is reversible. In others, early recognition and appropriate care may result in considerable improvement in quality of life.

The clinical findings in hepatic insufficiency are traditionally divided into those due to hepatocellular dysfunction and those due to portal hypertension. Recent studies have shown that such division is not only simplistic but incorrect. Thus this review will describe the features of hepatic insufficiency in roughly the order in which they would be encountered during the clinical examination of such patients (Table 1.1). Since acute liver failure, portal hypertension, ascites, bleeding esophageal varices and encephalopathy are described in detail elsewhere in this volume, they will only be mentioned in passing in this chapter.

Table 1.1 Features of hepatic insufficiency

---

1. General health and malnutrition

2. Fever, infection and inflammation

3. Cutaneous and peripheral manifestations
   White nails
   Palmar erythema
   Clubbing
   Arterial spiders

4. Jaundice

5. Bleeding tendency

6. Endocrine features
   Gynecomastia
   Testicular atrophy
   Amenorrhea

7. Circulatory changes and portal hypertension

8. Pulmonary complications

9. Retention of water and electrolytes

10. Clinical features
    Dilated vessels
    Liver size
    Splenomegaly

11. Central nervous system effects

12. Hepatoma

13. Cholestasis

GENERAL HEALTH AND NUTRITION

Patients with chronic liver disease and hepatic insufficiency frequently complain of being easily fatigued, tired and weak. While edema and ascites may give a false impression of normal or increased body size, careful examination will often reveal loss of muscle bulk. Prolonged anorexia may result in decreased intake of protein and calories while patients with alcoholic liver disease may substitute alcohol for carbohydrate and protein calories. Alcoholic patients may have folic acid, thiamine, nicotinic acid and pyridoxine deficiencies, while patients who have been jaundiced for some time may have signs of fat-soluble vitamin deficiencies including easy bruising, night blindness and osteomalacia. Severe cholestasis may be associated with malabsorption of fat and steatorrhea. Prolonged, severe cholestasis may lead to the appearance of xanthelasma and xanthomas.

FEVER

Up to one-third of patients with hepatic insufficiency and inflammation (hepatitis) may have a chronic low-grade fever. However, infections are so common in this group of patients that full investigation, including blood cultures and diagnostic paracentesis, is mandatory. Indeed, any unexplained deterioration must be investigated in this way since these patients are almost invariably in an immunocompromised state. The Kupffer cells normally remove blood-borne bacteria passing through the liver, particularly those absorbed from the gut. There is a high incidence of septicemia due to enterobacteria in cirrhosis, and endotoxemia from gut-derived bacteria may be a factor in the associated renal failure. There is also an increased incidence of bacterial endocarditis, pneumonia, spontaneous peritonitis and tuberculosis. These infections are also noted in alcoholic patients, as are aspiration pneu-

monia and lung abscesses. Organisms range from Gram-negative (coliform) and Gram-positive (pneumococci) bacteria to fungi. Fungemia may occur particularly in severely ill, hospitalized patients.

CUTANEOUS AND PERIPHERAL MANIFESTATIONS

Patients with hepatic insufficiency may present with cutaneous and peripheral manifestations which often aid in establishing the diagnosis.

Palmar erythema (liver palms) is a frequent finding in hepatic insufficiency. These patients have warm hands with a bright red color, especially marked in the thenar and hypothenar eminences and at the tips of the fingers. This red color, which blanches on pressure, is also seen in rheumatoid arthritis, thyrotoxicosis, during pregnancy and in certain normal people as a familial trait.

Clubbing of the fingers and toes, the cause of which is still not understood, may occur. This is characterized by loss of the angle between the nail bed and the nail with an increase in size of the distal phalanges.

White nails are frequently found in hepatic insufficiency. These opaque, pale nails which are abnormally soft, may also be seen in the nephrotic syndrome and in other conditions of chronic ill health.

Symptomatic arthropathy is a common association of both Wilson's disease and genetic hemochromatosis. In the latter, involvement of the first and second metacarpophalangeal joints and knees predominates.

Arterial spiders (spider nevi) occur in patients with hepatic insufficiency, viral hepatitis, normal pregnancy, users of the contraceptive pill, thyrotoxicosis and, occasionally, in normal people, especially young females. In the last two conditions they are usually transient. They consist of a central arteriole from which numerous vessels radiate – as

3

the name indicates, vascular nevi resemble spiders. As the radiating vessels draw their blood supply from the central arteriole, the spider's legs will blanche and disappear if a pinhead is gently pushed into the body. When the pin is lifted the legs fill rapidly with blood. Vascular spiders occur most commonly in the distribution of the superior vena cava but are not limited to this region. Spider nevi often disappear with improved liver function. Conversely, new spiders may appear with deterioration of liver function. Because of their occurrence in pregnancy and because estrogens cause similar changes in the endometrium, they have been attributed to disturbances in estrogen metabolism.

JAUNDICE

Approximately 200–250 mg of bilirubin are produced daily (Chapter 2). The unconjugated bilirubin formed from heme is relatively insoluble in water and is transported in serum bound to albumin. The pigment enters the liver cell at the sinusoidal membrane by carrier-mediated transport. Conjugation to glucuronic acid is catalysed by the microsomal enzyme glucuronyl transferase. Conjugated bilirubin excreted into the bile is reduced in the gastrointestinal tract by bacteria to form stercobilinogen, some of which is absorbed and undergoes an enterohepatic circulation. It is this pigment which, under abnormal conditions, appears in the urine as urobilinogen. Jaundice is observed clinically when serum bilirubin levels exceed 2.5 mg/dl (ca. 40 µmol/l). In hepatic insufficiency defects of uptake, conjugation and excretion result in increased levels of both conjugated and unconjugated bilirubin in the serum. The conjugated bilirubin appears in the urine. In addition, there is a defect in the enterohepatic circulation of stercobilinogen, and urobilinogenuria is frequently observed.

BLEEDING TENDENCY

Patients with hepatic insufficiency have multiple and complex abnormalities of hemostasis. These are described in detail in Chapter 3. Clinically this is seen as a tendency to bruise easily or to prolonged bleeding after minor procedures such as dental surgery. All patients with liver disease should have a full coagulation and hemostasis screen prior to any invasive procedure.

ENDOCRINE FEATURES

Endocrine changes are most commonly found in patients with hepatic insufficiency due to alcohol.

Gynecomastia, the enlargement of breasts due to true breast tissue in males, is a frequent finding in chronic liver disease. It may be unilateral or bilateral and is best felt with the palm as a fleshy, firm, well demarcated disk of tissue. It is usually associated with decreased libido and frequently with testicular atrophy which occurs in at least 50% of patients with cirrhosis. This is characterized by small testicles which are softer and less sensitive to pressure than usual. Men with alcoholic liver disease have been shown to have abnormal testicular, pituitary and hypothalamic function. The specific mechanism of testicular atrophy is thought to be related to a combination of an altered testicular energy metabolism due to alcohol (Chapter 7), a direct toxic effect of acetaldehyde produced from alcohol in the testis, and competitive inhibition of conversion of vitamin A to retinal by alcohol in the testis. The mechanism of the feminization that occurs in men with liver disease is less easy to explain and is probably multifactorial. However, this is at least in part due to shunting from the portal to the systemic circulation of gut-absorbed sex hormones, which normally undergo an enterohepatic circulation.

Alcoholic females with liver disease frequently develop amenorrhea and are relatively infertile. The pathogenesis of these changes is complex but many of the ovarian changes are thought to be due to factors similar to those operating in the testis.

CIRCULATORY CHANGES

Alterations in the systemic circulation are not infrequently seen in patients with hepatic insufficiency. The most common findings are those of a hyperdynamic circulatory state. These patients have warm skin, resting tachycardia, bounding pulses, low blood pressure, and an active cardiac apical impulse. On auscultation of the heart, flow murmurs may be heard. The cardiac output is increased in more than half of patients with hepatic insufficiency. Many of these patients have expanded plasma volumes and central venous pressure may be increased. Peripheral resistance is reduced. Tense ascites may reduce the cardiac output, presumably by decreasing venous return to the heart. In these patients large volume paracentesis is accompanied by an increase of cardiac output. The primary mechanism of the hyperdynamic circulatory changes in advanced liver disease appears to be a fall in systemic vascular resistance as a result of portal systemic shunting of vasodilator compounds generated in the splanchnic area (e.g. glucagon).

PULMONARY COMPLICATIONS

Arterial hypoxemia may occur in patients with hepatic insufficiency. Severe hypoxemia in this setting characterizes the hepatopulmonary syndrome. This appears to be due to a perfusion–diffusion defect. Here the alveolar capillaries are thought to be dilated to a point where the blood flowing close to their walls is oxygenated while that flowing near their

center is not. These patients may be dyspneic, especially when upright (platypnea).

A small percentage of patients with hepatic insufficiency develop clinically significant pulmonary hypertension. Right heart catheter and Doppler studies suggest that sub-clinical pulmonary hypertension is present in 2.5% of patients. This appears to be related to portal systemic shunting of blood rather than to liver disease *per se*.

RETENTION OF WATER AND ELECTROLYTES

This is described in detail in Chapter 12. However, a few points are worth re-emphasizing here. More patients die as a result of the treatment of ascites than die from ascites *per se*. In the presence of portal hypertension there is only a limited capacity for transferring fluid from the ascitic to the intravascular compartment per day. Thus, urinary or gastrointestinal fluid loss of more than 1 liter a day will be at the expense of the interstitial and intravascular compartments. When edema is present, this may be without hazard, but in the absence of edema such diuresis may lead to encephalopathy, renal impairment and death.

Many patients with ascites with low serum albumin concentrations have the capacity to synthesize normal amounts of this protein. However, albumin synthesis is very sensitive to dietary protein restriction and the combination of liver disease and an excessively low protein diet will aggravate the fluid retention seen in patients with hepatic insufficiency. Thus patients who have ascites and who are not encephalopathic should receive normal protein diets. Those with encephalopathy should be treated with lactulose and the minimum degree of protein restriction compatible with normal mental function.

Finally, spontaneous peritonitis is frequent in patients with hepatic insufficiency and, if untreated, is associated with a high mortality. This complication must therefore be actively looked for, as described in Chapter 12.

FEATURES ON ABDOMINAL EXAMINATION

Cirrhosis results in partial obstruction of the venous blood flow through the liver, and as venous pressure increases it is transmitted backwards and causes congestion and enlargement of the spleen. Decompression of this elevated portal pressure can only occur where the portal and systemic blood vessels meet, and thus dilated vessels resembling varicose veins are found at the gastroesophageal junction, around the ligamentum teres in the retroperitoneal area and between the inferior mesenteric and anal vessels. Clinical signs of portal hypertension may be minimal; conversely, an enlarged firm spleen as well as dilated superficial abdominal vessels which radiate out from the umbilicus may be found. In some cases a venous hum may be heard over the upper abdomen due to blood rushing through these large collaterals.

Signs of hypersplenism with reduced red blood cells, white blood cells and platelets are frequently associated with the finding of an enlarged spleen in portal hypertension (Chapter 3). The low white blood cell and platelet counts are not usually clinically significant and seldom require any treatment.

The liver may be impalpable and percussion may reveal a decreased liver span. When palpable, it is firm and occasionally nodular. Significant enlargement of the liver may suggest the superimposition of an acute alcoholic hepatitis, alcoholic cirrhosis alone or the development of a hepatocellular carcinoma. Also, cirrhosis secondary to chronic cholestatic diseases is often associated with hepatomegaly.

CENTRAL NERVOUS SYSTEM EFFECTS OF HEPATIC INSUFFICIENCY

Patients with advanced liver disease frequently manifest signs of hepatic encephalopathy.

Hepatic encephalopathy may be seen in both acute (Chapter 12) and chronic (Chapter 13) forms of liver failure and may range from virtually undetectable personality changes through intellectual impairment to deep coma with decerebrate or decorticate rigidity and central depression of the respiratory centers. This is typically preceded by central respiratory stimulation and alkalosis. In addition to the wide range of intensity of the symptoms, variability over time is characteristic of hepatic encephalopathy.

The mildest form of encephalopathy is a deterioration of intellectual function and this may not be noticed by the physician but only by the patient's colleagues or relatives. Next, the patient may develop a sleep disorder; either hypersomnia or an inversion of sleep rhythm. Movement becomes slower, the face expressionless and speech monotonous and slurred. At this stage, several diagnostic features may be present on examination. The earliest sign is constructional apraxia, an inability to reproduce simple designs. Deterioration of handwriting occurs and may provide an acceptable day-to-day progress record. In addition to all this, the patient develops a flapping tremor, seen also in other metabolic encephalopathies, including uremia and hypoxia as in respiratory failure. The tremor is seen when the patient stretches his or her arms forward, hyperextends the wrists and abducts the fingers. This maneuver results in jerky, irregular, flexion of the wrist and or metacarpophalangeal joints. In addition to tremor, some patients have myoclonic jerks of the entire arm which may be spontaneous. Another important physical finding is the fetor hepaticus, which may be detected in virtually all patients with hepatic encephalopathy. This odor is also present in patients with extensive spontaneous or surgical portal systemic shunting of blood.

In addition to the changes in intellect and consciousness and the physical signs described above, patients with hepatic encephalopathy may undergo personality changes ranging from irritability, childishness or apathy through to frank psychosis. As the condition worsens the patient's drowsiness may progress to coma. At first, the patient may respond to verbal stimuli but later only to painful stimuli, and finally there is a complete lack of response. At this stage the patient may lie quietly in bed with open eyes looking wide awake, but is in fact deeply unconscious. Hyperventilation due to a primary respiratory drive is a frequent finding. Finally there is depression of the respiratory center and death may occur from respiratory arrest.

HEPATOCELLULAR CARCINOMA

This occurs most commonly in hepatitis B surface antigen-positive chronic active hepatitis (HBsAg-positive) and hemochromatosis (42% and 36% respectively). A quarter of patients with alcoholic, or hepatitis C virus cirrhosis may develop tumor and an overall figure of about 24% is identified in all cirrhotics in North American and in British series. This condition usually presents as pain in the liver, refractory ascites or unexplained weight loss and clinical deterioration (Chapter 20).

CHOLESTASIS

Certain causes of biliary cirrhosis, including primary biliary cirrhosis and sclerosing cholangitis, may present with predominant features of cholestasis (Chapter 11). These patients develop severe itching (pruritus) and excoriation of the skin. Deposits of lipid in the skin may produce xanthelasma and xanthomas.

Patients also develop steatorrhea. As a result of defective lipid absorption, deficiency of fat-soluble vitamins is common. It is therefore very important to evaluate night blindness, skin changes and early bone disease in these patients.

PROGNOSIS

There are few unselected comparative studies on the prognosis of different forms of cirrhosis. In the usually quoted studies, less than half of the patients survive 1 year and only one-tenth survive 6 years. The prognosis in patients with cryptogenic cirrhosis appears to be better than that of patients with alcoholic cirrhosis. Cumulative 5-year survival figures appear to be about 25% in cryptogenic cirrhosis.

There is good evidence that the prognosis in alcoholic cirrhosis is greatly improved in those who stop drinking. Similarly, treatment of autoimmune chronic active hepatitis with steroids, hemochromatosis with venesection and Wilson's disease by copper chelation significantly improves the prognosis.

Of the many prognostic formulae the Child–Pugh classification appears to be most useful in predicting the outcome of patients with liver disease as well as their ability to survive various surgical procedures (Chapter 2)

TREATMENT

This is both specific and general. Specific treatment is aimed at the removal of the etiological agent such as alcohol, iron, copper or drugs. Recognition of early liver disease due to alcohol is important since rehabilitation may offer a greater chance of successful treatment than previously suggested. Autoimmune chronic hepatitis may respond to corticosteroids, although the effect on cirrhosis is less certain (Chapter 9). There are no proven specific 'effective long-term treatments' for primary biliary cirrhosis (Chapter 9) and only experimental treatment for HBsAg-positive and C chronic liver disease, which includes interferon and antiviral agents (Chapter 8).

Treatment of the complications of liver disease is difficult but may result in a significant improvement in quality of life in these patients. Encephalopathy may be managed by appropriate dietary measures with decreased protein intake and the use of lactulose (Chapter 13). Ascites and fluid retention may be managed appropriately by salt and fluid restriction and use of aldosterone antagonist and loop diuretics (Chapter 16). Gastrointestinal hemorrhage is managed appropriately by sclerotherapy, beta-blockers, interventional radiological or surgical procedures (Chapter 14). Prophylactic beta-blocker therapy may have a place in compliant patients who appear at high risk for repeated variceal bleeding. Prophylactic sclerotherapy, however, does not appear to be indicated prior to variceal bleeding because of an unacceptably high rate of complications and morbidity (Chapter 14).

Appropriate management of complicating superimposed bacterial infections is of benefit in all patients with cirrhosis. Prophylactic antibiotic therapy in patients who have experienced an episode of bacterial peritonitis may have long-term benefits. Prophylactic antibiotics (quinilones, semisynthetic penicillins and cephalosporins) may prevent or attenuate repeat episodes of peritonitis.

Early detection of hepatocellular carcinoma in a compensated cirrhotic patient, by maintaining a high degree of clinical suspicion, regular ultrasound examinations and alpha-fetoprotein screening, may select a group where surgical resection may be feasible (Chapter 20).

Recognition of potentially hazardous motor coordination abnormalities in patients with early encephalopathy will enable appropriate counseling regarding motor vehicle driving and occupational risks (Chapter 13).

However, liver transplantation offers the only hope for a cure in most advanced forms of chronic liver disease, and is recognized as the treatment modality of choice in these conditions (Chapter 27).

RECOMMENDED READING

Quiroga, J., Beloqui, O. and Castilla, A. (1992) Cirrhosis, in *Hepatobiliary Diseases* (eds J. Prieto, J. Rodes and D.A. Schafritz), Springer–Verlag, Heidelberg and Berlin, pp. 323–415.

Sherlock, S. and Summerfield, J.A. (1991) *Colour Atlas of Liver Disease*, Mosby Year Book Inc., St Louis.

2

Biochemical evaluation of liver disease

RALPH KIRSCH, NATHAN BASS and IRWIN ARIAS

INTRODUCTION

Ideally laboratory tests should assist in the diagnosis of liver disease, indicate the functional reserve of the diseased organ and accurately determine liver blood flow as well as the amount of blood bypassing the liver. Currently available tests partly fulfil the first requirement but do not yield sufficiently accurate information in respect of liver function, blood flow or portal systemic shunting. This chapter is divided into two parts: it will review those tests used to diagnose liver disease and assess liver function; it will then attempt to provide an approach to the use of these tests in patients with various forms of liver disease.

LIVER TESTS

Liver enzymes are the most widely used tests of liver dysfunction. They often provide useful information on the type of liver damage and are especially useful in separating cholestasis from hepatocellular necrosis. However, they do not distinguish between the various forms of hepatitis or between intrahepatic and extrahepatic cholestasis, nor can they be used to assess the degree of liver dysfunction and hence prognosis.

TESTS FOR HEPATOCELLULAR NECROSIS

SERUM TRANSAMINASES

Serum AST (aspartate aminotransferase) and ALT (alanine aminotransferase) activities are the most frequently measured indicators of liver disease. These enzymes are widely distributed in the body (Fig. 2.1), with large quantities present in liver, cardiac muscle and skeletal muscle.

While ALT is a cytosolic enzyme, four-fifths of AST is found in mitochondria and one-fifth in cytosol. Some elevation of AST and ALT is found in almost all forms of liver disease. Extremely high levels, more than 10 times the upper limit of normal, are found in toxic or viral hepatitis and in shock due to low cardiac output. In most disease states, serum ALT activity is greater than that of AST (Fig. 2.2).

An exception to this rule is found in alcoholic liver disease where hepatic ALT is reduced. This is reflected by modest increases in serum ALT activity with an AST : ALT ratio

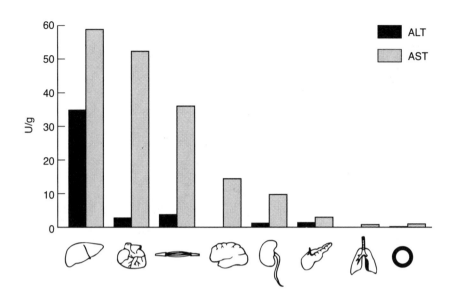

Figure 2.1 Aspartate aminotransferase (AST) and alanine aminotransferase (ALT) activity in human organs.

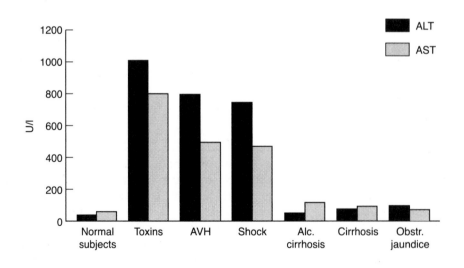

Figure 2.2 Serum transaminase activity in hepatobiliary disease. AVH, acute viral hepatitis.

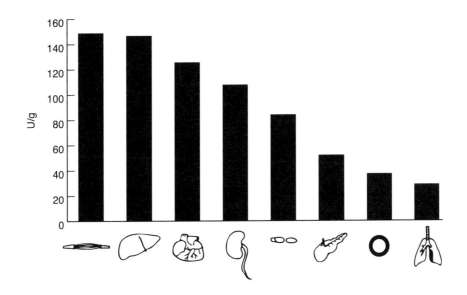

Figure 2.3 Lactate dehydrogenase (LDH) activity in human organs.

greater than 2. Higher elevation of the AST than ALT, however, is commonly observed in post-necrotic cirrhosis and chronic hepatitis.

Some laboratories can distinguish between mitochondrial and cytosolic AST isoenzymes. High mitochondrial : total AST ratios in serum have been found to be highly suggestive of alcohol-induced liver damage.

AST and ALT activities are relatively easy to measure and are usually not influenced by circulating inhibitors. An exception to this is found in uremic patients in whom a dialysable inhibitor may give rise to falsely low measurements of transaminase activity. Finally, the transaminases, although sensitive indices of hepatocellular damage, are not specific and cannot be used to predict the outcome of liver disease.

LACTATE DEHYDROGENASE (LDH)

This enzyme is widely distributed in human tissues (Fig. 2.3). It thus is extremely non-specific. The use of LDH isoenzymes is relatively expensive and of limited clinical use.

TESTS FOR CHOLESTASIS

ALKALINE PHOSPHATASE

Alkaline phosphatase activity as measured in serum represents the sum of the activity of several chemically distinct, unrelated, glycoproteins. The alkaline phosphatases are membrane-associated proteins. Most activity is associated with the plasma membrane but lower activities have been found in membranes of the endoplasmic reticulum,

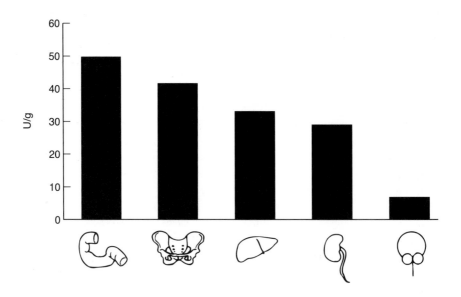

Figure 2.4 Alkaline phosphatase activity in human organs.

Golgi apparatus and nucleus. The enzymes are widely distributed in human tissues (Fig. 2.4).

More than one protein with alkaline phosphatase activity has been found in several organs, including the intestine and liver. Serum alkaline phosphatase activity is relatively high during the first two decades of life, declines to adult levels in the early 20s, and increases again in the later years of life. In health, most of the serum alkaline phosphatase activity is derived from liver and bone. High levels are found in diseases of most of the organs in which these enzymes are found. However, in liver disease the highest serum activities are found in cholestasis. These increases are thought to reflect an increased translation of mRNA stimulated by retained bile acids. High molec-ular weight forms of alkaline phosphatase appear in the serum of patients with cholestasis. These may represent complexes of alkaline phosphatase with lipoprotein X as well as activity associated with plasma membrane fragments which have been released into the circulation. Some patients with cirrhosis or chronic hepatitis have increased serum alkaline phosphatase activity of intestinal origin. The mechanism of this is not known. Most laboratories can distinguish alkaline phosphatase activity originating in liver, placenta and bone. Because serum activity originates from unrelated proteins with differing substrate specificities, laboratories using different methods tend to identify different components. The practice of expressing data from different laboratories in multiples of the upper limit of normal is therefore often invalid and may mislead clinicians monitoring the course of individual patients.

GAMMA-GLUTAMYL TRANSPEPTIDASE

Gamma-glutamyl transpeptidase (GGT) is a membrane protein which catalyzes the transfer of gamma-glutamyl groups from peptides such as glutathione to other amino acids. GGT also catalyzes the conversion of xenobiotic–glutathione conjugates to mercapturic acid. GGT is widely distributed in the tissues of the body. Serum GGT activity in neonates is five times that of adults. Serum GGT is higher in males than in females and increases with age. Increased serum activity is associated with cholestasis from whatever cause, but can also be found in alcoholic liver disease, patients on enzyme-inducing drugs, those with pancreatic disease and after myocardial infarction. GGT is a sensitive indicator of cholestasis but is extremely non-specific. GGT lacks both sensitivity and specificity in the diagnosis of alcoholic liver disease. The main value of GGT measurement in the evaluation of liver disease is in confirming the hepatic origin of an elevated alkaline phosphatase.

TESTS FOR METABOLISM AND SYNTHETIC FUNCTION

UREA SYNTHESIS

Under normal circumstances the urea cycle operates at less than its maximal capacity. This means that it can respond to dietary protein excess by increasing urea production. In cirrhosis, urea synthesis may be reduced and the adaptive response to dietary protein blunted. This results in a tendency to hyperammonemia and high amino acid concentrations, with a relatively low plasma urea.

ALBUMIN

Albumin is one of the most important plasma proteins produced by the liver. Serum levels represent the net result of synthesis, distribution (between the intravascular and extravascular compartments) and degradation. In normal, steady-state conditions, 12 g of albumin are synthesized and degraded daily and all newly synthesized albumin is released into the plasma pool from where it is distributed. Patients with cirrhosis and ascites frequently have low plasma albumin levels. However, many of these patients have been shown to have normal albumin synthesis rates and normal or increased total-body albumin pools. The plasma volume is frequently expanded but dilution alone does not account for all of the hypoalbuminemia. In fact, these patients have a maldistribution of albumin. Up to 80% of newly synthesized protein is delivered, via lymphatic vessels, directly into the ascitic compartment.

Because of its long half-life of 20 days, albumin levels in the plasma respond slowly to changes in synthesis and distribution. In addition, the latter are affected not only by liver disease but also by nutrition, hormonal balance, osmotic pressure, acute phase reaction stimuli and alcohol. Thus the serum albumin concentration *per se* is not an accurate prognostic indicator in liver disease although it is a useful component of the Child–Pugh classification, which is currently the best index of the severity of liver disease.

Certain coagulatory proteins may also be useful markers of hepatic synthetic function (Chapter 3).

IMMUNOGLOBULINS IN LIVER DISEASE

Patients with chronic liver disease and those with extrahepatic portal hypertension should be considered to be immunocompromised. Despite this, both groups have high levels of IgG, IgA and, to a lesser degree, IgM. Apart from IgM, which is frequently increased in primary biliary cirrhosis (Chapter 9), the increased globulins are of no diagnostic value. The increased immunoglobulin levels are probably due to the presence of both impaired Kupffer cell function and bowel-derived antigens in the portal blood bypassing the liver. Since these are not pronounced features of acute disease, the presence of increased immunoglobulins may be indirect indicators of chronic disease or inflammation.

CHOLESTEROL, LIPIDS AND LIPOPROTEINS

The liver plays a major role in lipid metabolism . Although there are well-defined abnormalities of triglyceride (increased) and lipoproteins (broad beta band) in acute liver disease, these are of little use in diagnosis and prognosis.

Cholestasis is almost invariably associated with increased plasma LDL cholesterol concentrations. Unfortunately this does not distinguish between the various causes of cholestasis and is thus of limited use.

INDICES OF LIVER CELL UPTAKE AND TRANSPORT

BILIRUBIN METABOLISM

Most (70%) of the 200–250 mg of bilirubin produced daily is derived from hemoglobin. Senescent red blood cells are engulfed by phagocytes and hemolyzed. Heme is dissociated from globin and transferred to the endoplasmic reticulum enzyme heme oxygenase in such a way that only its alpha-meso bridge is exposed to attack by activated oxygen. Biliverdin IX-alpha, iron and carbon monoxide are formed (Fig. 2.5).

All carbon monoxide produced in the body is derived from this reaction and its measurement in expiration can be used to assess heme

degradation. Biliverdin reductase catalyzes the reduction of the central meso-bridge of biliverdin to form the open-chain tetrapyrrole, bilirubin IX-alpha.

Bilirubin has eight side chains: two vinyl, four methyl and two propionic acid groups. These should, if accessible to the surrounding medium, confer water solubility to the molecule. However, in nature, both proprionic acid side chains are bound via their carboxylic acid groups to the hydrogen atoms attached to the nitrogen moeity of each of the four pyrroles (Fig. 2.6). This causes the molecule to fold in on itself, internalizing the side chains, and thus making bilirubin insoluble in water.

Unconjugated bilirubin in plasma is maintained in solution by binding to albumin. Due to its insolubility in water and tight binding to albumin, unconjugated bilirubin never appears in the urine, even when its plasma level is increased.

Bilirubin entering the circulation is taken up almost exclusively by the liver. There is increasing evidence that this process involves a carrier-mediated membrane transport system. Bilirubin uptake competes for uptake with sulfobromophthalein (BSP) and indocyanine green (ICG) but not with bile acids; and putative bilirubin transport proteins have been purified from liver cell plasma membranes.

Inside the liver cell bilirubin is bound to the glutathione S-transferases (GSH S-T) which constitute 2% of hepatic cytosol protein. The major effect of this binding appears to be to limit reflux of bilirubin from the hepatocyte into plasma.

Virtually all bilirubin excreted in bile is diglucuronide (90%) or monoglucuronide (10%). Conjugation of bilirubin to these water-soluble forms is catalyzed by an endoplasmic reticulum enzyme, uridine diphosphate (UDP) glucuronyl transferase, specific for bilirubin. Bilirubin glucuronyl transferase activity is extremely low in fetal livers. Its activity at term is 1% of adult values. This

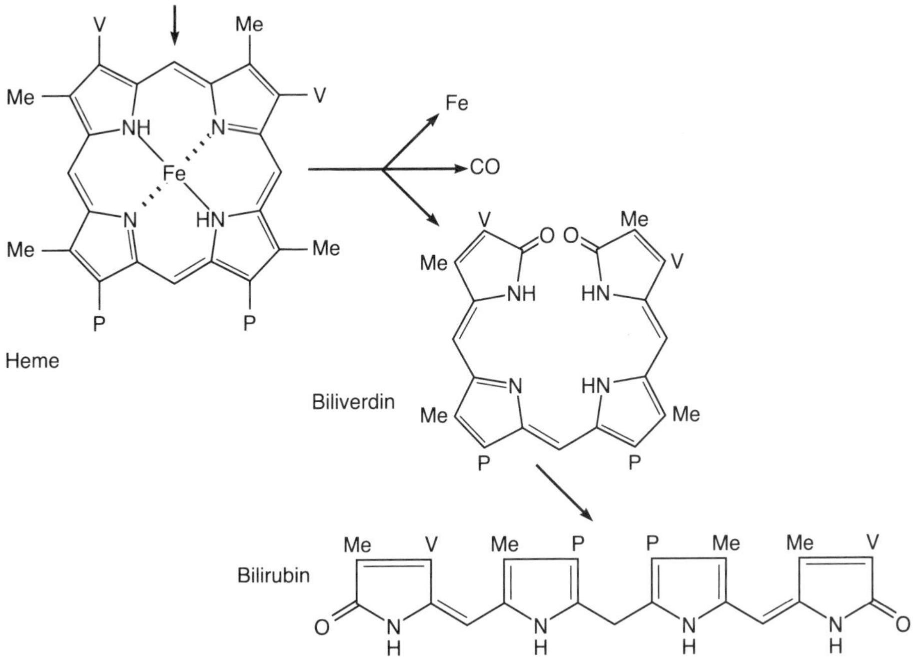

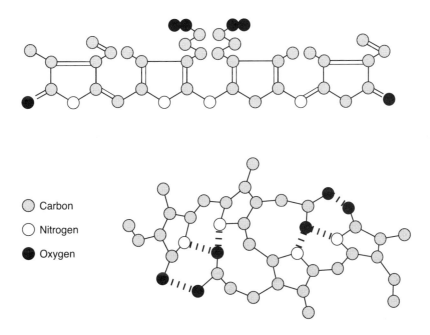

Figure 2.5 Bilirubin formation.

Figure 2.6 Chemical structure of bilirubin IX-alpha (top) and the molecular structure of internally hydrogen-bonded bilirubin IX-alpha (bottom). Intramolecular H-bonds are represented by broken lines.

Table 2.1 Urinary excretion of bile pigments in jaundice

	Bilirubin	Urobilinogen
Normal	→	↑
Gilbert's syndrome	→	↑
Hemolysis	→ – ↑ (may be ↑↑↑↑ in sickle cell disease)	↑↑↑ – ↑↑↑↑
Hepatocellular jaundice	↑↑ – ↑↑↑↑	↑↑ – ↑↑↑
Cholestatic jaundice	↑↑↑↑	→ – ↑ (absent in complete biliary obstruction)

rises rapidly after birth to reach adult values at 14 weeks. Bilirubin glucuronyl transferase activity is higher in the livers of females than in males. This finding has been used to explain the higher incidence of Gilbert's syndrome in males.

Thus, an increase in the unconjugated (or indirect-reacting) bilirubin fraction in the plasma may be accounted for by increased production of bilirubin (e.g. in hemolysis), impaired uptake (Gilbert's syndrome, liver disease) or impaired conjugation (Gilbert's syndrome, Crigler–Najjar syndrome, liver disease).

Transport from the hepatocyte into the bile canaliculus is thought to be the rate-limiting step in removal of bilirubin from the body. Secretion may involve an ATP-dependent membrane transport system shared with BSP and ICG. Although bile acids do not share this system, bilirubin secretion is increased by infusion of bile acids.

The entire transport system for bilirubin normally operates well within its maximal capacity. Indeed, normal livers are able to clear relatively large loads due to hemolysis without large increases in circulating bilirubin. Increases in serum unconjugated (indirect-reacting) bilirubin with otherwise normal liver function tests is typically found in hemolytic states or Gilbert's syndrome. In disease, hepatic clearance decreases with secretion being the rate-limiting step. Thus both conjugated and unconjugated bilirubin appear in the circulation, usually associated with abnormal liver function tests and bilirubinuria (Table 2.1).

With complete failure of bilirubin excretion (e.g. complete biliary obstruction), serum bilirubin levels tend to plateau at a maximum below 500 µmol/l (ca. 30 mg/dl) with excretion occurring mainly via the urine. Extreme levels of hyperbilirubinemia above this level are usually associated with severe neurological disease with concurrent hemolysis and/or renal impairment. Following an episode of cholestasis, it is not unusual to find an elevation in the concentration of conjugated bilirubin that persists for several weeks after clinical and biochemical resolution. This is due to some of the conjugated bilirubin having become chemically and irreversibly bound to albumin. The pigment persists in the blood until albumin is degraded and is of no clinical significance. Bilirubinuria is not found under these conditions.

BILE ACID SECRETION

The bile acids are the major organic anions excreted by the liver. Since their pool size and flux is much larger than that of bilirubin, their measurement should theoretically provide a sensitive index of hepatic dysfunction. Unfortunately measurement of bile acids is relatively difficult. Currently three methods are used: gas chromatography (slow and technically demanding), enzymatic assay (now available in kit form which can only measure total bile acids), and radioimmunoassay

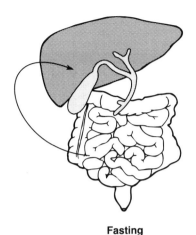 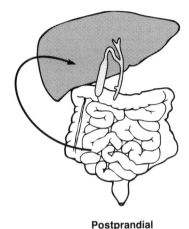

Fasting

Continuous secretion of small quantities of bile acid into duodenum; 70% of di- and 90% of tri-hydroxy BA extracted. Small amounts of BA in blood.

Postprandial

Gall bladder pool recycles to liver; 70% of di- and 90% of tri-hydroxy BA extracted. Increased BA concentration in blood.

Figure 2.7 Rationale for measuring postprandial bile acids (BA).

(available in kit form, measures total bile acids). Fasting bile acids are sensitive indicators of hepatic dysfunction (Fig. 2.7).

However, it may be argued that they do not add sufficiently to data obtained by routine testing to justify their use. Postprandial bile acids should theoretically be even more sensitive than fasting bile acids. Unfortunately this is not translated into a clinically useful advantage. Similarly, the ratio of cholic to chenodeoxycholic acid in the serum can be used to distinguish cholestasis from hepatocellular disease, but its accuracy is no greater than currently used tests.

SULFOBROMOPHTHALEIN (BSP) AND INDOCYANINE GREEN (ICG) EXCRETION

Apart from bilirubin and the bile acids, two exogenous organic anions, the dyes BSP and ICG, have been used to assess liver function.

Sulfobromophthalein (BSP)

For many years, BSP excretion was regarded as a sensitive index of liver dysfunction. Unfortunately BSP clearance is influenced by a variety of factors other than liver disease. In addition, local tissue damage due to extravascular dye at the site of injection and rare reports of severe, even fatal, allergic reactions have led to the virtual abandonment of BSP clearance as a test of liver function.

Indocyanine green (ICG)

There are several theoretical and practical reasons why ICG should be preferable to BSP. It does not appear to cause allergic reactions, is excreted unchanged into the bile (most BSP in bile is conjugated), has a higher hepatic extraction rate than BSP and can be measured by dichromatic ear lobe densitometry.

17

Unfortunately, minor changes in hepatic function can only be detected when the ICG clearance system is saturated. This would require large doses of ICG which are prohibitively expensive. Standard tests, with up to 5 mg ICG/kg body-weight, are relatively insensitive and are not often used.

HEPATIC DRUG METABOLISM

The concept of using a series of drugs to assess liver function, liver blood flow and portal systemic shunting is appealing. Such tests would give hepatologists equivalents to the nephrologist's glomerular filtration rate and renal blood flow. The information gleaned would also allow the rational adjustment of the doses of therapeutic agents.

The agent(s) used would have to be safe, when given intravenously in normal persons and in patients with liver disease. It should be removed entirely by the liver and elimination would have to be affected by liver disease.

Finally, the parent drug or its products must be easy to measure in blood, urine, saliva or breath.

Drugs taken up by the liver may be divided into two broad categories: those that have a low rate of entry into the liver cell and those where cell entry is so high that it is virtually all taken up during a single passage of blood through the liver (Fig. 2.8).

Since blood flow is so variable in liver disease a concept of intrinsic clearance, that is the clearance from whole blood that would be achieved if liver blood flow were not rate-limiting, has been evolved. The intrinsic clearance of a drug is influenced by its binding to plasma proteins as well as by uptake, metabolism and excretion. However, allowing for extrahepatic influences such as changes in protein concentration, two groups of drugs emerge. Those with low intrinsic clearance (antipyrine) and those with high intrinsic clearance (ICG, lidocaine, propanolol, galactose). Theoretically, drugs with low intrinsic

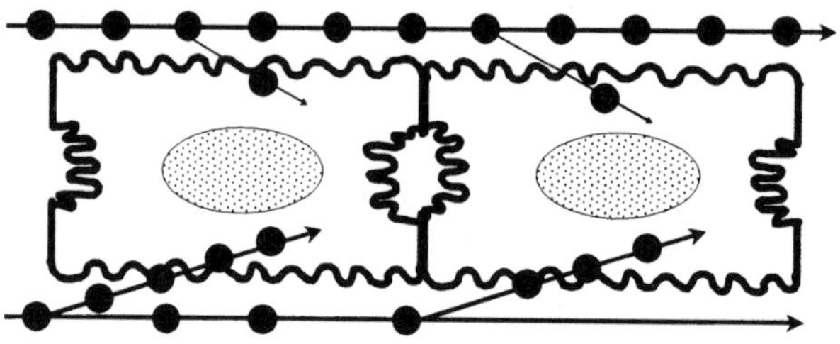

Intrinsic clearance (IC) = the clearance from whole blood which would be achieved if liver blood flow were not rate-limiting.

Drugs with low IC may indicate liver function.   (Antipyrine)

Drugs with high IC may indicate hepatic blood flow   (BSP)
(ICG)
(Lidocaine)
(Propanolol)
(Galactose)

Figure 2.8 Intrinsic clearance of drugs by the liver.

18

clearance could be used to study hepatocellular function, while those with high clearance would yield important information on hepatic blood flow. Unfortunately, the data obtained from these tests have been disappointing. Part of the reason is that the tests cannot discriminate between the effects of shunting (portal systemic and intrahepatic) and those of a reduced functional cell mass. Even if this could be achieved, inter-individual variations in the normal population may be too large to allow detection of minor hepatic dysfunction. Finally, most studies assume a linear relationship between their results and the degree of liver damage. All of these problems may still be overcome, but at present the use of drugs as measures of liver cell dysfunction remains a largely experimental procedure.

THE USE OF DIAGNOSTIC TESTS IN PATIENTS WITH LIVER DISEASE

It is vital that all investigations be appropriate and cost-effective. The clinical findings dictate the line of investigation to be followed. Before ordering any test, the practitioner should have a clear idea of why the test is being done,

what complications, if any, it may cause and what the test will cost. Tests may be done for either diagnostic or for monitoring purposes.

There are a few biochemical tests that are of value in the diagnosis of specific types of liver disease. These tests are described in detail in later chapters and are summarized in Table 2.2.

Accurate measurement of transaminase activity is required in patients with chronic active hepatitis where responses to steroids or interferon are being monitored. Tests used to monitor patients should be performed at optimal intervals. There is no need for daily liver tests (except in the case of the prothrombin international normalized ratio (INR, Chapter 3) after administration of vitamin K), and in most instances weekly, fortnightly or even monthly testing will suffice. Patients with stable disease may not need any tests at all other than monitoring for hepatocellular carcinoma (HCC). Finally, the predictive value of the test used must be borne in mind. This is influenced by the prevalence of the disease sought. A highly sensitive test – such as the anti-mitochondrial antibody, which is positive in the vast

Table 2.2 Tests for specific types of liver disease

Liver disease	Specific biochemical test	For detail see Chapter(s)
Hemochromatosis	Serum iron, transferrin, TIBC, ferritin	21
Alpha-1 antitrypsin deficency	Serum alpha-1 antitrypsin alpha-1 antitrypsin phenotype	9, 24
Chronic viral hepatitis	Hepatitis viral serology	8
Chronic autoimmune hepatitis	Anti-nuclear antibodies Anti-smooth muscle antibodies Anti-liver and -kidney microsomal antibodies	9
Primary biliary cirrhosis	Anti-mitochondrial antibodies	11
Hepatocellular carcinoma	Alpha-fetoprotein	20

TIBC, total iron-binding capacity

Test	Cholestasis	Hepatocellular disease
AST and ALT	N to ↑	↑↑↑
Alkaline phosphatase	↑↑↑	N to ↑
Cholesterol	N to ↑↑↑	N
Prothrombin index	N to ↓↓	N to ↓↓↓
Albumin	N	N to ↓↓↓
Bilirubin	N to ↑↑↑	N to ↑↑↑
Bile acids	↑ to ↑↑↑	↑ to ↑↑↑

Figure 2.9 The use of liver tests to discriminate between cholestasis and hepatocellular disease. N, normal.

majority of patients with primary biliary cirrhosis (PBC) – may also be positive in a small number of patients with much more common diseases. Thus, if used as a screening test for PBC it will be as likely to identify patients with other diseases as those with PBC. If, on the other hand, it is used in patients in whom there is clinical evidence to support the diagnosis of PBC (e.g. a cholestatic liver enzyme profile), it is much more likely to be of use to the clinician.

Liver tests are best at confirming the diagnosis of liver damage in the appropriate clinical setting (the high AST and ALT in hepatitis). They are also valuable in discriminating between cholestasis and hepatocellular disease (Fig. 2.9). They are extremely poor at screening the population for liver disease and, in their own right, are poor indicators of severity and prognosis.

The algorithms in Figures 2.10 and 2.11 may prove useful to those faced with the investigation of patients with hepatitis and/or cholestatic liver disease.

For prognosis we would recommend the Child–Pugh Classification (Fig. 2.12). It is of particular use in deciding whether to subject a patient to a surgical procedure and is becoming of increasing use in assessing the

need for liver transplantation. In the case of some types of liver disease, e.g. PBC, more accurate, disease-specific and biochemical parameters have been developed and Kaplan–Meier plots of survival determined.

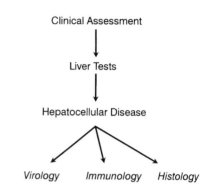

Figure 2.10 Algorithm for patients with hepatocellular disease.

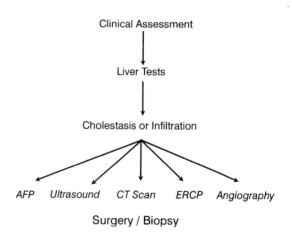

Figure 2.11 Algorithm for patients with cholestasis or infiltrating lesions of the liver. AFP, alpha-fetoprotein; CT, computed tomography; ERCP, endoscopic retrograde cholangiopancreatography.

Score	1	2	3
Ascites	None	Slight	Moderate to severe
Encephalopathy	None	Slight	Moderate to severe
Bilirubin (μmol/l)	< 2	34 – 51	> 51
Albumin (g/l)	> 35	28 – 35	< 28
Prothrombin (%)	> 70	40 – 70	< 40

> Grade A = 5 – 6
> Grade B = 7 – 9
> Grade C = 10 – 15

Figure 2.12 The modified Child–Pugh classification for patients with liver disease.

RECOMMENDED READING

Baker, A.L. (1992) Liver chemistry tests, in *Liver and Biliary Diseases* (ed. N. Kaplowitz), Williams and Wilkins, Baltimore, pp. 182–94.

Bass, N.M. (1992) An integrated approach to the diagnosis of jaundice, in *Liver and Biliary Diseases* (ed. N. Kaplowitz), Williams and Wilkins, Baltimore, pp. 588–609.

Johnson, P.M. (1989) Role of the standard 'liver function tests' in current clinical practice. *Ann Clin Biochem*, **26**, 463–71.

McIntyre, N. and Rosalki, S. (1992) Biochemical investigations in the management of liver disease, in *Hepatobiliary Diseases* (eds J. Prieto, J. Rodes and D. Schafritz), Springer–Verlag, Heidelberg and Berlin, pp. 39–71.

Reichling, J.J. and Kaplan, M.M. (1988) Clinical use of serum enzymes in liver disease. *Dig Dis Sci*, **33**, 1601–14.

3

Hematological evaluation in liver disease

SIMON ROBSON and MORAG CHISHOLM

INTRODUCTION

The liver is the major site of hemopoiesis in the fetus. It metabolizes and stores nutrients such as iron, folate and vitamin B_{12} which are crucial for blood cell proliferation and maturation. Under certain circumstances, it is capable of producing erythropoietin and colony stimulating factors, both of which will influence hemopoiesis. Finally, the liver synthesizes and regulates several major plasma proteins including those responsible for hemostasis. It is thus hardly surprising that liver disease may be associated with disturbances of red cells, white cells and platelets as well as with disordered hemostasis. While there is usually a considerable overlap between these disturbances, each will be dealt with separately in this chapter.

RED CELL ABNORMALITIES IN LIVER DISEASE

Some degree of anemia is usually present in patients with chronic liver disease. The causes are often multiple and include dilution (increased plasma volume), blood loss (gastrointestinal hemorrhage), impaired bone marrow production (folate, iron or pyridoxine deficiency, or chronic disease) and increased destruction (hypersplenism, altered red cell membrane lipids, disseminated intravascular coagulation (DIC)).

Where anemia is significant a clinical history of alcohol consumption, poor nutrition or blood loss is important. Evidence of nutritional deficiency, gastrointestinal blood loss and portal hypertension should be looked for. Red cell size, shape, volume and hemoglobin content are useful aids to the diagnosis. Mild macrocytosis usually implies that the anemia is due to chronic liver disease *per se*. Target cells are often seen in cholestasis as a consequence of bile salt fluxes. Significant macrocytosis, usually associated with alcoholic liver disease, may suggest folate and very rarely B_{12} deficiency. Acanthocytes are associated with an increased red cell membrane cholesterol to phospholipid ratio and have a shortened half life *in vivo*. Hypochromic microcytic cells denote iron and more rarely pyridoxine deficiency. The coexistence of liver disease and nutritional abnormalities such as iron deficiency may give rise to combinations of the above.

Serum B_{12} concentrations are often high due to release of stored vitamins in necrosed hepatocytes. Folate may be reduced in alcoholic liver disease and megaloblastic change noted in the bone marrow. The serum iron is usually normal but may be increased with active or acute liver damage. Transferrin saturation and ferritin may be influenced by liver disease as well as iron status and may thus be misleading. They are more useful at screening family members with no apparent liver disease for hemochromatosis where this diagnosis has been made in a first-degree relative.

WHITE CELL CHANGES IN LIVER DISEASE

Leukopenia, associated with neutropenia and lymphopenia, is a fairly constant feature of chronic liver disease. Hypersplenism contributes to this finding. Leukocytosis in response to sepsis, hemolysis and acute blood loss may be seen. High white cell counts, possibly due to release of colony stimulating factors from damaged hepatic parenchymal cells and probably related to the inflammatory process, are also found in acute alcoholic hepatitis.

PLATELETS IN LIVER DISEASE

Moderate thrombocytopenia, usually above the level associated with spontaneous bleeding, is common in cirrhotic patients. The low platelet counts may be due to increased splenic sequestration, destruction through immunological mechanisms associated with high levels of platelet-bound IgG and as part of disseminated intravascular coagulation (DIC). Abnormal platelet function may also occur. The bleeding time provides a clinically useful measurement of both quantitative and qualitative platelet function and interactions with vessel wall.

COAGULATION IN LIVER DISEASE

Hemostatic abnormalities develop in approximately 75% of patients with chronic liver disease and are particularly pronounced in the setting of acute liver failure. Features range from petechial hemorrhages, ecchymoses and bleeding around venepuncture sites, to epistaxis and life-threatening gastrointestinal hemorrhage.

Abnormalities of coagulation in liver disease are complex and wide-ranging and include the abnormal synthesis and clearance of clotting proteins and their inhibitors, production of abnormal proteins (deficient carboxylation of glutamic acid residues on prothrombin or abnormally sialylated fibrinogen), thrombocytopenia, abnormal platelet function and DIC.

Molecular biological techniques have shown that the liver is the main site of synthesis of almost all coagulation proteins. The liver also synthesizes the fibrinolytic proteins, the anti-proteases and the anti-coagulatory proteins – protein C, anti-thrombin III (AT III) and tissue factor pathway inhibitor which interact with endothelial cells, leukocytes and platelets (Fig. 3.1).

The vitamin K-dependent proteins (prothrombin, Factors VII, IX and X) are synthesized as precursor proteins in the rough endoplasmic reticulum of liver cells. To function in the coagulation cascade they require post-translational modification which facilitates the binding of calcium, an important cofactor in the coagulation process. This carboxylation of certain N-terminal domain glutamic acid residues, catalyzed by a vitamin K-dependent enzyme, is defective in the absence of vitamin K or in the presence of warfarin. Secretion of the vitamin K-dependent proteins is independent of this step and thus in vitamin K deficiency and in liver disease functionally abnormal (antigenic, immunologically reactive) forms appear in the plasma.

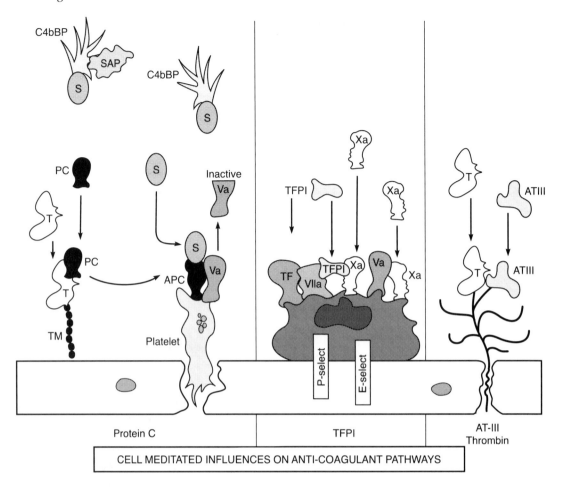

Figure 3.1 Anti-coagulant proteins: protein C and S, TFPI and anti-thrombin III. The major anti-coagulant pathways are illustrated above. Protein C is activated by thrombin bound to thrombomodulin which is depicted as an elongated multidomain protein on the endothelial cell surface. The activated protein C interacts with uncomplexed protein S and the new complex is bound by platelets or endothelial cells where the complex is responsible for the inactivation of Factor Va. Only free protein S is an active anti-coagulatory protein and the circulating protein S may be complexed to C4bBP, an inhibitory protein of the classical complement pathways. TFPI has three inhibitor domains, one of which interacts with Factor Xa and inhibits it. The resultant complex of Xa-TFPI interacts with the Tf-VIIa complex and results in reversible inhibition of its catalytic function. On the right-hand side of the monocyte membrane, Factors Xa and Va are preparing to bind prothrombin to form the prothrombinase complex. The balance of these opposing processes on the cell surface is influenced by the circulating and endothelial associated TFPI and its activation by Factor Xa. Finally the anti-thrombin activity may be localized on either thrombomodulin or on the heparin-like proteoglycans, depicted as an arboreal structure on the endothelial cell. Interestingly, anti-thrombin III when complexed to heparin is also capable of inhibiting the Tf-VIIa complex but not free VIIa (not shown). TF, tissue factor; TFPI, tissue factor pathway inhibitor; PT, prothrombin; T, thrombin; C4bBp, C4b binding protein; SAP, serum amyloid P; PC, protein C; APC, activated protein C; S, protein S; Tm, thrombomodulin; ATIII, anti-thrombin. 'Factor' is deleted before the Roman numerals for convenience.

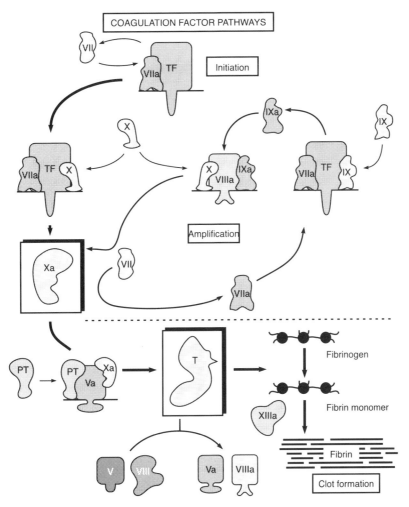

Figure 3.2 Coagulation pathways, the assembly and function of coagulation complexes. Inactive coagulation factors or zymogens interact on negatively charged cell membranes (the outer leaflet must contain aminophospholipid) with activation complexes comprising serine proteases, regulatory (activated) cofactors and calcium. In the initiation reaction, the Tf–Factor VIIa complex generates Factor Xa. Even though the protease Factor VII may interact with Tf, human Factor VII must be activated to attain function. Factors Xa and VIIa can generate more Factor VIIa which then interacts with Tf. In the amplification pathways, the Tf–VIIa complex binds IX and forms IXa which then binds to the activated cofactor VIIIa. This complex then generates functionally competent Factor Xa which augments that formed by the initial Tf–VIIa complex. The prothrombinase complex comprises the active cofactor Va, the protease Factor Xa and the zymogen prothrombin. The generated thrombin cleaves the fibrinopeptides A and B from fibrinogen proteins to form fibrin monomers which then interact and are cross-linked by the transglutaminase XIIIa. Note that thrombin also activates the pro-cofactors V and VIII which then permits their binding function as described above. The integrated 'to and fro' pathways depicted in the figure suggest that the initiation process is consolidated by the amplification pathways and that low levels of thrombin activation are crucial for the activation of the cofactors V and VIII. TF, tissue factor; PT, prothrombin; T, thrombin. 'Factor' is deleted before the Roman numerals for convenience.

Precursor forms can be detected by several methods including a difference between functional and immunological assays. In severe liver disease prothrombin synthesis may be reduced. This will be reflected by low values in both assay systems.

Vitamin K deficiency is unusual in hepatocellular disease, but may follow cholestasis or obstruction to the flow of bile salts. A 30% or greater improvement in the international normalized ratio (INR) within 24 hours of administration of parenteral vitamin K, confirms the diagnosis of prior depletion of vitamin K usually associated with cholestasis.

The two most widely used tests of coagulation are the INR and the activated partial thromboplastin time (APTT). The INR is abnormal in Factor VII deficiency. Both the INR and APTT are altered by deficiency of Factors I, II, V, VII and X. When other causes of an abnormal INR, such as DIC or vitamin K deficiency, have been excluded, the disturbances of the INR may serve as a useful measure of the severity of the liver disease process. Fibrinogen estimates by functional analyses and the determination of fibrin(ogen) degradation products, including the D-dimer, are of use in the diagnosis and monitoring of DIC. Recent advances have emphasized the importance of the extrinsic pathway and tissue factor (Fig. 3.2).

Apart from liver cell failure, portal systemic shunting of blood can cause disturbed coagulation. Patients with extrahepatic portal hypertension and normal liver function frequently have abnormal INR and APTT results. This may be due to chronic low-grade DIC, possibly caused by bowel-derived endotoxins in portal venous blood bypassing the liver.

The pathogenesis of DIC in liver disease is multifactorial and is more frequently observed when clinical decompensation occurs with complications such as sepsis and variceal hemorrhage. The release of tissue factor and

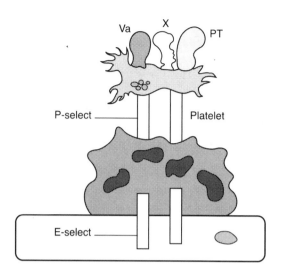

Figure 3.3 Cellular components of coagulation. Neutrophils (or monocytes) bind to endothelial cells by virtue of the leukocyte adhesion receptors, the selectins and integrins (not shown for simplification), which interact with carbohydrate moeities, the intercellular adhesion molecules (ICAM-1 and 2) and peptide sequences in matrix proteins and fibrin. Platelets interact with leukocytes and serve as additional loci for the formation of the prothrombinase complex, thrombin generation and fibrin formation. The fibrinogen (and other coagulation factor) content of platelets serve to further localize or focus clot formation. TF, tissue factor; PT, prothrombin; T, thrombin. 'Factor' is deleted before the Roman numerals for convenience.

expression of tissue factor on endothelial cells, impaired clearance of activated coagulation proteins and decreased synthesis of inhibitors (such as anti-thrombin III and protein C) are the postulated mechanisms. In addition, systemic endotoxemia may promote procoagulant activity in association with neutrophils and monocytes-macrophages, often in the context of platelet binding and assembly of the prothrombinase complex (Fig. 3.3).

Although the catabolism and turnover of fibrinogen is increased in liver disease, normal concentrations may be maintained by increased synthesis. The native protein may however be abnormal and be deficient in the A-alpha C terminal chains with excessive carbohydrate substitution elsewhere.

The incidence and severity of DIC in liver disease is controversial. Accurate diagnosis depends on demonstrating the simultaneous activation of both clotting and lytic systems. Most routine laboratories measure the presence of the terminal fibrin degradation product (FDP) D-dimer since generation of this product indicates both coagulation activation and plasminolysis. Where more sensitive and quantitative measurements have been used DIC has been found to be present in almost all patients with cirrhosis or with extra-hepatic portal hypertension and spontaneous portal systemic shunting. While this DIC is usually mild it becomes clinically significant in the presence of sepsis or gastrointestinal hemorrhage. Heparin therapy is controversial and may provoke further hemorrhage. Fresh-frozen plasma, coagulation factor concentrates (e.g. cryoprecipitate containing Factor VIII and fibrinogen) and platelet transfusions are used to replace specific deficiencies in the clotting mechanism. Anti-fibrinolytic therapy has limited utility at this time.

Coagulation tests and determinations of FDP and/or DD should be monitored regularly but intervention with coagulation factors or other modalities is indicated only if the patient is bleeding or requires an invasive procedure.

DISORDERED HEMOSTASIS AND IMMUNITY

Disturbances in coagulation and fibrinolysis may play an important role in the pathogenesis of the immunological abnormalities associated with severe acute and chronic liver disease. Proteolytic plasmin-derived fragments of fibrin and fibrinogen (FDP) have diverse biological properties. Apart from their well-known anti-coagulant effects, the FDP also have vasoactive and immunosuppressive properties. Catabolism of fibrinogen and fibrin may result in negative feedback pathways dampening down other effector limbs of the immune response or acute phase responses *in vivo*.

HEPATIC MANIFESTATIONS OF SPECIFIC HEMATOLOGICAL CONDITIONS

Patients with severe hemophilia or other individuals who required repeated blood component administration have traditionally run a high risk of contracting post-transfusional hepatitis. Because of their immunocompromised state and the levels of virus administered in unscreened blood previously, approximately 25% of patients have evidence of chronic viral hepatitis B or C (Chapter 8).

Hemolysis results in increased heme degradation and increased turnover of iron and bile pigments. Tissue siderosis with iron loading occurs in chronic hemolytic states such as the thalassemias and sideroblastic anemias. Pigment stones with choledocholithiasis is a well-recognized feature of chronic hemolysis as seen with hereditary spherocytosis or the various erythrocyte enzyme defects.

Acute hemolytic crises in sickle cell anemia with sickling episodes may be associated with hepatic infarcts and occasionally liver failure, characterized by coma, deep cholestatic jaundice and marked prolongation of the prothrombin time. This clinical picture may mimic fulminant viral hepatitis.

Up to 70% of patients with lymphoma have hepatic involvement. Needle biopsy of the liver for the confirmation of suspected hepatic involvement is usually positive in the setting of hepatosplenomegaly and abnormal liver tests.

Cholestatic disease may be observed in

Hodgkin's disease. Jaundice in this condition may also be due to bile duct obstruction secondary to hilar lymphadenopathy. In Hodgkin's disease, the demonstration of a normal liver on computed tomography (CT) scan suggests that a liver biopsy will most likely be normal.

In myeloproliferative states, bone marrow infiltration commonly leads to myeloid metaplasia in the liver, resulting in significant portal hypertension.

Hypercoagulable states including paroxysmal nocturnal hemoglobinuria, the antiphospholipid syndrome or the deficiency of protein C, predispose to both portal and hepatic vein thrombosis (Budd–Chiari syndrome). Latent myeloproliferative disorders have been reported to be a major etiological factor in 'idiopathic' extrahepatic portal venous obstruction.

Bone marrow transplantation is occasionally complicated by liver toxicity syndromes, graft-versus-host disease (GVHD) with cholestasis and veno-occlusive disorders. High levels of von Willebrand factor and serum angiotensin converting enzyme associated with decreases in Factor VII, which may be linked to endothelial cell damage, may predict this. Risk factors include the presence of viral hepatitis, high-dose anti-microbial therapy, mismatched allogeneic marrow grafts and the intensity of conditioning therapy prior to grafting. Low-dose heparin administered prophylactically may be given but is of uncertain benefit.

Histiocytosis X may be complicated by granulomatous hepatic infiltrates with the development of severe cholestasis and a picture comparable to primary sclerosing cholangitis.

Type II Gaucher's disease, in infants, is characterized by hepatosplenomegaly and early death. The adult Type I variant is usually associated with a reasonable prognosis.

HEMATOLOGICAL MANIFESTATIONS OF SPECIFIC LIVER DISEASES

VIRAL HEPATITIS

Anemia is rare but macrocytosis may occur. Leukopenia may occur in the preicteric phase but this is transient. Neutropenia, and the presence of virocytes (atypical mononuclear cells with cytoplasmic vacuoles, basophilic cytoplasm and large irregular nuclei often with nucleoli) may be seen. Patients with viral hepatitis B may rarely develop aplastic anemia, usually as a late extrahepatic manifestation of the infection. Severe aplastic anemia has been associated with seronegative, HCV RNA-positive, community-acquired hepatitis C infection. Novel non-ABC viral agents also appear to be implicated in instances of fulminant hepatitis with associated marrow aplasia. The mechanisms of marrow aplasia remain speculative but almost certainly involve stem cell destruction or suppression. Hepatitis B and C infections are both responsible for a significant proportion of the liver involvement associated with the mixed type cryoglobulinemias.

HEPATOCELLULAR CARCINOMA

Hepatocellular carcinoma is linked with the development of erythrocytosis (and thrombocytosis) secondary to the unregulated release of erythropoieitin and colony stimulating factors by the tumor cells. Hepatic malignancies are also associated with high plasma levels of abnormal hypersialylated fibrinogen and des-carboxy-prothrombin proteins which do not function normally (Chapter 20).

ALCOHOLIC LIVER DISEASE

Alcohol has a direct toxic effect on the blood and bone marrow. Alcohol decreases folate absorption, inhibits its metabolism and may increase its excretion. Furthermore, alcohol blocks conversion of pyridoxine to pyridoxal phosphate. While consumption of alcohol may deliver and enhance absorption of more iron, this may be countered by the increased incidence of upper gastrointestinal conditions associated with blood loss.

Macrocytosis is the hallmark of alcoholic liver disease and slowly responds to alcohol withdrawal. Folate deficiency plays a role. Pyridoxine deficiency leads to sideroblastic changes and should be considered when anemia is normo- or microcytic in the absence of blood loss.

Alcohol appears to impair the ability of granulocytes to combat bacterial infection. There is often a lymphopenia with reduced T cell numbers and impaired blastogenic responses *in vitro*.

Platelet production is often decreased. Thrombocytopenia, thought to be due to a direct toxic effect of alcohol or metabolites on megakaryocytes, responds to withdrawal of alcohol, often with transient rebound thrombocytosis.

SURGERY AND TRANSPLANTATION

Even minor surgery in patients with liver disease may precipitate major alterations in hemostasis. The precautions that should be taken with liver biopsy are detailed in Chapter 5. Liver transplantation for parenchymal liver disease with portal hypertension may be associated with major hemorrhage requiring massive blood transfusion. These changes are more pronounced in the anhepatic state and following reperfusion of the donor organ. This may be related to the pronounced fibrinolytic component of an ongoing DIC and in this situation the use of aprotonin may have some benefits in reducing the requirement for further blood transfusion. Transient deficiencies of protein C, anti-thrombin III and other anti-coagulant proteins may predispose to an initial hypercoagulable state which could be a factor in the development of arterial and portal venous thromboses observed in the immediate post-tranplantation period. Peritoneovenous shunting of ascites with the cellular associated tissue factors and endotoxins may precipitate DIC and lead to severe clinical complications and even death.

RECOMMENDED READING

Carr, J.M. (1989) Disseminated intravascular coagulation in cirrhosis. *Hepatology*, **10**, 103–10.

Chisholm, M. (1992) Hematological disorders in liver disease, in *Wright's Liver and Biliary Disease* (eds G.H. Milward-Sadler, R. Wright and M.J.P. Arthur), WB Saunders, Philadelphia, pp. 203–28.

Kruskal, J.B., Robson, S.C., Franks, J.J. and Kirsch, R.E. (1992) Elevated fibrin and fibrinogen related antigens in patients with liver disease. *Hepatology*, **16**, 920–3.

Leiber, C.S. and Salaspuro, M.P. (1992) Alcoholic liver disease, in *Wright's Liver and Biliary Disease* (eds G.H. Milward-Sadler, R. Wright and M.J.P. Arthur), WB Saunders, Philadelphia, pp. 899–964.

Mammen, E.F. (1992) Coagulation abnormalities in liver disease. *Hematol Oncol Clin North Am*, **6**, 1247–57.

Robson, S.C., Kahn, D., Kruskal, J.B. *et al.* (1993) Disordered hemostasis in extrahepatic portal hypertension. *Hepatology*, **18**, 853–7.

4

Radiological evaluation of liver disease

STEVE BENINGFIELD

INTRODUCTION

The marked progress in imaging of liver disease in the last few decades with the advent of ultrasound (US), computed tomography (CT) and magnetic resonance imaging (MRI) have provided greater insight into the anatomy, physiology and pathology of the liver. Improvements in surgical technique have placed an increased demand on the accuracy of imaging. The advent of liver transplantation has also widened the scope of imaging and the role of interventive biliary and vascular procedures.

In the evaluation of hepatic parenchymal disease, liver pathology may be broadly divided into diffuse and focal categories for imaging purposes.

DIFFUSE LIVER DISEASE

In general, imaging is not very accurate in the detection and characterization of diffuse liver disease.

HEPATITIS

Acute hepatitis may reveal non-specific findings such as hepatomegaly, reduced echo-genicity, minimal ascites and slight secondary gall bladder wall thickening on US.

Chronic hepatitis may reveal increased liver echogenicity, features of portal hypertension and possible secondary development of hepatocellular carcinoma (HCC).

FATTY INFILTRATION

This may occur as either diffuse or focal fatty infiltration. The radiological features in underlying causative conditions such as alcohol abuse and obesity are similar. The importance of this condition is that it may mimic other more significant lesions on US, CT and MRI. Initial small islands of fatty infiltration may spread and coalesce leaving residual areas of normal parenchyma, both of which may simulate focal disease. These areas often have geographic borders. The pattern may change within days.

Ultrasound scanning of fatty infiltration of the liver will reveal areas of increased echogenicity where fat is present within the hepatocytes. The fat accumulates in hepatocytes, creating a number of interfaces which reflect the ultrasound waves. In contrast to mass lesions, vessels running through areas of fatty infiltration are not displaced.

On CT scanning the overall density of the liver parenchyma is reduced and may be in the fat density range (<0 Hounsfield units, HU). If the liver density is ≥10 HU less than splenic density without contrast medium, or >25 HU less than splenic density after contrast medium administration, fatty infiltration is supported.

The sulfur colloid scan is usually normal in fatty infiltration, making it useful in the exclusion of other possible causes of the imaging findings.

Magnetic resonance imaging is not very sensitive to fatty infiltration, but an increase in intensity on the T1-weighted image is suggestive. A fat suppression sequence may be very useful to distinguish fatty tissue (which becomes low intensity) from other pathological tissue.

CIRRHOSIS

US, CT and MRI are relatively insensitive in the detection of cirrhosis. Clues include a nodular liver outline, enlarged caudate lobe (Fig. 4.1), areas of focal atrophy with adjacent hypertrophy, inhomogeneous liver, as well as spontaneous portosystemic collateral veins,

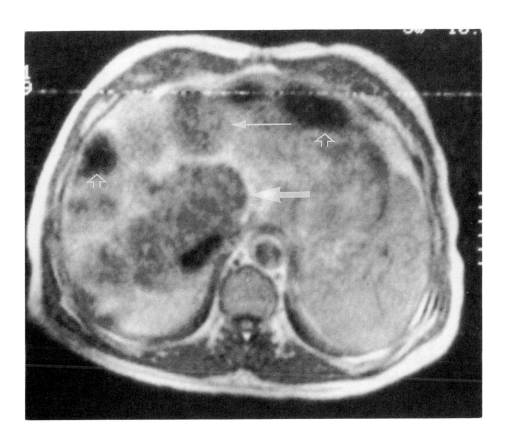

Figure 4.1 Magnetic resonance image (MRI) of cirrhotic liver showing hypertrophy of low signal intensity caudate lobe (thick arrow) and low signal intensity regenerating nodule (thin arrow) due to iron accumulation. Bowel gas is also present (open arrows).

31

portal hypertension, portal vein thrombosis and splenomegaly. The presence of an underlying hepatocellular carcinoma should always be excluded in cirrhotic livers.

Recently, high-frequency ultrasound probes (≥5 MHz) have been used to analyze the liver surface. A totally irregular surface is supportive of the diagnosis of cirrhosis whereas interspersed nodularity suggests malignant disease.

Portosystemic collateral veins may be well delineated on CT with enhancement following intravenous contrast medium administration, particularly with the use of the new spiral CT sequence which images a volume rather than a slice of the body, and allows computer reconstructions of the vascular systems.

MRI has the added advantage of sensitivity to iron accumulations which may occur within cirrhotic nodules (Fig. 4.1). MRI is also sensitive for the detection of hepatocellular carcinomas which may develop within these cirrhotic nodules.

The direction and velocity of blood flow in the portal venous system may be well demonstrated by using flow sensitive techniques including MRI angiography.

Angiography shows a 'corkscrew' pattern of the arterial branches reflecting the loss of volume of the liver, but is fairly non-specific.

PORTAL HYPERTENSION (PHT)

Imaging may reveal some of the causes and the effects of PHT. US may reveal clues to the diagnosis, such as features of portal vein thrombosis, cirrhosis or the Budd–Chiari syndrome. Effects of PHT include a distended portal vein, splenomegaly, ascites and spontaneous portosystemic collaterals including the coronary (left gastric) vein, recanalized umbilical vein and splenorenal veins. Gastro-esophageal varices may be seen as tubular structures adjacent to the esophagus. The use of Doppler US allows measurement of flow

direction and velocity as a guide to severity.

Portal vein thrombosis and portal cavernous transformation may be seen by US, CT with contrast medium and MRI.

MRI angiography with techniques to eliminate signals from other vessels can identify flow and direction in the portal veins.

PORTAL VEIN THROMBOSIS

This may be identified on US as an enlarged echogenic portal vein with no signal on Doppler interrogation. CT with intravenous contrast medium will also show lack of enhancement of the lumen of the occluded vessel.

Splenic or superior mesenteric artery injection with venous portography is usually definitive. Occasionally hepatofugal flow may create a pseudo-occlusion due to reversed flow in a patent splenic vein.

CONGENITAL HEPATIC FIBROSIS

This uncommon condition of children may reveal evidence of biliary dilatation and portal hypertension (PHT), as well as associated cystic disease in the kidney.

HEMOCHROMATOSIS

US has little role apart from detecting cirrhosis and portal hypertension. CT scanning may demonstrate an increase in the overall density of the liver in some patients with idiopathic hemochromatosis, and associated features of portal hypertension and cirrhosis.

Low signal intensity of the liver (due to paramagnetic effects of iron) and the spleen in secondary hemochromatosis are supportive features of the diagnosis on MRI, but are not consistently identified.

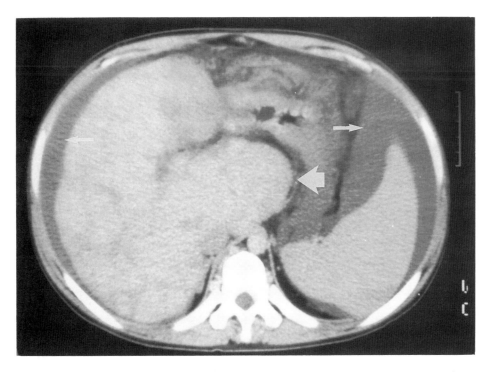

Figure 4.2 Chronic Budd–Chiari syndrome with caudate lobe hypertrophy (broad arrow) and ascites (thin arrows). Also note inhomogeneous appearance of liver on CT.

WILSON'S DISEASE

The abnormal accumulation of ceruloplasmin in the liver may be suggested on CT scanning by an increase in the density of the liver.

BUDD–CHIARI SYNDROME

The acute case presenting with hepatomegaly and ascites will benefit from imaging. Clot or obstructing tumor may be seen in the inferior vena cava (IVC) or hepatic veins, as may tumor in the liver. The use of duplex or color Doppler may show absent hepatic vein flow or reversed flow in vein branches.

Patchy perfusion of liver parenchyma due to the stagnant outflow may be seen on CT with contrast medium and angiography. Angiography may show stretched vessels indicating hepatomegaly. Inferior vena cavography showing a membrane, and

hepatic venography showing the classic 'spider web' pattern of new collaterals may be definitive. Direct injection of contrast medium into the hepatic parenchyma allows identification of outflow vessels.

In the chronic case, caudate lobe hypertrophy (Fig. 4.2), atrophy and regenerating nodules elsewhere may be seen with US, CT and MRI. Scintigraphy with sulfur colloid may show a 'hot spot' of uptake in the caudate lobe. Portal hypertension, ascites and nodular regeneration may all be seen.

FOCAL LIVER LESIONS

LIVER ABSCESSES

Amebic liver abscess

Amebic abscesses may be single or multiple. On US a surrounding rim of edema may be detectable. The content of the abscess ranges from fluid to markedly echogenic material simulating a solid lesion (Fig. 4.3). Careful observation in the latter cases may sometimes reveal slight internal movement of the thick echogenic fluid within the abscess. The inner lumen may be irregular. Attempted aspiration, if indicated, may assist in determining whether the abscess has liquefied or not.

On CT scanning the abscess is generally fairly well defined and of low density. The proximity of the abscess to the diaphragm, liver surface and pericardium are important prognostic and therapeutic pointers. Gas may be present in the abscess after secondary infection (rare), fistulation to the gastrointestinal tract or aspiration attempts.

Pyogenic abscesses

These range from large solitary abscesses to multiple abscesses. Ultrasound features range from fluid-containing cysts to fairly echogenic rounded lesions with gas (Fig. 4.4) or dependent debris which may appear to be solid. An associated biliary or gastrointestinal cause for the abscess may be identified.

On CT, abscesses appear as reasonably well-defined rounded low-density areas possibly containing gas. The wall of the abscess may enhance, and surrounding edema may be present. Septations may be apparent, but these do not always prevent drainage through a single catheter.

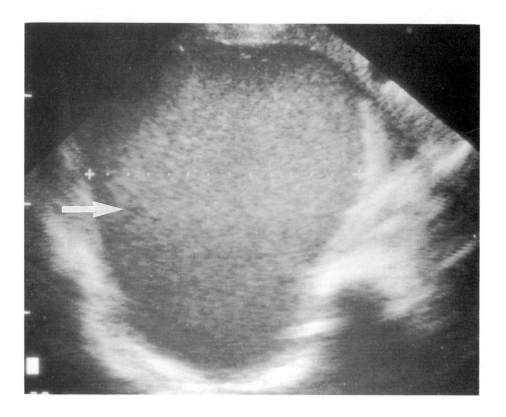

Figure 4.3 Echogenic fluid (arrow) in amebic abscess (cursors) simulating a solid lesion on US.

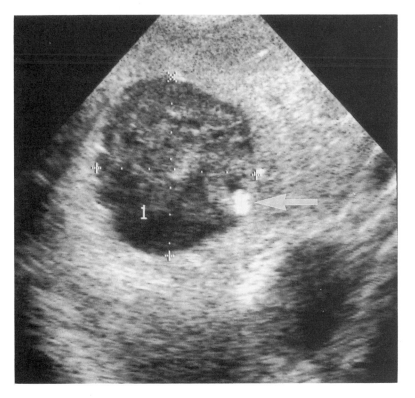

Figure 4.4 Pyogenic abscess (cursors) with echogenic fluid and gas bubble (arrow) on US.

Fungal abscesses

These uncommon abscesses may be suspected when they also occur in the spleen, or when they have central higher densities.

LIVER TRAUMA

Both blunt and penetrating injury to the liver can cause a wide range of appearances on imaging. Liver lacerations with intrahepatic, sub-capsular and/or intraperitoneal hemorrhage may be identified. Sub-capsular hematomas may be fairly extensive and have a characteristic lentiform or crescentic shape. It is important to consider whether an underlying pathological lesion or process is present precipitating the hemorrhage, particularly if the trauma was mild.

On ultrasound the intra- and peri-hepatic hemorrhage may appear inhomogeneous with a laminated appearance. As the hematoma ages and liquefies, central fluid areas are seen. The use of Doppler may facilitate identification of false aneurysms or arteriovenous (AV) fistulae. Hemobilia is suspected when a blood clot is seen in the gallbladder or main bile duct. The presence of blood in the peritoneal cavity may be suspected when echogenic ascites is seen.

CT scanning demonstrates hematoma in the early phase as a mixed, high-density appearance.

Angiography allows the accurate detection of extravasation, false aneurysms or AV fistulae and may allow for palliative or definitive embolization in association with surgery.

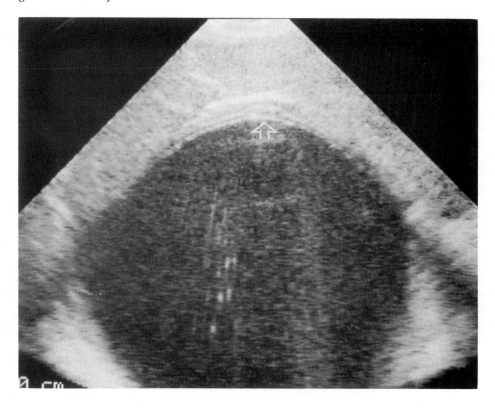

Figure 4.5 Hydatid cyst showing delamination of endocyst (arrow) from ectocyst on US.

The patency of the portal venous system should be established before embolization is performed.

LIVER CYSTS

Simple liver cysts

These common cysts may occur in isolation or associated with polycystic disease or tuberous sclerosis. Isolated cysts are usually single and may have fine septations. The wall is very thin and the contents have the imaging features of water. They may become fairly large, over 10 cm in diameter and may be symptomatic.

Hydatid cysts

The liver is the most common site for the development of the cysts of *Echinococcus gran-* *ulosus*. Characteristic cysts seen in other organs may support the diagnosis. The appearances range from that of a simple cyst to a complex 'mass'. Slight delamination of the endocyst from the ectocyst (Fig. 4.5), as well as the presence of internal membranes (Fig. 4.6) or daughter cysts (Fig. 4.7) seen on US, CT scanning or MRI are highly suggestive of the diagnosis. A more complex pattern may be seen with small daughter cysts, membranes and debris present. Dense curvilinear calcification may occur in older cysts. Segmental biliary fistulae and obstruction may occur. Membranes may enter the biliary tree and cause obstruction. These membranes are often not well seen by US, but can be detected by endoscopic retrograde cholangiopancreatography (ERCP) as undulating membranous filling defects.

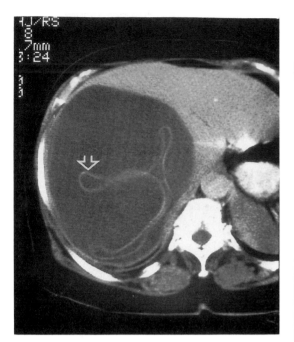

Figure 4.6 CT showing membrane lying (arrow) within hydatid cyst.

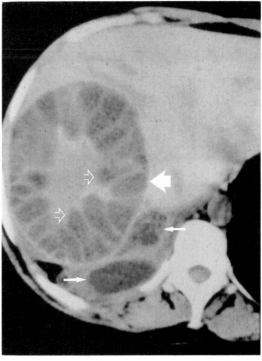

Figure 4.7 CT showing daughter cysts (open arrows) in hydatid cyst arranged around periphery of main cyst (broad arrows). Also note other cysts posteriorly (thin arrows).

BENIGN LIVER LESIONS

Cavernous hemangioma (CH)

This benign lesion is found in 4% of the population and is the most common benign tumor involving the liver. It consists of large vascular spaces lined by single layers of endothelial cells.

US detection of CH is good for lesions over 1–2 cm in diameter. Typically the smaller CH is a diffusely echogenic, well-defined lesion. The echogenicity is thought to be due to the interfaces created within the lesion by the endothelial-lined spaces. As the lesion enlarges it becomes inhomogeneous, with central hypoechoic areas due to scar formation following thrombosis. While the appearances may be highly suggestive of CH, caution should be exercised as primary or secondary malignancies may have similar features. However, in a patient with no history of malignancy and normal liver function tests a follow-up scan in 3–6 months has been recommended.

CT scanning without contrast medium typically shows a low-density, well-defined lesion within the liver. Larger lesions may have a lower density scar (Fig. 4.8a). A dynamic CT scan performed before, during and after the administration of contrast medium will give a diagnostic pattern in most CHs. A fairly dense peripheral nodular enhancement followed by gradual enhancement of the entire lesion, perhaps with the exception of a central scarred area, occurs (Fig. 4.8b).

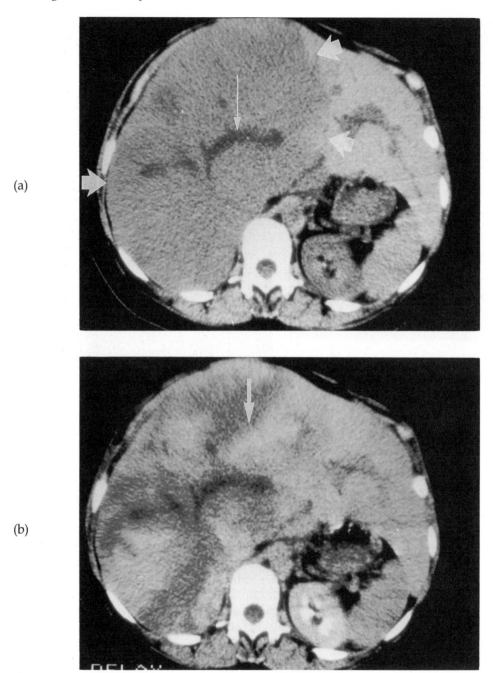

Figure 4.8 (a) CT of large right liver cavernous hemangioma (broad arrows) before contrast administration. Note central low-density scar (thin arrow). (b) A few minutes after contrast medium administration shows peripheral enhancement (arrow) of the cavernous hemangioma. The entire lesion subsequently became isodense with liver, apart form the central scar.

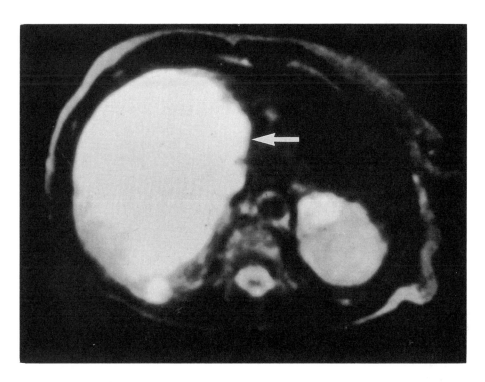

Figure 4.9 A T2-weighted MRI image showing the hyperintense 'light bulb' sign (arrow) of a cavernous hemangioma.

After several minutes, the lesion becomes the same density as liver (or the aortic lumen). This pattern reflects the diffusion of the contrast medium material into the blood-filled spaces of the CH. False positives for this type of appearance are rare but may occur with vascular malignancies. Unfortunately, a significant proportion of CH have atypical enhancement patterns, necessitating the use of other imaging strategies. During routine CT scanning with contrast medium, the lesion may be mistaken for other more sinister pathology.

MRI may show a characteristic pronounced T2 hyperintensity in CH. This is known as the 'light bulb' sign (Fig. 4.9). However, occasional cystic lesions can mimic CH on MRI. T2-weighted MRI is very sensitive for small CH and has a role particularly in diagnosis of those lesions closely related to the larger venous structures of the liver, which is a problem area for labeled red cell scans.

A labeled red cell isotope scan using technetium is another accurate way of diagnosing CH. The labeled red cells are injected intravenously; scanning over the liver will then show initial perfusion of the normal liver parenchyma with a photopenic defect representing the CH (Fig. 4.10a). Scanning over subsequent minutes shows the photopenic area filling in and gradually becoming increasingly active compared with the adjacent liver (Fig. 4.10b).

Angiography, previously the 'gold standard' for detection of CH, is infrequently used. The typical features are a normal feeding artery with peripheral irregular collections of contrast medium appearing in the late arterial phase and persisting well into the venous phase of the angiogram.

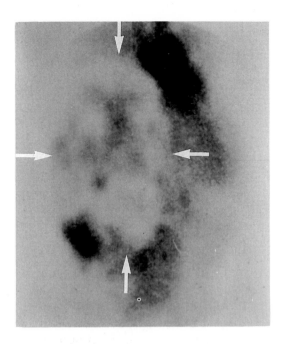 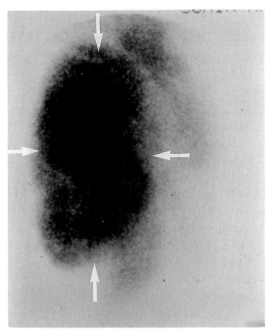

Figure 4.10 (a) Early phase of a labeled red cell scan showing photopenic area in the liver (arrows).

(b) Later scan showing filling in of the hemangioma with labeled red cells (arrows).

Hemangioendothelioma

This differs from CH in having multiple layers of endothelial cells lining the luminal surface. They may be hypervascular with an arteriovenous shunt, and tend to occur in children and neonates.

Hepatic adenoma

This uncommon benign neoplasm of hepatocytes is generally spherical in shape and fairly well defined with a pseudo-capsule. Adenomas occur most commonly in females in the third and fourth decades, often associated with the use of oral contraceptives. The major clinical problem of hepatic adenoma is the propensity of over one-third to bleed, sometimes fatally, either into the liver or, usually more seriously, into the peritoneal cavity.

The lesion is typically hyperechoic (due to cellular fat or glycogen content) or mixed without other distinguishing features on US. The use of color Doppler has been of limited value.

The lesion is close to the density of liver parenchyma on CT unless bleeding has occurred. Slight enhancement of the lesion may follow contrast medium administration.

On MRI the lesion may be hyperintense (due to fat) or isointense on T1-weighted images, and isointense on T2-weighted images with areas of hyperintense hemorrhage.

Angiography classically demonstrates a peripheral 'basket-weave' appearance of hypertrophied arterial vessels surrounding the tumor. Neovascularity is present with a slight capillary blush. No AV shunting is present. After a large hemorrhage the lesion may be compressed by the mass effect of the hemorrhage, with only an avascular area seen in the liver.

Focal nodular hyperplasia

This lesion is slightly more common than hepatic adenoma and is thought to arise on the basis of hamartomatous tissue or a small arteriovenous malformation. It may have a central stellate scar with radiating fibrous septae and possibly a pseudocapsule.

The lesion closely parallels the appearances of normal liver parenchyma on US, CT and MRI. There may be transient enhancement of the lesion with delayed enhancement of the scar after either iodine or gadolinium-containing contrast medium administration. The central scar tends to be hyperintense on T2-weighted images, probably due to the blood vessels and bile duct tissue within the fibrous scar.

Angiography typically demonstrates a central feeding vessel with branches radiating in fibrous septae into the hypervascular lesion with a prominent capillary blush. However, the angiographic features are frequently not specific.

Differentiating hepatic adenoma from focal nodular hyperplasia (FNH) is important clinically from a prognostic and therapeutic point of view as FNH is seldom a clinical problem, whereas the hepatic adenoma's tendency to hemorrhage necessitates resection in most cases.

Kuppfer cells are present both within FNH and hepatic adenomas and technetium sulfur colloid isotope uptake may occur in either. However, should uptake in the lesion exceed that of the adjacent liver parenchyma FNH is virtually certain as the Kuppfer cells in the hepatic adenoma do not function as well.

Hamartomas

Usually found in children, these often develop dominant cystic components.

MALIGNANT DISEASES OF THE LIVER

HEPATOCELLULAR CARCINOMA

Three patterns of hepatocellular carcinoma (HCC) have been recognized: single, multifocal or diffuse (Chapter 20). US is generally an accurate means of identification of HCC. Typically HCC are rounded hypoechoic lesions but a small percentage may be echogenic, possibly due to fatty change or dilated sinusoids in the tumor. Calcification is infrequent. Peripheral HCC typically bulges the liver capsule (Fig. 4.11). Pre-existing cirrhosis in the liver makes detection difficult by reducing the quality of scanning and making the liver appear inhomogeneous, limiting detection of small HCC. The features of portal hypertension may be present.

Most HCC are hypodense on CT without contrast medium. A small proportion are increased in density, possibly due to high copper binding protein content. Some HCC will have areas of very low density below 0 Hounsfield units, representing fatty metamorphosis. This is more commonly reported in the Far East, usually pathologically, and less frequently on imaging.

After intravenous contrast medium administration, there may be brief enhancement of the viable portion of most HCC but this rapidly reduces to the pre-contrast medium levels. The capsule may also enhance. Occasionally arterioportal shunting can be suspected by the prominent enhancement of adjacent portal vein branches. The detection of soft tissue density within portal vein branches (Fig. 4.12) or the biliary tree (Fig. 4.13) is highly suggestive of tumor infiltration, a typical feature of HCC. This may be seen both with ultrasound and CT, but is better seen in the smaller branches with US if carefully sought.

In general, CT scanning will detect lesions down to approximately 2 cm in diameter,

41

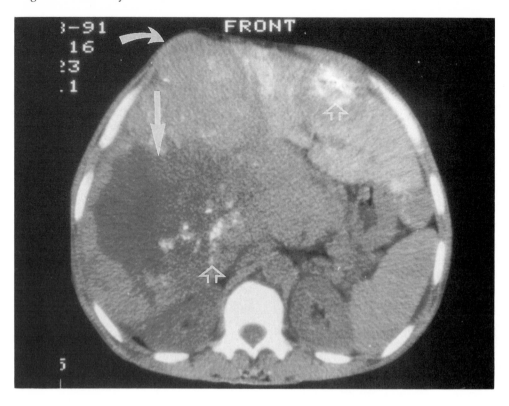

Figure 4.11 CT of large hepatocellular carcinoma after receiving intrarterial lipiodol and adriamycin (open arrows) for chemotherapy. Note the tumor bulging the anterior liver capsule (curved arrow). Also note central low-density necrosis (straight arrow).

with the size limit of US slightly better than this in good hands. Small HCC lesions may not be well seen on conventional contrast medium enhanced CT but the use of computerized tomographic arterial portography (CTAP) enhances their detection. The technique of CTAP entails the placement of an arterial catheter in the superior mesenteric artery during arteriography. This remains in position for the infusion of 100–150 ml of contrast medium given at a rate of 1–3 ml/sec. CT scanning is commenced 20–30 sec after starting this injection. By this time the portal venous return of contrast medium enhances the normal liver parenchyma but not the HCC. This provides excellent contrast between the HCC and liver. Lesions of 1 cm

or less can be accurately detected. However, false positives can occur with this technique, most notably perfusion defects which are usually characterized by their wedge-shaped configuration.

The use of lipiodol injection into the hepatic artery, followed by CT to detect smaller lesions is sometimes useful, but not specific (Fig. 4.11).

Magnetic resonance imaging is enjoying increased use in Japan in detection of HCC. Typically on T1-weighted imaging HCC are low intensity but in a small percentage may be higher intensity possibly due to fat, protein or copper content. T2-weighted imaging shows hyperintense lesions.

Morphological features that support the

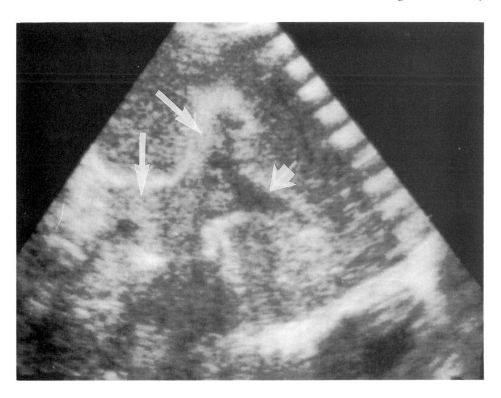

Figure 4.12 Transverse US investigation of left lobe of liver showing hepatocellular carcinoma infiltration (thin arrows) into left portal vein (broad arrow).

diagnosis of HCC on all imaging modalities include a fairly well-defined pseudocapsule consisting of fibrous tissue surrounded by compressed vessels and bile ducts. A central scar may be seen. Within the lesion a 'mosaic' pattern may be present. This is thought to arise as a result of new clones of tumor cells arising within the original lesion or by daughter cells being engulfed by the main lesion. Portal venous invasion may also be detectable on MRI.

Small HCC lesions remain difficult to detect. Angiographic features include large feeding arteries, hypervascularity and neovascularity (Fig. 4.14a) and arterioportal shunting. (Fig. 4.14b).

An important additional imaging point is that HCC may be associated with synchro-nous malignancies in other viscera, particularly the colon and stomach in up to 8% of patients.

A further finding may be evidence of rupture of the hepatocellular carcinoma with hemoperitoneum. This has been reported in 8% or more of patients in Japan and areas of Africa.

Fibrolamellar hepatocellular carcinoma

This infrequent variant of HCC is characterized by the amount of fibrous tissue within the stroma of the lesion. A fairly well-defined capsule and sometimes a central scar may be present.

The lesion may be difficult to distinguish from liver parenchyma on imaging, but may

43

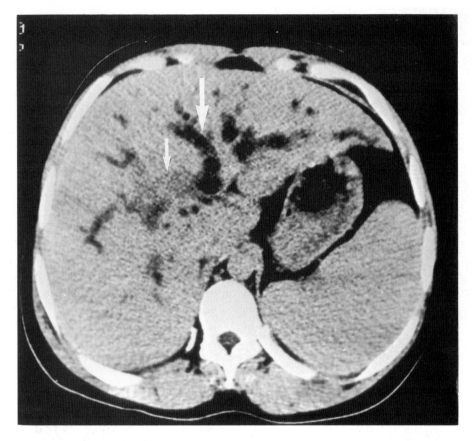

Figure 4.13 CT showing hepatocellular carcinoma (small arrow) infiltrating into the bile ducts causing biliary dilatation (large arrow).

have central calcification. After administration of contrast the central scar and capsule may enhance. On MRI scanning, the scar typically is hypointense on T2-weighted images. This is in contrast to the scar in FNH which is hyperintense due to the presence of vessels and ducts.

Hepatoblastoma

Found in children, these rare tumors tend to appear heterogeneous with cystic areas, calcification and/or hemorrhage. They are hypervascular on angiography.

Angiosarcoma

These very rare hypervascular lesions are often of a mixed solid and necrotic nature.

Metastases

Metastases are by far the most common malignancy in liver. The most common site of origin is the gastrointestinal tract. The large majority are multiple. Metastases may be hypoechoic, cystic (e.g. ovarian, colon and squamous), hyperechoic (e.g. colon) or mixed on US. Fine calcification may occur in mucinous adenocarcinoma metastases.

44

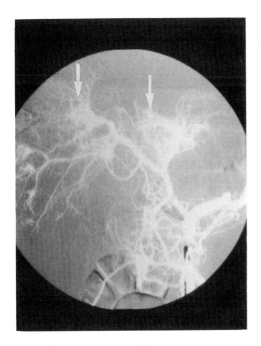

Figure 4.14 (a) Early arterial phase of an arteriogram showing marked neovascularity in hepatocellular carcinoma (arrows).

On CT scanning metastases are typically hypodense but calcification may be clearly seen. After contrast medium administration a variety of enhancement patterns including peripheral, mixed and central types occur. Hypervascular metastases enhance strongly and include renal, carcinoid and islet cell tumors. There is a risk that enhancing lesions may mask themselves by becoming equal in density to the liver. About one-third of metastases do not enhance. CT performed with a dynamic incremental bolus technique (DIBCT) using an intravenously injected bolus of contrast medium is more accurate than unenhanced CT. CTAP provides an even more accurate method. This is important where resection of colon carcinoma metastases is contemplated. Generally up to four of these metastases may be resected with an improved prognosis. This resection may be assisted by intraoperative ultrasound, which is one of the most accurate methods of imaging.

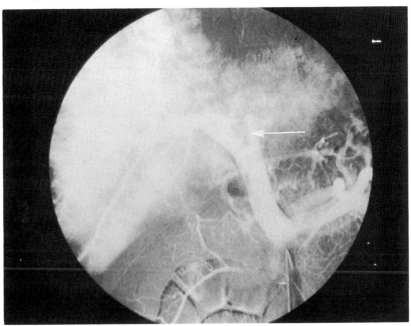

Figure 4.14 (b) Later film showing marked arterioportal shunting and tumor occluding left portal vein and protruding into the main portal vein (arrow).

MRI is sensitive for the detection of metastases showing hypointense lesions on T1-weighted imaging and hyperintense lesions on T2-weighted imaging. Occasionally a halo may be seen. The newer fast sequences and gradient echo and echo planar imaging techniques may provide advantages. Injection of gadolinium either intravenously or as with CTAP also has benefit in some cases. The dynamic contrast medium behavior is as for CT.

Lymphoma

This may occur as a solitary mass, as nodules or as a diffuse process. It can simulate liver metastases on imaging, appearing as hypoechoic or low-density lesions. Ancillary features such as splenomegaly, para-aortic adenopathy and bowel wall thickening are helpful in suggesting the diagnosis.

CONCLUSIONS

At a practical level ultrasound is generally the first investigation of choice. It is cost-effective and accurate if performed correctly. It generally easily separates solid and cystic lesions. Intraoperative ultrasound is one of the most accurate imaging methods reserved for resection of HCC and metastases.

CT is an excellent second line investigation provided that contrast medium is given rapidly and in large enough amounts. CT arterial portography (CTAP) is a further improvement in accuracy mainly reserved for pre-operative staging of metastases or HCC.

Magnetic resonance scanning is useful in the detection of CH and malignant lesions, with promising improvements in scanning times and contrast medium usage.

Nuclear medicine is generally reserved for detection of CH and for separating FNH and hepatic adenoma from other lesions.

The supportive role of fine needle aspiration biopsy under US or CT guidance is critical in speeding up the histological diagnosis in these cases.

BILIARY DISEASE

IMAGING ANATOMY

The central intrahepatic biliary tree can normally only be seen parallel to the portal vein branches. With dilatation there is an increase in slightly tortuous tubular structures in the liver. The common hepatic and bile ducts are jointly referred to as the main bile duct, as the entrance of the cystic duct is not seen clearly enough on US to allow distinction of these two sections. The main bile duct normally measures less than 6 mm in diameter and is located directly anterior to the portal vein in the porta hepatis. The gallbladder normally measures <4 cm in transverse diameter and its wall is <3 mm in thickness.

OBSTRUCTIVE JAUNDICE

Imaging is able to diagnose the obstruction, its level and its cause in the majority of cases. An abrupt irregular termination of a duct suggests malignancy; a smooth gradual taper or smooth rounded filling defect favors benign disease. Extrahepatic dilatation tends to occur first. Left duct dilatation may precede right duct dilatation. Focal atrophy and hypertrophy may be seen due to vascular or biliary compromise. US is the first recommended investigation.

Biliary calculi

US is the modality of choice for evaluation of gallbladder calculi. The accuracy is excellent provided that visualization is adequate. A well-distended gallbladder, achieved by fasting the patient prior to the ultrasound, greatly facilitates visualization. A mobile echogenic focus casting an acoustic shadow is diagnostic of a biliary calculus. There are a number of appearances of calculi; small floating stones, pigment stones, mixed stones and cholesterol stones all have varying appearances. Positioning of the patient is critical in detecting the more difficult to see calculi. A repeat scan after a few days is often useful. Biliary sludge may mask small calculi.

Gas in the biliary tree may be seen on plain film, US and CT. Causes include fistulae, sepsis and surgery. Once calculi have entered the common bile duct they are far more difficult to detect accurately by US. Overlying duodenal gas frequently obscures the lower portion of the common bile duct.

The next step in investigation, if needed, is ERCP. This is very sensitive for the detection of biliary calculi both in the gallbladder and in the remainder of the biliary tree. The further advantage of ERCP is the ability to perform a sphincterotomy and remove biliary calculi if indicated.

CT scanning may detect stones in the main bile duct as densities in the duct, and help resolve problem cases. The 2,6-dimethyl-phenylcarbamoylmethyl iminodiacetic acid (HIDA) scan may also be useful.

Intrahepatic calculi

Relatively common in the Far East and in parts of Africa, these are probably due to *Clonorchis sinensis* in the former and *Ascaris lumbricoides* in the latter. These may not be well seen by either US or CT, possibly due to their pigment nature, but ERCP or percutaneous transhepatic cholangiography (PTC) usually demonstrate them well.

Pancreatitis

Chronic pancreatitis often produces a smooth tapered narrowing of the distal main bile duct. Calcification in the pancreas on CT and a dilated pancreatic duct with abnormal side

branches on US, CT and ERCP are supportive features.

Ascariasis

Biliary ascariasis can be common where this infestation is frequent. Generally seen in the main bile duct on cholangiography (Fig. 4.15) or US (Fig. 4.16), they can also be seen intrahepatically, in the gallbladder or the pancreatic duct. On US they are seen as parallel echogenic lines, which may appear like short tubes.

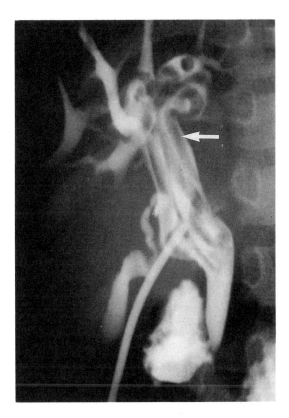

Figure 4.15 Ascaris worms (arrow) noted in common hepatic duct during T-tube cholangiogram.

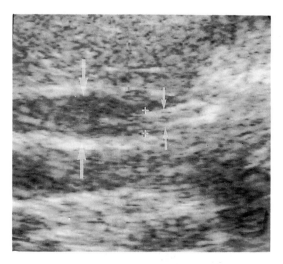

Figure 4.16 Longitudinal US of a dilated main bile duct (large arrows) showing ascaris as parallel echogenic lines (small arrows and cursors).

Post surgical complications

These are generally in the form of biliary stenoses or bile leaks with biliary dilatation, jaundice and/or cholangitis.

Pancreatic head carcinoma

This is the commonest cause of malignant biliary obstruction. Features of biliary dilatation will be seen upstream of the tumor but frequently the pancreatic head lesion is underestimated or poorly seen, if at all. CT scanning improves the detection of pancreatic head carcinoma, particularly with the use of a rapidly given bolus of intravenous contrast medium to enhance the adjacent normal parenchymal pancreas and vascular structures.

ERCP has a cardinal role in this diagnosis, showing duct abnormalities such as irregular narrowing and the 'double duct' sign of adjacent irregular occlusions of pancreatic and bile ducts.

Cholangiocarcinoma

Cholangiocarcinoma is less common than HCC and occurs in two main pathological forms:

1. A sclerosing type.
2. A less common nodular type.

Predisposing causes include stones, sepsis, choledochal cysts or sclerosing cholangitis.

The more common sclerosing form often causes extrahepatic duct or bifurcation obstruction (Fig. 4.17). These are often poorly detectable on US and CT imaging (Fig. 4.18) and the evidence of the biliary dilatation in both lobes without significant extrahepatic dilatation is usually the clue. MRI is also not able to demonstrate clearly these sclerosing cholangiocarcinomas. ERCP and percutaneous transhepatic cholangiography clearly demonstrate the involvement of the ducts by the

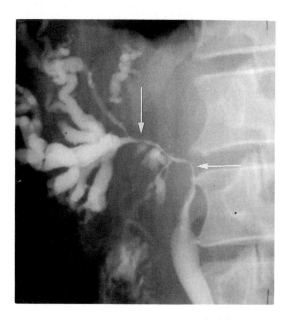

Figure 4.17 Cholangiogram showing extensive cholangiocarcinoma (arrows) extending well into the right ducts.

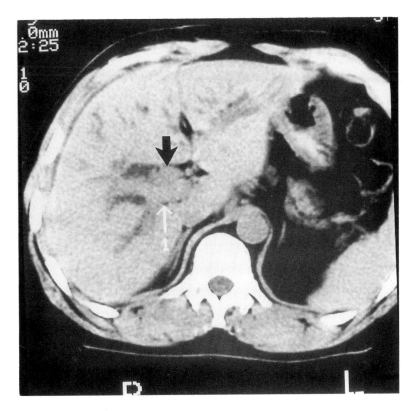

Figure 4.18 CT showing small cholangiocarcinoma (black arrow) anterior to portal vein (white arrow).

cholangiocarcinoma and also allow the possibility of therapeutic intervention.

The nodular type may simulate a liver parenchymal mass such as HCC. A rarer type of cholangiocarcinoma is the papillary intraluminal type.

Periampullary carcinoma

This rare condition, offering a significantly better outlook than pancreatic head carcinoma, is generally diagnosed by ERCP.

Hilar metastases

Nodal involvement in the hepatic hilum can closely simulate cholangiocarcinoma, as may benign disease.

INFLAMMATORY CONDITIONS

Acute cholecystitis

Ultrasound provides an accurate means of assessing the gallbladder in suspected acute cholecystitis. Cardinal features of this condition include gallbladder wall thickening (>3 mm), pericholecystic fluid, calculi within the lumen, debris and membranes in the lumen, gallbladder distension (>40 mm transversely), a pericholecystic halo and abnormalities of the gallbladder wall including lucencies and gas (Fig. 4.19). Diffuse thickening of the gallbladder wall may be due to intrinsic causes such as cholecystitis, sepsis, perforation, carcinoma or AIDS. Extrinsic causes include hepatitis, congestive cardiac failure, hypoalbuminemia, fluid overload or cirrhosis. Irregular thickening of the gallbladder wall may be due

49

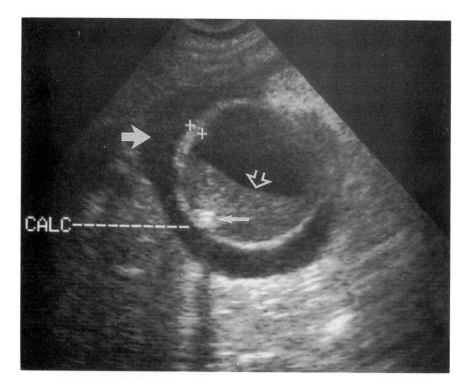

Figure 4.19 Transverse US of the gallbladder showing calculus (small arrow), sludge (open arrow), thick wall of gallbladder (cursors) and pericholecystic fluid (large arrow).

to polyps, carcinoma, metastases, chronic cholecystitis or an adherent stone. Causes of gallbladder distension include obstructive or non-obstructive conditions, the latter including hyperalimentation, bedridden patients, diabetes mellitus, AIDS and narcotics.

CT scanning may provide additional information in complicated acute cholecystitis.

The iminodiacetic acid scans (e.g. HIDA) may be useful ancillary tests for cholecystitis, showing no gallbladder uptake in the acute case, and delayed uptake in chronic cholecystitis.

Chronic cholecystitis

These cases tend to have shrunken, thick-walled gallbladders on imaging that may easily be overlooked. Stones in the gallbladder may be misinterpreted as bowel gas.

Sclerosing cholangitis

This condition is generally poorly evaluated by US and CT but thickening and irregular caliber variation of bile duct walls may be noted. Features of biliary cirrhosis may be superimposed.

This condition may be either primary, including that associated with inflammatory bowel disease, or secondary, due to sepsis, stones or surgery.

ERCP is the definitive test for the detection of sclerosing cholangitis and clearly demonstrates the intra- and extrahepatic involvement (Fig. 4.20). The irregular narrowing of the

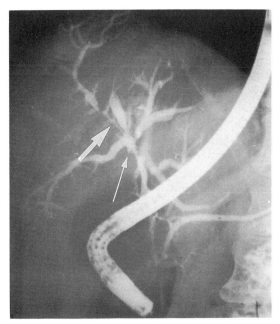

Figure 4.20 ERCP showing irregular narrowing (large arrow) and diverticulum formation (thin arrow) in sclerosing cholangitis.

ducts with occasional diverticuli and shortening are all suggestive features. The development of cholangiocarcinomas in these patients should be anticipated.

CONGENITAL BILIARY CONDITIONS

Choledochal cysts

Perhaps more accurately termed choledochectasia, this uncommon condition is more often seen in the pediatric population. Ultrasound is an excellent means of assessing both the intra- and extrahepatic involvement. Caroli's disease is well evaluated by US and CT (Fig. 4.21) showing duct involvement and stones. Stones can be mistaken as gas in the bile ducts on US. ERCP and PTC also provide useful information concerning the extent of this condition. CT allows the assessment of liver atrophy and hypertrophy. The development of cholangiocarcinoma may be identified by any of these modalities.

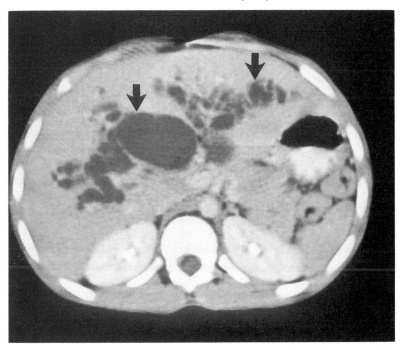

Figure 4.21 CT showing markedly dilated ducts (arrows) in Caroli's disease.

Benign biliary tumors

These are rare, but include biliary cystadenoma which is often a cystic mass with an irregular thickened wall and many septa.

Biliary fistulae

These may occur in the duodenum or colon from the gallbladder or main bile duct. Sinograms, barium studies or ERCP may demonstrate the abnormality.

HEPATIC TRANSPLANTATION

The potential complications of liver transplantation include problems of leaks or obstructions at any of the anastomotic sites:

- the biliary anastomosis (either to bowel or bile duct);
- the portal vein anastomosis;
- the hepatic artery anastomosis;
- the IVC anastomoses.

The use of Doppler US facilitates screening for vascular complications, but angiography may be needed.

Focal liver lesions including lymphoceles occur fairly frequently. Bile lakes and biliary dilatation or narrowing may follow rejection or vascular compromise, and may be seen by US, CT, ERCP or PTC.

CONCLUSIONS

In general, US scanning is the primary imaging modality for detection of biliary disease. It is accurate and effective, and is generally able to assess the intra- and extrahepatic systems including the gallbladder.

CT scanning may be a useful ancillary imaging modality for complex cases. ERCP and PTC are extremely informative, as well as providing the option of treatment in various biliary conditions.

RECOMMENDED READING

Choi, B.I., Takayasu, K. and Han, M.C. (1993) Small hepatocellular carcinomas and associated nodular lesions of the liver: pathology, pathogenesis, and imaging findings. *AJR*, **160**, 1177–87.

Di Lelio, A., Cestari, C., Lomazzi, A. and Beretta, L. (1989) Cirrhosis: Diagnosis with sonographic study of the liver surface. *Radiology*, **172**, 389–92.

Drane, W.E. and Van Ness, M.M. (1988) Hepatic imaging in diffuse liver disease. *Clin Nucl Med*, **13**, 182–5.

Freeny, P.C. (1988) Hepatic CT: state of the art. *Radiology*, **168**, 319–23.

Freeny, P.C. (1990) Radiological diagnosis of hepatic neoplasms. *Postgrad Radiol*, **10**, 265–86.

Golli, M., Mathieu, D., Anglade, M.-C. *et al.* (1993) Focal nodular hyperplasia of the liver: value of color Doppler US in association with MR imaging. *Radiology*, **187**, 113–17.

Harned, R.K., Chezmar, J.L. and Nelson, R.C. (1992) Imaging of patients with potentially resectable hepatic neoplasms. *AJR*, **159**, 1191–4.

Heiken, J.P., Brink, J.A., McLennan, B.L. *et al.* (1993) Dynamic contrast-enhanced CT of the liver: comparison of contrast medium injection rates and uniphasic and biphasic injection protocols. *Radiology*, **187**, 327–31.

Joseph, A.E.A. and Saverymuttu, S.H. (1991) Ultrasound in the assessment of diffuse parenchymal liver disease (Editorial). *Clin Radiol*, **44**, 219–21.

Lindberg, C.-G., Lundstedt, C., Stridbeck, H. and Tranberg, K.-G. (1993) Accuracy of CT arterial portography of the liver compared with findings at laparotomy. *Acta Radiologica*, **34**, 139–42.

Low, R.N., Francis, I.R., Sigeti, J.S. and Foo, T.K.F. (1993) Abdominal MR imaging: comparison of T2-weighted fast and conventional spin-echo, and contrast-enhanced fast multiplanar spoiled gradient-recalled imaging. *Radiology*, **186**, 803–11.

Numata, K., Tanaka, K., Mitsui, K. *et al.* (1993) Flow characteristics of hepatic tumors at color Doppler sonography: Correlation with arteriographic findings. *AJR*, **160**, 515–21.

Procacci, C., Fugazzola, C., Cinquino, M. *et al.* (1992) Contribution of CT to characterization of focal nodular hyperplasia of the liver. *Gastrointest Radiol*, **17**, 63–73.

Rubin, R.A., Lichtenstein, G.R. and Alvi, A. (1993) Hepatic scintigraphy in the evaluation of solitary solid liver masses. *J Nucl Med*, **34**, 697–705.

Saini, S. (1992) Contrast-enhanced MR imaging of the liver. *Radiology*, **182**, 12–14.

Soyer, P., Roche, A., Levesque, M. and Legmann, P. (1991) CT of fibrolamellar hepatocellular carcinoma. *J Comput Assist Tomogr*, **15**, 533–8.

Soyer, P., Elias, D., Zeitoun, G. *et al.* (1993) Surgical treatment of hepatic metastases: impact of intraoperative sonography. *AJR*, **160**, 511–14.

Soyer, P., Van Beers, B., Grandin, C. *et al.* (1993) Primary lymphoma of the liver: MR findings. *Eur J Radiol*, **16**, 209–12.

5

Biopsy of the liver

RICHARD HIFT

INTRODUCTION

Though biochemical and serological tests and hepatic imaging all provide useful information about the cause and extent of hepatic disease, it is often important to assess liver histology directly in order to diagnose a patient's illness and manage it correctly. Where the indication is appropriate and an acceptable technique is employed, closed percutaneous needle biopsy is a safe and useful diagnostic procedure.

INDICATIONS

Biopsy is invaluable in the diagnosis of hepatic disease in cases where the cause of the illness is not otherwise apparent, or where more than one cause may be operative. Thus biopsy may help define the cause of hepatomegaly, abnormal transaminase levels or a hepatic mass. An assessment of liver histology is also useful in monitoring the progress of chronic liver disease and in assessing the need for specific therapy (such as interferon for viral hepatitis or immunosuppression for autoimmune chronic active hepatitis) as well as in assessing the degree of response to therapy. It also provides prog-

nostic information in many disorders. After transplantation it may help in the diagnosis of rejection or infection in the grafted liver. Biopsy may also aid the diagnosis of systemic disease by demonstrating the presence of specific pathological features in the liver as part of a generalized illness; examples are malignant infiltration in lymphoma and caseating granulomas in tuberculosis. Liver biopsy may also confirm a diagnosis of some inherited metabolic conditions, such as hemochromatosis and Wilson's disease.

CONTRAINDICATIONS

There are few absolute contraindications to percutaneous liver biopsy but a number of relative contraindications exist. The decision to perform a biopsy on a patient is always an individual one, and, in general, the more contraindications a patient has, the more reluctantly the biopsy should be performed.

ABSOLUTE CONTRAINDICATIONS

Where the patient is confused or uncooperative percutaneous biopsy should not be undertaken except under general anesthesia as sudden movements during the procedure may lead to laceration of the liver. Focal lesions that may represent vascular tumors such as a hemangioma must not be needled until they have been proved not to be vascular by angiography, dynamic computed tomography (CT) scanning or labeled erythrocyte studies. Hydatid cysts must not be punctured, to avoid soiling the peritoneal cavity with cyst contents which may result in anaphylaxis and metastatic seeding of the disease. Biopsy must not be undertaken in the presence of dilated intrahepatic bile ducts since these increase the risk of a biliary leak and consequent peritonitis. Refractory ascites is also a contraindication as the interposition of fluid between the abdominal wall and liver makes direct pressure and hemostasis less effective.

RELATIVE CONTRAINDICATIONS

A coagulopathy, conveniently defined as an international normalized ratio in excess of 1.4, a platelet count of $<60 \times 10^9/l$ or a prolonged bleeding time, and also significant anemia are contraindications to biopsy until such time as they have been corrected because of the risk of hemorrhage. Ascites should be cleared before biopsy is undertaken. Though biopsy may be helpful in the diagnosis of the Budd–Chiari syndrome, both this and severe congestive heart failure are relative contraindications since the engorged venous system of the liver may predispose to hemorrhage. Two infiltrative conditions, myelofibrosis and amyloidosis, are also regarded as relative contraindications since in these disorders the liver is stiff and inflexible and bleeding may be severe and prolonged.

Biopsy should also be avoided in suspected focal malignant disease which is potentially curable by resection, particularly where the tumor lies near the liver surface and cannot be approached through a margin of normal liver. Malignant seeding may occur down the needle track and on to the peritoneal surface, with earlier dissemination and a lower chance that surgery will be effective. In such a case consideration should be given to making the diagnosis by frozen section during laparotomy rather than by a needle biopsy.

INAPPROPRIATE INDICATIONS

There are also some circumstances in which biopsy is inappropriate. If the cause of an acute viral or toxic hepatitis is obvious and the disease is likely to be self limiting, the diagnosis can be confirmed by serological tests and the progress of the disease monitored biochemically. It is here not necessary to obtain histological confirmation. As with many other interventions in medicine, there is little point in performing a biopsy if the result is unlikely to influence outcome or management.

PREPARATION OF THE PATIENT FOR BIOPSY

One area of medicine in which a defensive approach to practice is justifiable is in the performance of a liver biopsy. Complications should be foreseen and conditions optimized so as to reduce their likelihood.

The hemoglobin concentration, platelet count and prothrombin time should be assessed before the biopsy. It is wise to have the patient's blood cross-matched or at least have blood screened for unusual antibodies, so that compatible blood can be transfused without delay in an emergency.

It is useful to have a recent assessment of the liver by ultrasound or CT before embarking on the biopsy. This will exclude some contraindications to liver biopsy such as the presence of dilated ducts, may allow one to choose an approach that will avoid large veins or an aberrant gallbladder, and may give an indication of which area of the liver to sample for focal disease. The radiologist may be asked to indicate a suitable point of entry, depth and direction of biopsy to increase the yield and minimize the risk. Under some circumstances, it is appropriate to perform the biopsy under direct ultrasonic or tomographic guidance.

Details of the procedure must be explained fully to the patient who should then provide written, witnessed consent for the procedure. The biopsy should be carried out on a weekday morning wherever possible so that nursing and medical staff are available to observe the patient in the early post-biopsy period and to intervene in the event of complications. It is not advisable to perform a biopsy on a fasting patient since the gallbladder is more likely to be distended and will thus be more easily punctured. Thus the patient should have a light breakfast on the morning of the procedure and the biopsy should be performed within 2 hours of eating.

An intravenous line should be established in the left arm before the biopsy. This facilitates the administration of pre-medication, and will allow fluid replacement without delay in the event of a severe vasovagal episode or a catastrophic hemorrhage, as a result of which veins may collapse and cannulation will be difficult when it is needed most.

Adequate analgesic pre-medication is essential for a safe and satisfactory biopsy, though the patient should be awake enough to co-operate during the procedure. Intramuscular or oral narcotic analgesics are not nearly as satisfactory as intravenous narcotics given immediately before the biopsy as their absorption may be irregular and the patient's sensitivity to the medication is impossible to predict. Though pethidine alone often has sufficient sedative effect, a short-acting anxiolytic may be useful for the particularly anxious patient. Antibiotic prophylaxis is seldom indicated.

During the biopsy, the patient should lie obliquely with the right chest wall uppermost. The liver is usually biopsied through the pleural and intercostal spaces. Where it is enlarged, it may be possible to enter it through the abdominal wall, but this is always risky as the gallbladder or bowel may be punctured. Such an approach is best reserved for biopsy under ultrasonic guidance. Forced full inspiration or expiration are uncomfortable positions for the patient to hold and are in most cases unnecessary. The biopsy should be performed at the end of a gentle exhalation after which the patient should hold his or her breath. This position should be held during percussion of the chest to identify the area of liver dullness, during the administration of local anesthetic and while the biopsy is performed. It should be practiced with the patient once or twice before the biopsy commences. For blind biopsy, the liver should be entered via an intercostal space over the point of maximum liver dullness. This is assessed by percussing the upper and lower margins of the liver. A point just off the mid-axillary line (avoiding the lateral intercostal vessels) should be selected and marked with a pen. Once the biopsy site has been selected, the skin should be cleaned with iodine and alcohol. A sterile technique should be employed from here on.

Local analgesia is an important and often neglected part of the procedure. Adequate analgesia will not only reduce the patient's discomfort, but will also avoid the risk of a sudden gasp or movement, which may lead to laceration of the liver, as the biopsy needle is introduced. A common mistake is to infiltrate large amounts of local anesthetic subcutaneously, leaving the most important pain sensitive structures, the pleura and hepatic capsule, inadequately anesthetized. Following anesthetization of the skin through a small subcutaneous needle, a larger needle should be placed on the syringe and the patient asked to hold his or her breath at the end of a quiet exhalation. The needle is then inserted deeply enough to reach the capsule and pleura. This can be assessed by having the patient breathe gently with the needle *in situ*. Movement of the needle with respiration will confirm that it has penetrated the pleura. Conventional hypodermic needles may not be sufficiently long in obese patients or those with thick, muscular chests; a lumbar puncture needle may be a useful alternative. Following gentle aspiration to ensure that a blood vessel has not been entered, the local anesthetic is infiltrated widely both at this level and during withdrawal of the needle.

BIOPSY TECHNIQUE

Two techniques of percutaneous closed biopsy are in standard use. Both have advantages and disadvantages.

MENGHINI TECHNIQUE

In its simplest form, this needs only a syringe and Menghini needle, a reusable hollow metal needle with a sharp bevel and a plug at the proximal end. The technique is simple but requires some coordination. The needle is plunged into the liver substance while the plunger is simultaneously withdrawn, creating a vacuum in the syringe and withdrawing a core of liver tissue into the needle. This is cut off by the sharp edge of the needle, a process which may be aided by slight rotation. The introduction of a disposable plastic Menghini set (the Hepafix® kit) has greatly simplified the procedure. This set consists of a needle and syringe. The interior of the needle contains a small plastic stopper which prevents the biopsy specimen from being withdrawn into the syringe. This should not be removed. Around the needle is a plastic guard to prevent the needle being inserted too deeply. It is important to remove this when performing

the biopsy on a very obese patient, otherwise the needle may not prove long enough to reach the liver tissue. One side of the syringe is fitted with a stopper. As the plunger is withdrawn from the barrel of the syringe, the stopper springs out and prevents return of the plunger into the syringe. Thus, a vacuum is maintained within the syringe during performance of the biopsy without the need to coordinate the hands to prevent the plunger returning into the syringe.

Technique

A few milliliters of saline are drawn into the syringe and the needle is flushed. A skin incision just large enough to accept the needle is made. The needle is then advanced through the incision to the subcutaneous tissues and pleura. Half the saline is then expelled to clear the needle lumen. The patient is instructed to hold his or her breath at the end of a quiet expiration. The plunger is withdrawn and locked to create a vacuum. Taking care to advance the needle perpendicularly, i.e. directly towards the center of the right lobe of the liver, the needle is advanced firmly and quickly several centimeters into the liver. The whole assembly is then smartly withdrawn. A slight rotation as the needle is withdrawn may aid separation of the specimen. A gauze swab is placed over the incision to control superficial bleeding and the patient is turned on to his or her right-hand side.

The core is then expelled from the Hepafix® needle by unlocking the stopper, which will release the vacuum, and gently squirting a small amount of saline through the needle. This may have to be done several times before the specimen appears. The major advantage of the Menghini technique is that the diameter of the needle is smaller and the risk of hemorrhage correspondingly less. The disadvantages are that the core is smaller, and that a very fibrotic or cirrhotic specimen may fragment.

VIM SILVERMAN TECHNIQUE

The Vim Silverman needle uses a cutting sleeve to slice off a core of liver tissue which is then withdrawn into the needle. It has largely been replaced by the disposable TruCut® needle which uses a modified form of the same technique. It gives a somewhat larger and more reliable core than the Menghini needle, particularly in the fibrotic liver, but may carry a slightly higher risk of complications.

The needle has a sharp closed point behind which is an open chamber which will hold the specimen. Around the needle is a sliding sleeve with a sharp cutting edge which will slice off the sample as it moves down over the chamber. This cutting sleeve is operated by manipulating the two plastic handles of the instrument.

Technique

The initial anesthetization and incision of the skin and subcutaneous tissues are the same as that for the Menghini technique. At the end of a quiet expiration, the patient is instructed to hold his or her breath. The upper part of the needle should be guarded with the left hand to prevent it advancing too far into the liver. The needle is introduced perpendicularly to the skin and is directed towards the center of the right lobe of the liver. With the needle in the closed position, the assembly is plunged deep into the substance of the liver. The central needle is now advanced smartly, bringing the chamber out from within the sleeve. A piece of liver will prolapse into the chamber. Holding the needle firmly in this position, the lower handle is pushed sharply downwards which will cause the cutting edge to slide over the specimen chamber, slicing off a core which will then lodge in the chamber. A common error is to withdraw the point into the sleeve rather than to advance the sleeve towards the point. The whole assembly is now withdrawn with the handles

in this position. The TruCut® needle remains in the liver appreciably longer than the Menghini needle and requires more coordination for correct use. Provided the patient has been adequately anesthetized, is cooperative and holds his or her breath, excessive speed is unnecessary and it is better to perform the three stages of the technique correctly and deliberately rather than to fudge them by excessive haste.

Automatic triggering devices such as the TruCut® gun are available to make coordination of these three actions easier; consequently the needle spends less time in the liver, which is safer. Whichever technique is employed, practice and initial performance under supervision are essential.

POSTOPERATIVE CARE OF THE PATIENT

Following the biopsy, the incision is cleaned, dried and a simple wound dressing placed over it. For 2 hours, the patient should lie on his or her right side, which will apply pressure to the puncture site and promote hemostasis. Bedrest should be maintained for 6 hours. In many instances patients may return home the same day, though those at higher risk of complications, including patients with established cirrhosis, should be observed overnight. Nursing staff should be instructed in writing to perform adequate and frequent observations to detect the onset of complications at an early stage. They may, for instance, be ordered to monitor the pulse, blood pressure and degree of pain every 15 minutes for the first hour, every 30 minutes for the next 2 hours, hourly for the next 4 hours and then 4-hourly thereafter. The hemoglobin concentration or hematocrit should be checked twice in the first 8 hours. Nursing staff should be explicitly instructed to report a rise in pulse rate, a drop in systolic blood pressure or any abdominal pain to the doctor.

COMPLICATIONS OF CLOSED NEEDLE BIOPSY

The procedure has an overall morbidity of 1–2% with a reported mortality from 0.02–0.2%, which is marginally higher with use of cutting needles such as the Vim Silverman or TruCut® technique. The most common complications are pain and hemorrhage. The pain is often pleural and results from the passage of the needle through the pleural space. It may be minimized by adequate pre-medication and local anesthesia. It often responds well to narcotics such as tilidine or pethidine. Non-steroidal anti-inflammatory drugs and aspirin should be avoided after biopsy as they may inhibit platelet function, and indeed should not be administered for 7 to 10 days before biopsy.

Hemorrhage is common after biopsy but is minor in most cases. More severe hemorrhage is marked by the occurrence of pain over the liver itself (suggesting a sub-capsular hematoma) or by peritoneal pain indicating a bleed into the peritoneal space, or by tachycardia and hypotension. Management is by adequate analgesia, fluid replacement, and, if necessary, transfusion.

Where pain is particularly severe, or there is evidence of continuing blood loss, an ultrasonographic examination should be performed to delineate the extent of a hematoma. In most cases, bleeding will cease spontaneously, but it is wise to call in the assistance of a surgeon early as operation may be required. Obviously, it is essential that abnormalities in the prothrombin time or platelet count be corrected where these may contribute to the bleeding.

Other complications include vasovagal reactions, which will respond to fluid administration and atropine, a biliary leak with peritonitis, hemopneumothorax, and puncture of the abdominal or thoracic viscera.

The risk of hemorrhage has been shown to correlate with the number of attempts at biopsy. It is generally not advisable to perform more than two or at most three passes through the liver with a needle. Where an initial attempt with the Menghini technique fails, particularly where one suspects the liver is fibrotic or cirrhotic, it may be advisable to perform the second pass with a TruCut® needle.

HANDLING OF THE SPECIMEN

A single core may be divided into smaller specimens for different tests. This should be done by dividing the specimen on a wooden spatula with a sharp blade. Specimens for histology are placed in formalin, those for electron microscopy are best preserved in glutaraldehyde, and those for microbiology or frozen section in a small volume of normal saline which must not contain bacteriostatic chemicals, as do many vials of saline. It cannot be stressed enough that the utility and reliability of a histologist's report increases in proportion to the amount of clinical and laboratory information supplied to him or her. A knowledge of the background to the case greatly facilitates histological diagnosis. The request form for the histologist should always contain full clinical and laboratory information including relevant biochemical, hematological, serological and radiological findings.

OTHER TECHNIQUES OF LIVER BIOPSY

A transvenous liver biopsy is performed by catheterizing a hepatic vein (usually via the internal jugular vein), wedging the catheter in the hepatic substance and taking several small biopsies with a catheter-mounted needle. Its major advantage is that there is minimal risk of free hemorrhage. It also allows the estimation of pressure gradients across the inferior vena cava and the hepatic wedge pressure, and makes contrast-enhanced visualization of the inferior vena cava and hepatic veins possible. This is particularly useful in making the diagnosis of hepatic vein or vena caval obstruction as in the Budd–Chiari syndrome. It is also a useful technique where conventional needle biopsy is contraindicated as a result of ascites or coagulopathy. Unfortunately, the cores obtained by this route are often fragmented, contiguous acini are frequently not seen and histological interpretation may be less reliable than with the percutaneous biopsy. This technique should not be used where a percutaneous biopsy is feasible.

Open liver biopsy, such as a wedge biopsy during laparotomy, yields optimal samples for histology. Technique is important; the surgeon must provide more than just subcapsular material (which is often fibrous and may be misleading), and must avoid traumatizing the sample by traction or compression. Laparotomy should not be undertaken where needle biopsy is feasible. Under some circumstances, laparoscopic biopsy is ideal (often performed by the percutaneous TruCut® technique under direct laparoscopic vision) as it allows for directed sampling of a focal area of interest and also because post-biopsy hemorrhage can be controlled by cauterization.

A newer modification of the percutaneous needle biopsy technique is becoming more widely practiced and may reduce the risk of post-biopsy bleeding, particularly in patients with disturbed hemostasis. In this technique, a cannula is inserted into the liver, the needle biopsy is performed through the cannula and the needle then withdrawn. The needle track is embolized with a substance such as Gel Foam®, thus sealing the track, before the cannula is removed.

'Fine needle' techniques are also described to obtain much thinner cores with the use of fine bore needles. Although the risk of hemorrhage is obviously reduced, so too is the size of the specimen, which may lead to inadequate samples and unhelpful assessment.

Cytological examination of the fine needle aspiration sample is now widely practiced. This is particularly useful for the diagnosis of hepatic malignancy. However, as individual cells are seen rather than representative tissue, architectural assessment of the liver is impossible and this technique has no place in the diagnosis or monitoring of structural liver disease such as hepatitis or cirrhosis.

CHOICE OF BIOPSY TECHNIQUE

To some extent the choice of technique is determined by the nature of the liver disease. Where a focal lesion is under investigation, the biopsy must be appropriately directed so as to sample the area of interest. A guided fine needle aspiration biopsy or percutaneous needle biopsy should be performed under direct ultrasonic or computed tomographic guidance. Alternatively, laparoscopic or open biopsy may be performed. The risk of seeding of malignant material from a hepatocellular carcinoma as a result of the procedure must be considered.

With diffuse liver disease, blind percutaneous biopsy is suitable provided that any coagulation abnormalities and ascites have been corrected. The plugged biopsy technique is useful for borderline coagulation abnormalities. Where these are uncorrectable, transvenous biopsy may be undertaken.

RECOMMENDED READING

Chezmar, J.L., Keith, L.L., Nelson, R.C. *et al.* (1991) Liver transplant biopsies with a biopsy gun. *Radiology*, 179, 447–8.

Froehlich, F., Lamy, O., Fried, M. and Gonvers, J.J. (1993) Practice and complications of liver biopsy. Results of a nationwide survey in Switzerland. *Dig Dis & Sci*, 38, 1480–4.

Hopper, K.D., Abendroth, C.S., Sturtz, K.W. *et al.* (1993) Blinded comparison of biopsy needles and automated devices in vitro: 1. Biopsy of diffuse hepatic disease. *AJR*, **161**, 1293–7,

Janes, C.H. and Lindor, K.D. (1993) Outcome of patients hospitalized for complications after outpatient liver biopsy. *Ann Intern Med*, **118**, 96–8.

McGill, D.B., Rakela, J., Zinsmeister, A.R. and Ott, B.J. (1990) A 21-year experience with major hemorrhage after percutaneous liver biopsy. *Gastroenterology*, **99**, 1396–400.

Sbolli, G., Fornari, F., Civardi, G. *et al.* (1990) Role of ultrasound guided fine needle aspiration biopsy in the diagnosis of hepatocellular carcinoma. *Gut*, **31**, 1303–5.

Zins, M., Vilgrain, V., Gayno, S. *et al.* (1992) US-guided percutaneous liver biopsy with plugging of the needle track: a prospective study in 72 high-risk patients. *Radiology*, **184**, 841–3.

6

Histopathological assessment of liver disease

KASIMIR JASKIEWICZ and PAULINE HALL

INTRODUCTION

The examination of liver tissue provides information vital for the diagnosis of liver disease and the assessment of the stage of injury, and it is being used increasingly to monitor the efficacy of therapy.

In recent years, as the mechanisms of hepatocellular dysfunction, degeneration and death have become clarified, examination of liver biopsy specimens has yielded increasing amounts of information on the pathogenesis of liver disease. Liver biopsy specimens may help in the identification of etiological agents associated with liver injury. The various patterns of liver injury reflect the interaction between etiological agents, the hepatocytes, and the non-parenchymal cells within the liver, as well as the interactions between the parenchymal and non-parenchymal cells. The assessment of liver pathology is the mainstay for monitoring both the natural history of liver disease and the effects of therapy.

LIVER BIOPSY

The indications, contraindications, techniques and complications of liver biopsies are discussed in detail in Chapter 5.

TECHNICAL PROCEDURES AND STAINS

Biopsy specimens for routine histology should be fixed in 10% neutral buffered formalin (pH 7); needle biopsy samples require 2–3 hours of fixation at room temperature, while wedge biopsies, even when cut into 2 mm slices require rather longer. Most liver biopsy samples are processed overnight but in urgent cases, e.g. liver transplant patients or liver disease in pregnancy, the small size of the tissue sample makes it possible to process the tissue more rapidly, i.e. in 4 hours. In cases where electron microscopic study is indicated a 1 mm piece of tissue should be taken from one end of the fresh specimen and fixed in a cold (4°C) 4.5% solution of glutaraldehyde. In some situations fresh tissue allows a frozen section for rapid histological diagnosis; an 'oil red O' stain for suspected fatty liver of pregnancy; culture of microorganisms; enzyme assays; assay of metals (iron, copper, etc.); histochemistry; immunohistochemistry; DNA or RNA examination; and fluorescence of porphyrins and vitamin A. Many of these procedures can fortunately be performed on fixed, processed tissue. If the investigation of the fresh tissue is to be performed at a subsequent time the tissue should be wrapped in foil, snap frozen, e.g. in liquid nitrogen, and stored in a freezer. Tissue for hepatic iron measurement should not be placed in formalin or saline since the iron will leak out of the tissue into the fluid leading to erroneously low results.

The standard hematoxylin and eosin (H and E) stain allows assessment of the liver pathology. Other stains that should be performed routinely on every liver include: a connective tissue stain such as Masson's trichrome or sirius red; Gordon and Sweet's reticulin method (silver impregnation), for evaluation of the acinar architecture and detection of piecemeal necrosis and/or bridging necrosis; the periodic acid–Schiff stain after diastase digestion (D/PAS) to demonstrate mucin in biliary epithelial cells and tumors, intracytoplasmic inclusions such alpha-1 antitrypsin (AAT) globules, ceroid-laden Kupffer cells, *Mycobacterium avium–intracellulare* in Kupffer cells and basement membranes of bile ducts; Perls' Prussian blue reaction for iron is essential for the diagnosis of hepatic iron overload including genetic hemochromatosis; finally, the periodic acid–Schiff stain shows intranuclear pseudoinclusions of glycogen as well as cytoplasmic glycogen in hepatocytes which can be useful when assessing the severity of hepatocyte necrosis.

The orcein stain can be used for the non-specific detection of HBsAg in hepatocytes; to detect copper-associated protein in periportal hepatocytes in primary (Wilson's disease) and secondary copper accumulation (e.g. primary or secondary biliary cirrhosis); and to demonstrate the presence of elastic tissue in areas of bridging necrosis. Other useful stains include the rhodanine stain for copper, and chromotrope–aniline blue for Mallory bodies (blue) and giant mitochondria (pink). Suspected fatty change, particularly microvesicular fat which must be distinguished from hydropic change, can be confirmed by post-fixing a portion of the formalin-fixed tissue in osmium tetroxide if no fresh or frozen tissue is available. The tissue can be processed normally and the fat will be seen as black droplets in unstained sections; H and E and special stains can also be performed on sections of the osmicated tissue.

Newer immunohistochemical techniques allow the detection of viral antigens such as hepatitis B virus (HBV) both core and surface antigens, cytomegalovirus (CMV) and Epstein–Barr virus (EBV) in paraffin sections. Detection of HBsAg and HBcAg in tissue is routinely used in diagnostic laboratories while markers for hepatitis C virus (HCV) are under investigation in research laboratories; it is hoped that suitable HCV antibodies will soon be available commercially. In the meantime, detection of HCV RNA in hepatic tissue is possible using polymerase chain reaction technique. Monoclonal antibodies, e.g. for the recognition of B and T lymphocytes, histiocytes, immunoglobulins (IgG, IgM, IgA, etc.), are helpful in the differentiation of inflammatory infiltrates, which are polymorphous, from malignant monoclonal lymphomatous infiltrates. Tumor markers such as AAT, alpha-fetoprotein (AFP), human chorionic gonadotrophin (HCG), carcinoembronic antigen (CEA) and markers for various high- and low-molecular weight cytokeratins may allow the classification of metastatic tumors and differentiation of primary hepatic tumors. Extracellular matrix protein markers, e.g. fibronectin, can be used for the detection of sinusoidal capillarization. Epithelial markers and cytokeratins 7 and 19 may be used to detect remnants of bile ducts in primary biliary cirrhosis, primary sclerosing cholangitis and in the 'vanishing duct syndrome', while endothelial markers (the lectin *Ulex europaeus* and anti-Factor VIII) may be used in the recognition of vascular tumors or even the angiomatosis in non-cirrhotic portal hypertension.

63

Other special techniques that deserve mention include fluorescence microscopy to detect excess vitamin A (ideally using frozen sections) which exhibits rapidly fading yellow–green autofluorescence; orange–yellow autofluorescent lipofuscin granules and porphyrin crystals which are red in color. Scanning electron microscopy can be used to demonstrate particulate matter such as Thorotrast®, silicone ('spallation'), talc and other foreign material injected by intravenous drug users.

Either semi-quantitative grading systems, e.g. the four-point grading for iron overload or recently developed computerized morphometric analysis using a video image system, have a growing role in the attempted quantitation of features such as iron, collagen, fat, etc. in the liver. Morphometry can be used in the assessment of progressive liver injury, e.g. progressive hepatic fibrosis in patients on long-term methotrexate for psoriasis; to establish a diagnosis, e.g. measurement of hepatic iron when tissue is not available for chemical measurement of iron concentration, and to monitor benefits of therapy or progression of disease e.g. interferon in patients with chronic B or C hepatitis.

ASSESSMENT OF THE LIVER BIOPSY

Macroscopic examination of the liver core can provide useful information. Normal liver tissue is tan-colored, sometimes with pale mottling, while a fatty liver is pale yellow in color. Abnormal yellow–green to dark green pigmentation may be seen in cholestasis, a rusty-brown color in hemochromatosis and almost black tissue in Dubin–Johnson syndrome. Gray–white tissue, particularly in a fragmented biopsy with a nodular appearance, is suggestive of cirrhosis. A fragmented specimen with a variegated appearance and pale to pearly-gray with yellow necrotic areas may suggest a tumor. The wedge biopsy may, in addition to the features described above, show the characteristic features of a micronodular cirrhosis or a localized nodular lesion with normal adjacent liver.

Microscopic examination of all liver biopsies should be done in a standardized manner. This should start with an evaluation of the lobular/acinar architecture, followed by assessment of the hepatocytes, the terminal hepatic venules, sinusoids, Kupffer cells, portal tracts including the bile ducts, portal veins and hepatic arteries, and limiting plates.

PATTERNS OF LIVER INJURY

INFLAMMATION AND NECROSIS

The architecture of the liver can be markedly distorted by massive, submassive, zonal necrosis, e.g. zone 3 necrosis due to paracetamol (acetaminophen) (Plate 1), bridging necrosis, e.g. portal–portal linkage (Plate 2), mild lobular disarray due to focal hepatocyte necrosis, and piecemeal necrosis. Necrotic hepatocytes undergo lysis; this loss of hepatocytes is identified by finding collapsed or condensed reticulin framework and enlarged ceroid-laden Kupffer cells, which have ingested cell debris.

The entire spectrum of liver injury can be seen in association with a wide variety of drugs and viruses. Some agents such as herpes viruses produce spotty coagulative hepatocyte necrosis and/or small confluent areas of necrosis with a mixed inflammatory infiltrate. Necrosis of single hepatocytes may be seen as eosinophilic bodies termed apoptotic bodies (Plate 3). This pattern of cell death is seen frequently in both acute and chronic viral hepatitis but may also be seen in other types of hepatitis, e.g. due to drugs or alcohol. Hepatocyte necrosis seldom occurs in the absence of an inflammatory process, other than in the immunocompromised patient. In most situations hepatocyte necrosis is accompanied by resorptive, inflammatory and regenerative processes. Characteristically, an infiltrate of neutrophil polymorphs is seen in alcoholic hepatitis, while in viral hepatitis the cellular infiltration is predominantly lymphocytic. A necroinflammatory process involving zone 3 (centrilobular necrosis) is highly suggestive of hepatotoxic liver injury.

Piecemeal necrosis, which occurs at the interface of the hepatic parenchyma with the portal tracts, is characterized by focal liver cell necrosis with portal and periportal inflammation. The limiting plate becomes irregular due to lysis of the necrotic hepatocytes and associated collapse of the reticulin framework. Focal infiltrates of lymphocytes and plasma cells are seen in association with the hepatocyte necrosis. In cases of chronic hepatitis, increased amounts of fibrous tissue are seen in the portal tracts and extend into the hepatic parenchyma, often surrounding and isolating small islands of regenerating liver cells termed rosettes. Apoptotic bodies, deeply eosinophilic bodies, with or without pyknotic nuclear remnants, may be seen but the dead hepatocytes rapidly fragment and disappear.

In primary biliary cirrhosis (PBC) the 'non-suppurative destructive inflammation' of the bile ducts is sometimes described as 'piecemeal necrosis' of the biliary epithelial cells. The formation of lymphoid aggregates, with or without follicles, often with epithelioid granulomas near damaged bile ducts, and sometimes also in the parenchyma, are characteristic features of early PBC.

Granulomas are observed in many pathological conditions of the liver and can be produced by local irritants, mycobacterial and other infections, infestations such as schistosomiasis and hypersensitivity to drugs. Granulomas may reflect liver involvement in widespread infections such as miliary tuberculosis or in systemic diseases. For example, disseminated *Mycobacterium avium-intracellulare* infection frequently occurs in patients with acquired immune deficiency syndrome (AIDS). The non-caseating granulomas have a characteristic gray–blue color in H and E sections (Plate 4); the epithelioid cells are packed with D/PAS positive mycobacteria which are readily seen in Ziehl–Neelsen stained sections (Plate 5). In contrast, *Mycobacterium tuberculosis* is only seen in 15% of liver granulomas in non-immunocompromised patients. It is often impossible to establish the etiological diagnosis on histological criteria alone; thus close cooperation of the pathologist and clinician is particularly important in determining the etiology of granulomatous hepatitis.

FIBROSIS AND CIRRHOSIS

Classically, cirrhosis is characterized by distortion of the acinar architecture of the liver due to the presence of regenerative nodules of hepatocytes which are completely surrounded by bands of fibrosis tissue (Plate 6). These nodules typically have abnormally thick liver cell plates and an abnormal vasculature. Difficulties in interpretation may be encountered when biopsies are fragmented or distorted and torn by blunt biopsy needles.

Approximation of terminal hepatic venules to fibrotic portal tracts and fibrous tissue septa, the abnormal thickness and arrangement of plates of hepatocytes with absence of ceroid or lipofuscin in hepatocytes all suggest cirrhosis. The primary classification of cirrhosis by the descriptive terms 'micronodular' or 'macronodular' is often of little value in needle biopsy specimens since estimation of the size of nodules can be difficult and misleading, particularly when only fragments or tangential sections of a nodule are available. Nevertheless, it is usually easy to diagnose an established micronodular cirrhosis on the basis of a needle biopsy specimen. Cirrhosis is often initially micronodular, e.g. alcoholic cirrhosis, hemochromatosis, Wilson's disease, but may become macronodular following abstinence from alcohol or other appropriate forms of treatment.

The liver biopsy is central to the diagnosis of cirrhosis, the assessment of activity of hepatocyte injury, determination of the etiology of the liver disease and the early detection of hepatocellular carcinoma arising in regenerative nodules. The histological distinction between fibrosis and cirrhosis is important because of possible reversal of fibrosis, e.g. after relieving biliary obstruction. The diagnosis of incomplete septal cirrhosis can be made in the presence of irregular fibrous septa dividing hepatic parenchyma that show a partially preserved acinar/lobular arrangement, and when regenerative nodules are absent.

Occasionally the impression may be gained that acinar architecture is undisturbed with normal structural relationships and with regular spacing of portal tracts and terminal hepatic venules. The portal tracts themselves may be enlarged and linked by fibrous septa. This is a common finding in biliary tract disease, both primary and secondary biliary cirrhosis, and other conditions, such as schistosomiasis and congenital hepatic fibrosis, in which portal changes predominate. Progressive portal fibrosis and portal-to-portal fibrous linkage eventually lead to cirrhosis with a geographic or jigsaw-puzzle pattern. Bile ductular proliferation is common in biliary cirrhosis while abundant copper-associated protein in adjacent hepatocytes is typical of chronic cholestasis.

Cirrhosis is the end result of hepatic disease irrespective of the etiologies. The pattern of fibrosis and regeneration, the state of bile ducts and blood vessels, and the presence of piecemeal necrosis, steatosis, alcoholic hepatitis, and steatohepatitis, are important clues to the etiology. Special stains should be used to exclude the presence of viral antigens,

iron (Plate 7), AAT globules (Plate 8), copper, and copper-associated protein before labeling cirrhosis as 'cryptogenic'.

Chronic venous congestion can lead to hepatocyte necrosis with perivenular and pericellular fibrosis in zone 3 but progression to 'cardiac cirrhosis' is rare.

CHOLESTASIS

Cholestasis is identified histologically by the presence of bile pigment in the liver. Canalicular cholestasis near terminal hepatic venules is found in acute liver injury of various etiologies including cholestatic drug reactions (Plate 9) and as one of the complications of parenteral nutrition. Intrahepatic cholestasis is seen in benign recurrent cholestasis, in pregnancy, sepsis and lymphomas, especially Hodgkin's disease. The accumulation of copper-associated protein may be seen in periportal hepatocytes in any form of chronic cholestasis but is most marked in diseases that lead to loss of bile ducts, e.g. primary biliary cirrhosis.

Pure or bland perivenular cholestasis without hepatocyte necrosis and with little or no portal inflammation suggests drug-induced or other forms of intrahepatic cholestasis, but large bile duct obstruction should always be considered in the differential diagnosis. However, the characteristic features of extrahepatic biliary obstruction, as discussed below, are usually seen. The presence of hepatocyte necrosis and inflammation indicates a cholestatic hepatitis (Plate 10); however, many drugs and some viruses injure both the hepatocytes and the biliary epithelial cells. Substantial portal inflammation with parenchymal cholestasis but a poorly developed acinar reaction may result from infection with hepatitis A virus.

Dense bile plugs in the canaliculi or ductules suggest sepsis or hepatic failure. Bile can also be seen in large bile duct structures in congenital hepatic fibrosis, microhamartomas and in the liver adjacent to space-occupying lesions such as a hepatocellular carcinoma.

SPECIFIC PATHOLOGICAL ENTITIES

LARGE BILE DUCT OBSTRUCTION

The early stage of cholestasis due to large bile duct obstruction is characterized by the presence of bile plugs in canaliculi, particularly in the perivenular regions, sometimes with occasional apoptotic bodies and enlarged bile and ceroid-laden Kupffer cells. This is followed by portal tract edema and inflammation with a predominance of neutrophil polymorphs. When neutrophil polymorphs are seen in the walls and lumens of bile ducts together with bile plugs in bile ducts, the diagnosis should be regarded as that of extrahepatic biliary obstruction until excluded (Plate 11).

If the biliary obstruction continues for weeks to months, portal fibrosis, sometimes with a periductal predominance, and ductular proliferation may become apparent. Secondary alterations occur in the hepatocytes that are due to bile retention; the cells become swollen and rarified or foamy. In cases of prolonged, severe biliary obstruction the hepatocytes may show 'feathery degeneration' and 'bile infarcts' which are small confluent areas of necrosis of bile-laden hepatocytes, accompanied by an inflammatory reaction which includes numerous bile and ceroid-laden Kupffer cells. Sometimes collections of foamy Kupffer cells form aggregates; the term 'pseudoxanthomatous' can be used to describe the appearance of these cells. Unrelieved biliary obstruction leads to progressive portal fibrosis and fibrous linkage of adjacent portal tracts, and may develop into a true biliary cirrhosis.

In biliary obstruction, the inflammatory infiltrate in and around bile ducts is characteristically neutrophilic. However, the presence of acute cholangitis does not necessarily mean bacterial infection. Ascending cholangitis is a life-threatening complication of extrahepatic biliary obstruction and should be suspected when neutrophils are found in the lumens of bile ducts. Septicemia with hepatic microabscess formation is a frequent terminal event in cases of undiagnosed or unrelieved biliary obstruction.

PRIMARY SCLEROSING CHOLANGITIS

The diagnosis of primary sclerosing cholangitis is made primarily on the basis of the radiological findings (Chapters 4 and 11). The disease usually affects both the extrahepatic and intrahepatic biliary system but in the early stages may be patchy. The characteristic hepatic lesion is a dense concentric, periductal 'onion skin' fibrosis (Plate 12). However, this lesion will not be seen if the intrahepatic ductal system is not involved or may be missed by a needle biopsy if the lesion is focal. In these instances, the liver biopsy may be unhelpful or may only show the features of bile duct obstruction due to extrahepatic and/or intrahepatic biliary strictures. An infiltrate of mononuclear cells may be seen in the portal tracts and some cases show mild piecemeal necrosis sometimes leading to confusion with chronic active hepatitis. The presence of periductal 'onion-skin' fibrosis and fibrous cylinder-like structures in the place of bile ducts may be helpful in the differential diagnosis which includes chronic active hepatitis, primary biliary cirrhosis and other forms of chronic biliary tract disease. The finding of substantial amounts of copper-associated protein in periportal hepatocytes is unhelpful since this is also seen in primary biliary cirrhosis

Another feature commonly seen in these two biliary diseases, which is not usual in chronic active hepatitis (unless the liver is cirrhotic), is that of focal proliferation of bile ductules. A history of inflammatory bowel disease, usually ulcerative colitis, will be obtained in 50–70% of patients with primary sclerosing cholangitis.

PRIMARY BILIARY CIRRHOSIS

This chronic progressive cholestatic disease of unknown cause is characterized in its early stages by a non-suppurative destructive cholangitis and ultimately by portal fibrosis and biliary cirrhosis (Chapter 11). The histological progression of primary biliary cirrhosis has been divided into four overlapping stages:

1. The florid duct lesion 'non-suppurative destructive cholangitis' (portal hepatitis).
2. Ductular proliferation (periportal hepatitis).
3. Scarring (fibrosis).
4. Cirrhosis.

Distribution of the lesions within the liver is uneven. Therefore staging based on needle biopsy material is notoriously unreliable.

In the early stages of the disease there is destruction of septal and interlobular bile ducts. This involves segments of individual ducts and tends to be focal within the liver. Bile ducts are surrounded by a mononuclear cell infiltrate which frequently extends into the biliary epithelial cells. Portal tracts are expanded by an inflammatory infiltrate consisting of lymphocytes, monocyte-macrophages and plasma cells. The portal inflammation may spill over into the hepatic parenchyma but little or no hepatocyte necrosis is seen. Lymphoid follicles and epithelioid granulomas may be found in the region of interlobular ducts (Plate 13). In the second stage there is proliferation of ductules in the portal tracts and a gradual disappearance of the interlobular ducts. In stage 3 the inflammatory changes decrease and now the major lesion is the disappearance of small and medium-sized bile ducts and the formation of fibrous septae which link adjacent portal tracts. Finally cirrhosis – usually biliary in type – but sometimes indistinguishable from other causes, supervenes.

The histological finding of ductopenia (vanishing bile ducts) with features of chronic cholestasis, requires careful study of clinical data and differential diagnostic considerations. This observation may be made in chronic hepatitis, particularly due to HCV, primary biliary cirrhosis, primary sclerosing cholangitis, drug-induced bile duct destruction (e.g. flucloxacillin), idiopathic adult ductopenia, autoimmune cholangiopathy, graft-versus-host disease and liver allograft rejection.

CHRONIC HEPATITIS

Chronic hepatitis may be defined clinically as inflammation of the liver of at least 6 months' duration (Chapter 9). The known causes include viruses – HBV, HCV and other non-B, non-C (NBNC) viruses, drugs, metabolic defects (Wilson's disease, AAT deficiency, etc.), and autoimmune processes. The classification of chronic hepatitis is based on morphological criteria; thus a liver biopsy is essential for the diagnosis.

Chronic hepatitis has been traditionally divided into chronic persistent hepatitis (CPH), chronic active hepatitis (CAH) and chronic lobular hepatitis (CLH). CPH is characterized by the presence of portal tracts which are expanded by a mononuclear cell infiltrate, without piecemeal necrosis, and little or no lobular hepatitis. CAH is characterized by the presence of piecemeal necrosis (Plates 14(a) and (b)) and/or bridging necrosis (Plate 2) with a variable component of lobular hepatitis. Portal fibrosis is usually present at the time of initial diagnosis, and some will already be cirrhotic at the time of presentation. CLH is the term used to describe cases of chronic hepatitis in which the predominant feature is focal hepatocyte necrosis within the liver lobules/acini.

The identification of the hepatitis B, D and C viruses, together with the use of serial liver biopsies, sometimes as part of controlled studies of antiviral agents, have yielded increasing amounts of data which have led to a need to re-evaluate the classification of chronic hepatitis. Scheuer (1991) has pointed out that CPH, CAH and CLH cannot be regarded as separate diseases but rather represent 'snapshots' of the histological pattern of disease at a given moment of time. Sampling variability in chronic hepatitis is such that more than one of these patterns of injury may be present in different parts of the same liver, as well as occurring at different times in the evolution of the disease. The presence of HBcAg, HBeAg and DNA polymerase in the serum, and the tissue expression of HBcAg indicate viral replication.

The diagnosis of chronic hepatitis should include the etiology when known; descriptive or semi-quanitative information about the activity (mild, moderate, severe) and localization of necroinflammatory lesions; the degree of fibrosis, using the zero- to four-point scoring system of Scheuer (1991), and the immunohistochemical data.

In most cases of chronic hepatitis the etiology cannot be deduced from the histological appearances. The finding of HBsAg-rich 'ground-glass' hepatocytes is a useful exception (Plates 15(a) and (b)). In 'healthy' HBV carriers the only histological abnormality may be the presence of 'ground-glass' hepatocytes. 'Ground-glass' hepatocytes are also found in patients taking enzyme-inducing drugs, e.g. phenobarbitone, which cause proliferation of the smooth endoplasmic reticulum giving the cytoplasm a glassy, deeply eosinophilic appearance. Immunostaining for HBV antigens readily distinguishes the HBV-related 'ground-glass' cells from enzyme-induced cells and also from oncocytic hepatocytes which have deeply eosinophilic cytoplasm due to the presence of large numbers of mitochondria.

Chronic hepatitis C viral infection

Features such as: portal tract lymphoid follicles, sometimes with germinal centres; bile duct inflammation, degeneration and loss; activated sinusoidal lymphocytes; fatty change together with focal hepatoctye degeneration and necrosis with acidophil body formation and a mononuclear cell infiltrate, are highly suggestive but not specific for HCV infection (Plate 16). The diagnosis of chronic HCV has largely been resolved by the advent of serological tests but the diagnosis of acute hepatitis C is difficult because serology is negative in the early stages of infection.

ALCOHOLIC LIVER DISEASE

A broad spectrum of ethanol-induced liver injury has been described (Chapter 7). The mildest and most common is alcohol-induced steatosis, an early non-specific form of injury that is rapidly reversible if alcohol is withdrawn. More distinctive patterns of liver injury include perivenular fibrosis in association with fatty liver, alcoholic hepatitis (Plate 17), and micronodular cirrhosis (Plate 6).

Steatosis in alcoholic patients ranges from involvement of a few hepatocytes near the terminal hepatic venules in zone 3 to involvement of hepatocytes in all zones. Typically the fat droplets are macrovesicular but microvesicular fatty change (alcoholic foamy degeneration) is sometimes seen and may be fatal (Plate 18). It is not uncommon to see a mixture of macro- and microvesicular fat droplets. Lipogranulomas are a common finding in hepatic steatosis and are usually located near the terminal hepatic venules.

Alcoholic hepatitis is characterized by the presence of hepatocyte necrosis and an infiltrate of neutrophils (Plate 17). Mallory bodies are often present but are not pathognomonic of, or obligatory for, the diagnosis of alcoholic hepatitis. Other features that may be present include fatty change, enlarged hepatocytes showing ballooning degeneration, apoptotic bodies, cholestasis, giant mitochondria and excess iron. Perivenular and focal pericellular fibrosis are often present. Mild, focal fibrosis can be missed in sections stained by hematoxylin and eosin, consequently a special stain for collagen, e.g. the sirius red stain should be available to assist in the evaluation of hepatic fibrosis. The Ito cell (lipocyte or fat-storing cell) which stores vitamin A is now considered to be the main cell responsible for collagen deposition in the perisinusoidal space of Disse.

The evolution of alcoholic hepatitis to cirrhosis is characterized by progressive pericellular fibrosis and the formation of fibrous tissue septa linking perivenular to portal areas. At the same time hepatocyte regeneration, which follows episodes of necrosis, results in the formation of regenerative nodules. Thus the normal acinar architecture becomes disrupted throughout the liver and the terminal hepatic venules become incorporated in the bands of fibrous tissue that surround the regenerative nodules. Contraction of these fibrous tissue bands, due to the presence of contractile myofibroblasts, contributes to the nodular appearance of the liver and to the development of portal hypertension.

The spectrum of alcohol-associated liver injury includes 'microscopic cholangitis', 'occlusive central venous lesions', and alcoholic siderosis which must be differentiated from genetic hemochromatosis occuring in a drinker. Alcoholic cirrhosis is typically micronodular in type but may become macronodular, particularly in association with abstinence, but may then be complicated by the formation of dysplastic nodules and hepatocellular carcinoma.

Non-alcoholic steatohepatitis (NASH)

NASH may be seen in association with obesity, diabetes mellitus, following jejunoileal bypass surgery and with a variety of drugs including amiodarone, perhexiline maleate, glucocorticoids, diethystilbestrol, thioridazine and nifedipine. The liver injury may be mild and non-specific but can also mimic alcoholic hepatitis (Plate 19) and a preferred term may be 'pseudo alcoholic liver disease'. NASH is being recognized more frequently in men as well as women and often causes diagnostic and therapeutic problems if the liver injury is incorrectly attributed to alcohol. Nevertheless, the alcohol history should be known before liver injury can be designated as NASH. Steatohepatitis from causes other than alcohol is usually relatively mild but slow progression to cirrhosis has been observed in some patients..

HEPATIC INJURY DUE TO DRUGS AND TOXINS

Traditionally, drug and toxin-associated liver injury has been classified as being due to a direct hepatotoxic mechanism or to idiosyncratic mechanisms which are poorly understood (Chapter 10). Intrinsic hepatotoxins produce predictable, dose-related liver injury, e.g. paracetamol (acetaminophen) (Plate 1). Idiosyncratic drug reactions are unpredictable, i.e. liver injury does not occur in every individual or experimental animal exposed to the drug and the injury does not appear to be dose- or time-related. These clear-cut distinctions are useful clinically but may in fact be simplistic. A wide variety of morphological responses are described in association with hepatotoxins. Patterns of injury include hepatoctye necrosis, which can range from mild focal necrosis to fatal massive necrosis (e.g. halothane hepatitis) and/or cholestasis with and without hepatocyte and bile duct injury (e.g. chlorpromazine) (Plate 9). The latter may also lead to the 'vanishing bile duct syndrome' (e.g. flucloxacillin), extensive fibrosis and cirrhosis (e.g. methotrexate; peliosis hepatis), liver cell adenoma (e.g. estrogens) and hepatocellular carcinoma (e.g. anabolic steroids).

Drug-induced hepatocyte necrosis is more often acidophilic or coagulative than lytic; however, drugs such as isoniazid and α-methyldopa can cause liver injury which resembles acute viral hepatitis. Cholestasis is usually canalicular and is seen maximally in zone 3 areas. When due to steroids there is little or no inflammatory reaction. In contrast, cholestasis due to chlorpromazine may be associated with mild focal hepatocyte necrosis and sometimes also bile duct injury accompanied by portal inflammation. Sometimes cholestasis is prolonged and bile ductular proliferation and fibrosis may occur. Eosinophils are occasionally abundant but do not constitute proof of drug etiology.

Drug-induced granulomas (e.g. phenylbutazone, sulfonamides) may be portal, parenchymal or both. Allopurinol has been reported to cause 'fibrin-ring' granulomas that resemble those of Q fever. Granulomas sometimes are the only manifestation of drug reaction, but can also form part of a hepatitic or cholestatic picture.

A variety of drugs, e.g. α-methyldopa, isoniazid and nitofurantoin, have been associated with chronic hepatitis. Drug-induced chronic active hepatitis must be differentiated from chronic viral hepatitis and other causes of this pattern of liver injury.

BENIGN TUMORS

Hepatocellular adenoma

Hepatocellular adenomas are circumscribed, often encapsulated, yellow–brown tumors, usually single but occasionally multiple, composed of hepatocytes arranged in cords. Rosette formation and bile production are sometimes seen; hemorrhage, areas of necrosis, and rupture are frequent in larger tumors. Liver cell adenoma can be difficult to distinguish from a well-differentiated hepatocellular carcinoma.

Focal nodular hyperplasia

Unlike hepatocellular adenomas, focal nodular hyperplasia does not appear to be caused by oral contraceptives but the hormones may make the lesion more vascular and prone to hemorrhage. The lesion, which is thought to be hyperplastic rather than neoplastic, must be differentiated from hepatocellular adenomas and carcinomas. Focal nodular hyperplasia usually has a characteristic macroscopical appearance. The nodular lesion is usually solitary and visible from the capsular suface of the liver; the cut surface is light-tan in color and thin septa radiate from a central scar dividing the lesion into smaller nodules. The lesion is clearly demarcated from the surrounding liver but is usually unencapsulated. The central scar contains proliferating bile ducts and thick-walled arteries and blood vessels (Plate 20). The microscopic features of the lesion resemble cirrhosis and the synonym focal cirrhosis is sometimes used. Other common features include cholestasis, rosette formation and the accumulation of copper-associated protein.

Nodular regenerative hyperplasia

Nodular regenerative hyperplasia is a diffuse nodularity of the liver which is due to the presence of small regenerative nodules that are not associated with any fibrosis. Nodular regenerative hyperplasia is associated with a wide variety of diseases, including rheumatoid arthritis and diabetes mellitus, as well as being drug-related. The regenerative nodules vary in size from a few millimeters to 1 cm. The hyperplastic parenchymal nodules are surrounded by compressed reticulin framework but no fibrosis is seen. The hyperplastic foci are sometimes periportal and surround a portal tract. Partial nodular transformation is a similar process but is limited to the hilar region of the liver and is associated with portal hypertension

Bile duct adenoma

Bile duct adenoma is a benign, usually solitary, subcapsular nodule composed of small well-formed ducts embedded in mature fibrous tissue. They differ from microhamartomas (von Meyenburg complexes) and from biliary cystadenomas in that the ducts are smaller, more numerous and do not show microcystic features.

Miscellaneous

These include hemangiomas, lipomas, mesenchymal hamartomas, myxomas and inflammatory pseudotumors. These lesions are usually incidental findings and show a similar histology to that described in other organs.

PRIMARY MALIGNANT TUMORS

Hepatocellular carcinoma

A needle biopsy specimen from a well-differentiated hepatocellular carcinoma may have striking resemblances to normal hepatocytes arranged in trabeculae; however, the trabeculae are thicker than normal and the reticulin framework is scanty or absent. Indeed, connective tissue is uncommon except in fibrolamellar carcinomas, although focal areas of fibrosis may soon follow tumor necrosis. Over 60% of hepatocellular carcinomas are associated with pre-existing cirrhosis. Tumors may originate within hyperplastic/adenomatous nodules within the cirrhotic liver. Small hepatocellular carcinomas show small

crowded pleomorphic nuclear, trabecular and/or microacinar differentiation and cytoplasmic basophilia.

Hepatocellular carcinomas are usually well or moderately differentiated and are readily diagnosed as primary hepatocellular neoplasms by the pseudoglandular arrangement of cells resembling hepatocytes (Plate 21). Less common and less well-differentiated variants, particularly spindle-cell, clear-cell, giant-cell and sclerosing tumors, must be distinguished from metastatic tumors.

In general, grading of hepatocellular carcinoma appears to have little value in establishing the prognosis. The microscopic appearance of a tumor can show considerable variation in differentiation; thus a needle biopsy sample may not always include the most malignant component of the tumor. Nevertheless, high-grade tumors have an extremely poor prognosis (Chapter 20). Fibrolamellar hepatocellular carcinomas tend to have a better prognosis but are uncommon and usually present late. Hepatocellular carcinomas invade directly into vessels and bile ducts. This is frequently seen in advanced lesions.

Cholangiocellular carcinoma

Carcinoma of the bile ducts can arise anywhere between the papilla of Vater and the smaller branches of the biliary tree within the liver. Hilar adenocarcinomas (Klatskin's tumor) arise from the region of the junction of the left and right hepatic bile ducts. Characteristic features of cholangiocarcinomas include an abundance of sclerotic stromal tissue and perineural invasion. Microscopically, cholangiocarcinomas are mucin-secreting adenocarcinomas composed of cuboidal or columnar cells arranged in a small gland pattern or as single non-cohesive cells in a dense fibrous tissue stroma; it is unusual to see a papillary pattern of differentiation within a duct. It is always necessary to search for a primary extrahepatic gastrointestinal tract adenocarcinoma before considering an adenocarcinoma in the liver to be a cholangiocarcinoma.

Other malignant epithelial lesions, such as bile duct cystadenocarcinoma, combined hepatocellular and cholangiocellular carcinoma, carcinosarcoma and carcinoid tumors are uncommon. Hepatoblastomas, a malignant tumor of embryonic or fetal hepatocytes (often with mesenchymal elements), are restricted to young children.

MALIGNANT NON-EPITHELIAL TUMORS

Angiosarcoma

This rare tumor is the most common malignant mesenchymal tumor of the liver. The tumor has a variable macroscopic appearance ranging from small or diffuse to large hemorrhagic masses. Positive staining of tumor cells for Factor VIII-related antigen confirms the endothelial differentiation of the tumor. The tumor cells characteristically grow along the sinusoids surrounding the cords of hepatocytes which then appear to become hypoplastic. The outline of the tumor is usually indistinct because of the diffuse infiltration of sinusoids. The non-neoplastic liver tissue is usually non-cirrhotic, but may show fibrosis or other lesions related to the predisposing factors such as Thorotrast®, arsenic, vinyl chloride, copper-containing sprays, and rarely androgenic/anabolic steroid hormones.

Epithelioid hemangioendothelioma

This rare tumor may be confused histologically with cholangiocarcinoma, metastatic signet ring cell carcinoma and angiosarcoma. The microscopic appearance of the tumor is identical to that of the intravascular bronchiolar and alveolar tumor of the lung. The centre of the tumor is densely fibrotic and contains scattered elongated cells with vacuolated cytoplasm – called dendritic cells; plump epitheliod cells are seen at the periphery of the fibrotic mass and extend into the adjacent sinusoids. The tumor cells stain positively with Factor VIII. Vascular invasion and occlusion with tumor infarction in areas is a characteristic feature.

LIVER TRANSPLANT PATHOLOGY

HARVESTING INJURY

This is due to ischemia/hypoxia before harvesting or during preservation (Chapter 27) and is seen predominantly as perivenular ballooning degeneration of hepatocytes or, in severe cases, as a peculiar sub-capsular necrosis.

'Surgical hepatitis'

'Surgical hepatitis', characterized by a focal infiltrate of neutrophils is usually seen in the perivenular regions and sometimes throughout the acini. This pattern of injury, which is seen in association with abdominal surgery – including liver and gallbladder surgery – is rapidly reversible.

ACUTE REJECTION

Hyperacute and massive hemorrhagic rejection reactions in the liver graft are rare. Hyperacute rejection develops within days of transplantation and is characterized by massive necrosis of the transplanted liver.

Acute, reversible cellular rejection commonly occurs between 4 and 14 days after transplantation but may present several months later. The main histological features are a mixed inflammatory cell infiltrate within portal tracts, active bile duct damage and endothelialitis (Plate 22). Other causes of hepatic dysfunction in the early post-transplant period, such as infection and biliary obstruction may need to be distinguished, on clinical and radiological grounds, from rejection.

CHRONIC REJECTION

Chronic, irreversible rejection affects between 10% and 15% of patients, predominantly children, and may necessitate re-transplantation. This process may in fact commence as early as 9 days after transplantation and is one of the causes of the vanishing bile duct syndrome (VBDS). Portal tract inflammation involves the bile ducts which then become degenerate and disappear. Other features of chronic rejection include obliterative arteriopathy and centrilobular ischemic damage. However, these specific histological features, including the presence of foam cells in vessels, may not be detected in percutaneous biopsies, partly because of the caliber of the vessels involved in the rejection process. Other liver disorders common to transplant patients may overlap with those of chronic rejection. Features that may be seen in a liver removed for chronic rejection include marked cholestasis due to loss of bile ducts, fibrosis and sometimes cirrhosis.

OPPORTUNISTIC INFECTIONS AND RECURRENCE OF THE ORIGINAL DISEASE

The complications in liver allograft patients are the same as those described in other immunocompromised hosts. The most common viral infections are CMV, HBV, HCV, herpes simplex, adenoviral and non-B, non-C hepatitis. Major additional difficulties, however, are the differentiation of these infections from acute cellular rejection and drug-induced hepatitis.

Hepatitis B infection usually recurs where the transplant was performed for chronic HBV infarction. The pattern of injury ranges

from mild acute hepatitis, through chronic active hepatitis to cirrhosis. Fulminant hepatic necrosis sometimes occurs, while in other patients the syndrome of 'cholestatic fibrosing hepatitis' (Plate 15(a)) may progress rapidly to cirrhosis. In contrast, recurrent hepatitis C runs a more insidious course and fatal massive necrosis has not been described. Recurrence of primary biliary cirrhosis has been described but the distinction from rejection with bile duct loss is particularly difficult.

CONCLUSION

The recognition that a variety of etiological agents can produce similar patterns of liver injury, for example hepatotoxins inducing the entire spectrum of liver injury, and the growing awareness of conditions grouped together as 'pseudoalcoholic liver disease', highlight the need for closer clinicopathological discussions and correlation of all information. Close collaboration between clinicians and histopathologists is required to maximize the diagnostic value of liver biopsies. Where possible, the liver pathology should be reviewed on a regular basis by a team of clinicians and pathologists.

RECOMMENDED READING

Adams, D.H. and Neuberger, J.M. (1990) Patterns of graft rejection following liver transplantation. *J Hepatol*, **10**, 113–19.

Anthony, P.P., Ishak, K.G., Nayak, N.C. *et al.* (1978) The morphology of cirrhosis. *J Clin Pathol*, **31**, 395–414.

Bach, N., Thung, S.N. and Schaffner, F. (1992) The histological features of chronic hepatitis C and autoimmune chronic hepatitis: a comparative analysis. *Hepatology*, **15**, 572–7.

Bacon, B.R. and Briton, R.S. (1990) The pathology of hepatic iron overload: a free radical-mediated process? *Hepatology*, **11**, 127–37.

Baptista, A., Bianchi, L., De Groote, J. *et al.* (1988) The diagnostic significance of periportal hepatic necrosis and inflammation: Review. *Histopathology*, **12**, 569–79.

Bianchi, L., De Groote, J., Desmet, V. *et al.* (1974) Guidelines for diagnosis of therapeutic drug-induced liver injury in liver biopsies. *Lancet*, **i**, 854–7.

Britton, R.S., Tavill, A.S. and Bacon, B.R. (1994) Mechanisms of iron toxicity, in *Iron Metabolism in Health and Disease* (eds J. Brock, J.W. Halliday, M. Pippard and L.W. Powell), Ballière Tindall, London (in press).

Comer, G.M., Mukherjee, S., Scholes, J.V. *et al.* (1989) Liver biopsies in the aquired immune deficiency syndrome: influence of endemic disease and drug abuse. *Am J Gastroenterol*, **84**, 1525–31.

Desmet, V.J. (1985) Intrahepatic bile ducts under the lens. *J Hepatol*, **1**, 545–59.

Diehl, A.M., Goodman, Z. and Ishak, K.G. (1988) Alcohol-like liver disease in non-alcoholics. *Gastroenterology*, **95**, 1056–62.

Edelstone, A.L.W.F. (1985) Immunology of chronic active hepatitis. *Q J Med*, **55**, 191–8.

Ferrell, L.D., Crawford, J.M., Dhillon, A.P. *et al.* (1993) Proposal for standardized criteria for the diagnosis of benign, borderline, and malignant hepatocellular lesions arising in chronic advanced liver disease. *Am J Surg Pathol*, **17**, 1113–23.

Gerber, M.A. and Thung, S.N. (1987) Histology of the liver. *Am J Surg Pathol*, **11**, 709–22.

Hadchouel, M. (1992) Paucity of interlobular bile ducts. *Semin Diag Pathol*, **9**, 24–30.

Hall, P. de la M. (1991) Pathologic features of alcohol liver disease, in *Portal Hypertension* (eds K. Okuda and K.-P. Benhamou) Springer–Verlag, Tokyo, pp. 41–68.

Hall, P. de la M. (1992) Genetic and acquired factors that influence individual susceptibility to alcohol-associated liver disease. *J Gastroenterol Hepatol*, **7**, 417–26.

Hall, P. de la M. (1994) Alcoholic liver disease, in *Pathology of the Liver*, 3rd edn (eds R.N.M. MacSween, P.P. Anthony, P.J. Scheuer, B. Portmann and A.D. Burt), Churchill Livingstone, Edinburgh.

Hall, P. de la M. (1994) *Alcoholic Liver Disease: Pathology, and Pathogenesis*, Edward Arnold, London.

Hall, P. de la M. (1994) Histopathological spectrum of drug-induced liver injury, in *Drug-induced Liver Disease* (ed. G.C. Farrell), Churchill Livingstone, Edinburgh, pp. 115–51.

Knodell, R.G., Ishak, K.G,. Black, W.C. *et al.* (1981) Formulation and application of a numerical scoring system for assessing histological activity in asymptomatic chronic active hepatitis. *Hepatology*, **1**, 431–5.

Lai, C.L., Wu, P.C., Lam, K.C. and Todd , D. (1979) Histologic prognostic indicators in hepatocellular carcinoma. *Cancer*, **44**, 1677–83.

Lefkowitch, J.H. and Apfelbaum, T.A. (1989) Non-A, non-B hepatitis: characterisation of liver biopsy pathology. *J Clin Gastroenterol*, **11**, 225–32.

Lefkowitch, J.H. and Fenoglio, J.J., Jr. (1983) Liver disease in alcoholic cardiomyopathy: evidence against cirrhosis. *Hum Pathol*, **14**, 457–63.

Lefkowitch, J.H., Schiff, E.R., Davis, G.L. *et al.* (1993) Pathological diagnosis of chronic hepatitis C: a multicenter comparative study of chronic hepatitis C. *Gastroenterology*, **104**, 595–603.

MacSween, R.N.M., Anthony, P.P., Scheuer, P.J. *et al.* (eds) (1994) *Pathology of the Liver*, 3rd edn, Churchill Livingstone, Edinburgh.

Mak, K.M. and Lieber, C.S. (1988) Lipocytes and transitional cells in alcoholic liver disease: a morphometric study. *Hepatology*, **8**, 1027–33.

Nagore, N. and Scheuer, P.J. (1988) The pathology of diabetic hepatitis. *J Pathol*, **156**, 155–60.

Phillips, M.J. and Poucell, S. (1981) Modern aspects of the morphology of viral hepatitis. *Hum Pathol*, **12**, 1060–84.

Popper, H. (1981) Cholestasis: the future of a past and present riddle. *Hepatology*, **1**, 187–91.

Pritchard, D.J. and Butler, W.H. (1989) Apoptosis – the mechanism of cell death in dimethylnitrosamine-induced hepatotoxicity. *J Pathol*, **158**, 253–60.

Rappaport, A.M., MacPhee, P.J., Fisher, M.M. and Phillips, M.J. (1983) The scarring of the liver acini (cirrhosis). Tridimensional and microcirculatory considerations. *Virchows Arch [A]*, **402**, 107–37.

Rapper, R.M., Bathal, P.S. and Mackay, I.R. (1983) Chronic active hepatitis in alcoholic patients. *Liver*, **3**, 327–37.

Scheuer, P.J. (1991) Classification of chronic viral hepatitis: a need for reassessment. *J Hepatol*, **13**, 372–4.

Scheuer, P.J. (1994) *Liver Biopsy Interpretation*, 5th edn, WB Saunders, Philadelphia.

Scheuer, P.J., Asbrafzadeh, P., Sherlock, S. *et al.* (1992) The pathology of hepatitis C. *Hepatology*, **15**, 567–71.

Takase, S., Takada, N., Enomoto, N. *et al.* (1991) Different types of chronic hepatitis in alcoholic patients: does chronic hepatitis induced by alcohol exist? *Hepatology*, **13**, 876–81.

Thung, S.N., Gerber, M.A. and Popper, H. (1984) Basic morphological patterns of viral hepatitis A, B, non-A, non-B and delta agent in animal and man, in *Advances in Hepatitis Research* (ed. F.V. Chisari), Masson, New York, pp. 293–302.

Worner, T.M. and Lieber, C.S. (1985) Perivenular sclerosis as precursor lesion of cirrhosis. *JAMA*, **254**, 627–30.

7

Alcohol and the liver

RICHARD HIFT and CHARLES TREY

INTRODUCTION

Alcohol-related illnesses account for about 100 000 deaths per year in the USA and about 28 000 per year in the UK, where 7 million people are believed to drink sufficient quantities to jeopardize their health. About 20% of these deaths are due to liver disease.

FACTORS CONTRIBUTING TO THE DEVELOPMENT OF ALCOHOLIC LIVER DISEASE

Approximately 10–15% of alcoholics will develop cirrhosis. The risk is dependent on the degree and duration of alcohol consumption. In men, consumption of more than 80 g of alcohol/day, and in women, more than 40 g/day, appears to predispose to liver disease. Quantitatively, 10 g of alcohol is equivalent to approximately 30 ml of whisky, 100 ml of wine and 250 ml of beer.

The importance of the duration of alcohol consumption is shown by the observation that a high intake for 5 years was associated with a low incidence of cirrhosis whereas a similar intake over approximately 21 years resulted in cirrhosis in half of the subjects studied.

There is, however, no absolute dose or time threshold above which liver disease is inevitable. Recent evidence suggests that both may be influenced by as yet unknown genetic factors.

Though liver disease is thought to be induced largely as a result of the toxic effect of the alcohol or its metabolites other factors may play an additional role. Poor nutrition *per se* is not responsible for alcohol-related liver disease, as was once thought. However, it may play a part in the development of some complications such as cirrhosis.

METABOLISM OF ALCOHOL

Ethanol is metabolized by two major enzyme systems: the alcohol dehydrogenases (ADH) and the microsomal ethanol oxidizing system (MEOS) (Fig. 7.1). Less important contributions to the metabolism of ethanol are made by the enzyme catalase and by a process of non-oxidative esterification.

The alcohol dehydrogenases are non-specific cytosolic enzymes. There are about 20 isoenzymes which differ in the arrangement of their eight sub-units. ADH are responsible for the oxidation of ethanol to acetaldehyde

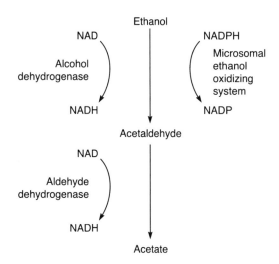

Figure 7.1 The metabolism of ethanol. NAD, nicotinamide-adenine dinucleotide; NADH, nicotinamide adenine dinucleotide (reduced form); NADP, nicotinamide adenine dinucleotide phosphate; NADPH, nicotinamide adenine dinucleotide phosphate (reduced form).

by transferring hydrogen atoms from ethanol to the cofactor nicotinamide adenine dinucleotide (NAD), which in turn is reduced to NADH. This NADH is then recycled back to NAD, making hydrogen ions available to other compounds in the process.

Though enzyme activity is largely expressed in the liver, the stomach wall also has some ADH activity. Several factors determine ADH activity. It is reduced in females, in Oriental people and in the presence of *Helicobacter pylori*. The enzyme is also inhibited by cimetidine and some related H_2 receptor blockers. Women are said to have a lower gastric alcohol dehydrogenase activity than men; less alcohol is metabolized during passage through the stomach, with more reaching the portal circulation. This may account in part for the lower threshold for alcohol-related liver disease observed in women.

The second metabolic pathway, the MEOS, comprises a specific sub-fraction of the cytochrome P450 family. The most active frac-

tion has been labeled P450IIE1 and is associated with the microsomes of the smooth endoplasmic reticulum. The MEOS oxidizes ethanol to acetaldehyde using molecular oxygen and nicotinamide adenine dinucleotide phosphate (NADP) as cofactors.

When alcohol is present in low concentrations, the ADH system is responsible for 90% of its metabolism. The ADH system is however saturable, and above a certain threshold the MEOS oxidizes a proportionately greater load of alcohol. The MEOS, like most cytochromes of the P450 group, is inducible. When exposed to high concentrations of ethanol for a period as short as a week, considerably more enzyme is synthesized and the metabolic capacity of the system is increased.

Following its production by either pathway, acetaldehyde is further converted to acetate by a family of enzymes known as the aldehyde dehydrogenases (ALDH). Chronic alcohol consumption leads to increased synthesis and decreased metabolism of acetaldehyde. The latter is thought to be due to a reduction in the capacity of mitochondria to oxidize acetaldehyde and a decrease in ALDH activity.

MECHANISM OF ALCOHOL-INDUCED LIVER DAMAGE

ACCUMULATION OF ACETALDEHYDE

The accumulation of acetaldehyde has been shown experimentally to have many deleterious effects. These include increased membrane permeability and fluidity, impaired protein assembly, disorganization of microtubular structures, disturbed export protein secretion, enhanced display of altered cell surface antigens (claimed by some to give rise to an immune response directed against the liver), inhibition of enzymes responsible for the metabolism of drugs and toxins, and stimulation of fibrogenesis.

Table 7.1 Some drugs that may interact acutely with alcohol

With potentiation of their effect		With an increase in blood alcohol levels
Amphetamines	Griseofulvin	Cimetidine
Antihistamines	Methyldopa	Haloperidol
Antipsychotics	Monoamine oxidase inhibitors	
Aspirin	Oral hypoglycemic agents	
Barbiturates	Propoxyphene	
Benzodiazepines	Tricyclic antidepressants	
Bromocriptine		

ALTERED INTRACELLULAR REDOX STATE

Greatly increased amounts of NADH are generated by the ADH-catalyzed metabolism of alcohol during chronic exposure. In order to regenerate NAD large quantities of hydrogen ion need to be handled by the body. This is achieved by a combination of immediate, short-term and delayed long-term responses. In the short term pyruvate is converted to lactate. This diversion of pyruvate away from the citric acid cycle is accompanied by decreased gluconeogenesis and, in the face of depleted glycogen stores, results in a tendency to hypoglycemia. In the long term, the excess hydrogen is handled by the kidneys. This is associated with reduced uric acid excretion, hyperuricemia and gout. Protein synthesis may also be impaired and lipid peroxidation increased. This may damage the membranes of cells and organelles, especially in areas of low oxygen tension which surround the central vein, and thus account in part for the selective perivenular effects of ethanol, which manifest histologically as perivenular necrosis, inflammation and fibrosis.

The altered redox state may also alter the balance between synthesis, export and breakdown of hepatic lipid thus contributing to the fatty liver which characterizes alcoholic liver disease.

EFFECTS OF ETHANOL ON DRUG METABOLISM

The metabolism of many drugs is altered by acute or chronic exposure to alcohol. Many of these may be of clinical importance (Tables 7.1 and 7.2).

ALCOHOL–DRUG INTERACTIONS MEDIATED BY ADH

ADH are non-specific in their use of ethanol as a substrate and will metabolize many other compounds including paraldehyde, whose clearance may be delayed in the presence of ethanol. The ADH also metabolize methanol and ethylene glycol to their toxic aldehydes. Ethanol will compete with these compounds for ADH, thus reducing the production of their harmful products. This interaction is used in emergency treatment of poisoning with these substances. The effects of ethanol are potentiated by cimetidine and ranitidine, which inhibit ADH.

Table 7.2 Some drugs that may be affected by chronic alcohol use

With reduction of their effect	With potentiation of their toxicity	Drugs that may interact with disulfiram
Barbiturates	Bromobenzene	Amitryptiline
Benzodiazepines	Isoniazid	Benzodiazepines
General anesthetics	Paracetamol (acetaminophen)	Cephalosporins
Meprobamate	Phenylbutazone (butazolidin)	Metronidazole
Propranalol		Phenytoin
Rifampicin		Warfarin
Tolbutamide		

ALCOHOL–DRUG INTERACTIONS MEDIATED BY ALDH

Disulfiram (Antabuse) inhibits ALDH, preventing the metabolism of acetaldehyde to acetate. In the presence of disulfiram, alcohol ingestion results in accumulation of acetaldehyde and a syndrome of tremor, nausea, vomiting, diarrhea, headache, facial flushing, tachycardia and hypertension or hypotension. Severe reactions may result in respiratory depression, collapse, arrhythmias, seizures, coma and death. Disulfiram is used in aversion therapy for alcoholics. Several other drugs, particularly metronidazole, chlorpropamide and cephalosporins, also inhibit ALDH and may cause disulfiram-like reactions when taken with alcohol.

ALCOHOL–DRUG INTERACTIONS MEDIATED BY THE MEOS

Regular drinkers display an increased tolerance of the effects of alcohol. This tolerance seems to extend to other drugs, notably sedatives such as barbiturates, benzodiazepines and general anesthetics, all of which may be required in higher than normal doses to achieve a given effect. This arises in part from a behavioral adaptation, but more importantly from the induction of MEOS. In response to the large amounts of ethanol, more enzyme is synthesized and its metabolic capacity is increased. This effect extends to closely associated isoforms of cytochrome P450, and the metabolism of other agents such as anti-convulsants, rifampicin and propanolol will thus be enhanced in subjects chronically primed with alcohol.

Induction of enzyme activity may exert either an aggravating or protective effect when hepatotoxic compounds are ingested. It will be protective if the effect of metabolism is to convert a potentially harmful agent to harmless metabolites. However, where the metabolites are themselves toxic, the risk of toxicity is greatly increased in the alcoholic since they will be formed more rapidly. Thus the hepatotoxicity of paracetamol (acetaminophen) is substantially increased in the alcoholic. Under normal circumstances, paracetamol is safely removed by conjugation with glucuronides and sulfates. Only when this pathway is saturated is it metabolized (to any extent) by cytochrome P450 to toxic intermediates, which are in turn detoxified by

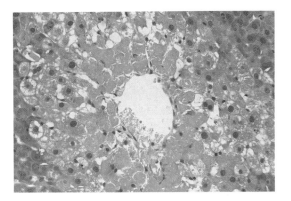

Plate 1 Coagulative necrosis of zone 3 due to paracetamol (acetaminophen). (Hematoxylin and eosin.)

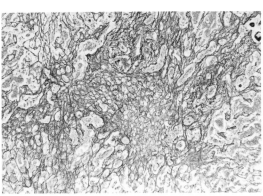

Plate 2 Bridging necrosis in chronic active hepatitis B (Gordon and Sweet's reticulin method). (Hematoxylin and eosin.)

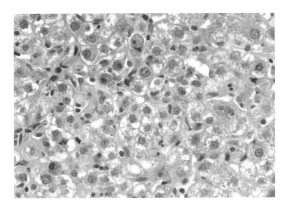

Plate 3 Apoptotic bodies in acute viral hepatitis. (Hematoxylin and eosin.)

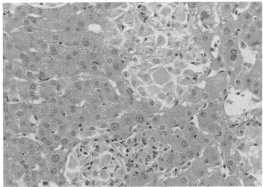

Plate 4 *Mycobacterium avium-intracellulare.* Several large granulomas are apparent. (Hematoxylin and eosin.)

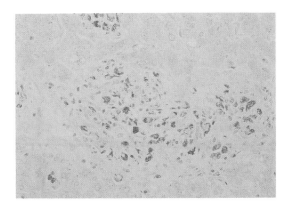

Plate 5 Numerous acid-fast bacilli in epithelioid cells (the same liver as in Plate 4a). (Ziehl-Neelsen stain.)

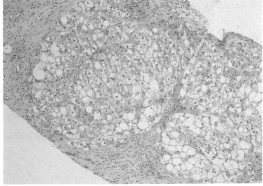

Plate 6 Micronodular cirrhosis and marked fatty change occuring in association with excess alcohol. (Hematoxylin and eosin.)

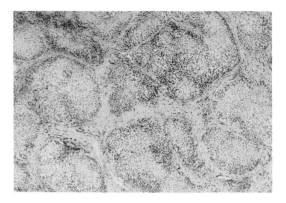

Plate 7 Cirrhosis due to genetic hemochromatosis. The hepatocytes show grade 4 siderosis (Perls' method for iron.)

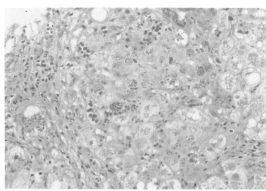

Plate 8 Cirrhosis due to alpha-1 antitrypsin deficiency. Numerous diastase/periodic acid – Schiff stain (D/PAS)-positive globules are seen in the hepatocytes.

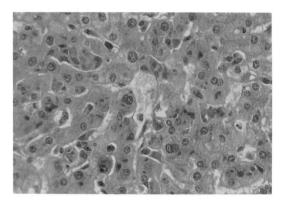

Plate 9 Cholestasis due to chlorpromazine. Bile is seen in canaliculi in the region of a terminal hepatic venule. (Hematoxylin and eosin.)

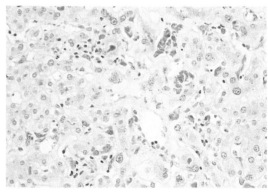

Plate 10 Cholestatic hepatitis due to flucloxacillin. Cholestasis, focal hepatocyte necrosis and numerous ceroid-laden Kupffer cells are seen. (Diastase/periodic acid – Schiff staining.)

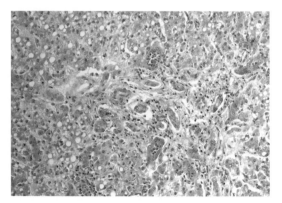

Plate 11 Extrahepatic biliary obstruction. Note the expanded, edematous portal tract and the heavy infiltrate of neutrophil polymorphs. Polymorphs are seen in the walls and lumens of proliferating bile ductules. (Hematoxylin and eosin.)

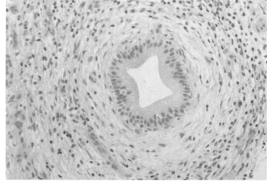

Plate 12 Primary sclerosing cholangitis. Edematous fibrous tissue, which contains an infiltrate of mononuclear cells, is forming concentric rings around a bile duct. (Hematoxylin and eosin.)

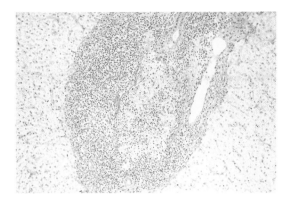

Plate 13 Primary biliary cirrhosis. A portal tract is expanded by a heavy infiltrate of mononuclear cells. The collapsed basement membrane of an injured bile duct is seen (center) with an adjacent epitheliod granuloma. (Diastase/periodic acid – Schiff staining.)

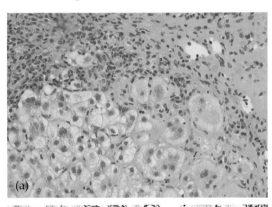

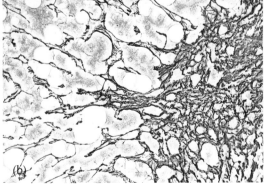

Plate 14 (a) Chronic active hepatitis due to hepatitis B virus. Piecemeal necrosis, a mononuclear cell infiltrate and portal fibrosis are seen. (Hematoxylin and eosin.) (b) The same liver showing focal collapse of the reticulin framework (Gordon and Sweet's reticulin method.)

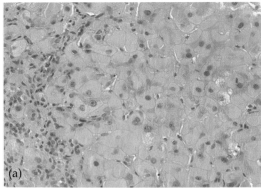

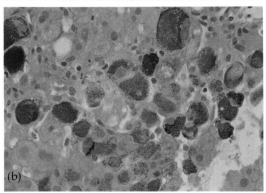

Plate 15 (a) Recurrent hepatitis B in an allograft liver. Large numbers of "ground glass" hepatocytes are apparent. (Hematoxylin and eosin.) (b) Hepatocytes containing large amounts of hepatitis B surface antigen. (Peroxidase-antiperoxidase stain.)

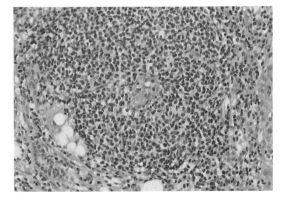

Plate 16 Chronic hepatitis C. A heavy infiltrate of mononuclear cells surrounds and extends into a small bile duct. (Hematoxylin and eosin.)

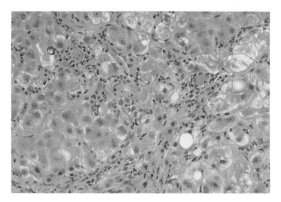

Plate 17 Alcoholic hepatitis. Focal hepatocyte necrosis. A prominent infiltrate of neutrophil polymorphs and Mallory bodies is seen. (Hematoxylin and eosin.)

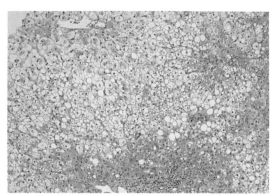

Plate 18 Alcoholic foamy degeneration. All but a few periportal hepatocytes (bottom right) show microvesicular fatty change. (Hematoxylin and eosin.)

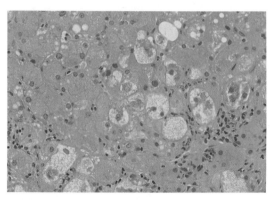

Plate 19 Non-alcoholic steatohepatitis in an obese, middle-aged diabetic female patient. The liver injury resembles alcoholic hepatitis but the patient did not drink alcohol. (Hematoxylin and eosin.)

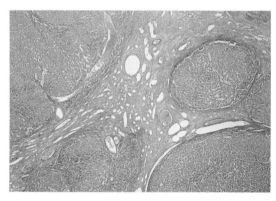

Plate 20 Focal nodular hyperplasia. Portion of a localized nodule which contains a central scar and radiating fibrous septa. (Hematoxylin and eosin.)

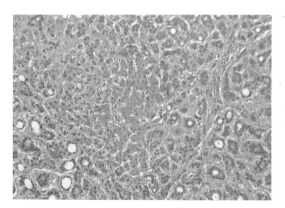

Plate 21 Hepatocellular carcinoma showing trabecular and acinar differentiation. (Hematoxylin and eosin.)

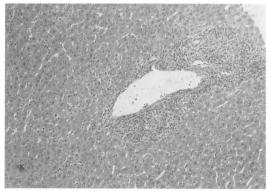

Plate 22 Liver allograft showing acute cellular rejection. A mixed inflamatory cell infiltrate surrounds and extends into a bile duct. Mild endotheliatitis is present but not well shown at this low magnification. (Hematoxylin and eosin.)

binding to glutathione. In chronic alcohol abuse, the increased cytochrome P450 will metabolize paracetamol (acetaminophen) sooner; more metabolites are produced and their toxicity may be compounded by pre-existing glutathione depletion frequently encountered in heavy drinkers. Thus quantities of paracetamol which are harmless in normal people may cause hepatic necrosis and death in the alcoholic. Such reactions have been reported both for 'accidental' over-doses and even for large therapeutic doses. Whereas a dose of approximately 12 g is necessary to induce hepatic necrosis in non-drinkers, as little as 2–6 g/day for several days has resulted in hepatic necrosis in alcoholics. The most dangerous circumstances arise when paracetamol is taken a few days after the cessation of drinking. Here the accelerated metabolism of paracetamol is completely unopposed. A similar mechanism may be responsible for an increased risk of hepatic necrosis following overdoses of ferrous sulfate or carbon tetrachloride in alcoholics. This heightened propensity of the regular drinker to drug-induced hepatic necrosis seems to have its counterpart in an increased sensitivity to the more chronic hepatotoxic effects of other drugs metabolized by the liver, particularly those showing affinity for ethanol-related forms of cytochrome P450, such as isoniazid, phenylbutazone (butazolidin) and bromobenzene.

Though acute alcohol intoxication leads to a rapid induction of the cytochrome P450 enzymes, with an increase in the therapeutic dose requirement for sedatives such as phenobarbitone, benzodiazepines and other sedatives metabolized by cytochrome P450, this phenomenon is temporary. Once the ingestion of alcohol ceases, P450 activity returns to normal, usually within a week, and continued administration of sedatives in high doses may lead to their accumulation and to potentiation of their effects.

CLINICAL SYNDROMES OF ALCOHOLIC LIVER DISEASE

Classically three forms of alcohol-induced liver disease are described: fatty liver, alcoholic hepatitis and cirrhosis. These should not be regarded as being mutually exclusive. Indeed, histological features of two or of all three often coexist on liver biopsy

ALCOHOLIC FATTY LIVER

This is the most common abnormality found in alcoholic subjects. It can be produced experimentally in both animals and man by the administration of alcohol. Indeed, accumulation of fat in the liver has been observed in experimental subjects exposed to alcohol for less than 1 week. The accumulation of fat may be due to a combination of: alcohol-induced lipolysis of peripheral adipose tissue with increased delivery to the liver; increased hepatic synthesis using acetate generated by the metabolism of alcohol; and inhibition of hepatic fatty acid oxidation.

Clinical features

Fatty liver is usually asymptomatic. Hepatomegaly is the most important clinical sign, and is often an incidental finding on routine examination. Liver function tests are often within normal limits. An isolated increase in γ glutamyl transpeptidase may reflect ongoing drinking, but this test is both insensitive and non-specific.

Prognosis

Alcohol-induced fatty liver itself is a mild disorder. It is usually reversible once drinking ceases. However, recent studies suggest that fibrogenesis may be stimulated even at this early stage in susceptible individuals. The clinical importance of finding a fatty liver is to alert both physician and patient to the need to moderate drinking before more serious liver damage occurs.

It should be stressed that these various categories of liver disease will often not be seen in isolation. In our experience, biopsy of an apparent fatty liver will often show mild to moderate inflammatory infiltrates in the portal tracts and pericellular fibrosis in addition to steatosis. These are harbingers of more serious conditions such as hepatitis and cirrhosis. A liver biopsy is thus often useful even in apparent fatty liver, and will confirm the need for urgent attempts to change the patient's drinking habits.

ALCOHOLIC HEPATITIS

Alcoholic hepatitis is, in the strictest sense, a histological diagnosis that should be made only on biopsy. The terminology is confusing: to be consistent, the term should be applicable to any biopsy revealing inflammatory activity within the hepatic parenchyma. Typical histological findings include fatty change, hepatocyte degeneration and necrosis, polymorphonuclear cell infiltration, Mallory bodies, giant mitochondria and pericellular fibrosis. These changes are most marked in the centrilobular area (acinar zone 3), and range from the minimal changes seen in association with fatty liver to severe necrosis and fibrosis in which it is easy to visualize cirrhosis as an inevitable outcome.

While few would argue with the need for a histological diagnosis, many patients with alcoholic hepatitis are severely ill and a biopsy is often precluded by a profound coagulopathy. Thus in practice, the diagnosis of alcoholic hepatitis is often based on a clinical syndrome supported by compatible laboratory findings.

Clinical features

The clinical presentation is that of an acute or fulminant hepatitis with anorexia, nausea, vomiting and abdominal pain. Hepatomegaly is almost invariable and is often tender because of distension of the hepatic capsule by fatty infiltration; fever, jaundice and leukocytosis are common, as are features of liver failure such as bleeding and encephalopathy. Ascites may be present and may denote some degree of established cirrhosis.

Absolute diagnostic indicators, other than a typical biopsy with a history of alcohol abuse, are lacking. Other pointers to alcohol abuse such as delirium tremens, Wernicke's encephalopathy, peripheral neuropathy, myopathy or cardiomyopathy may be present. Biochemical tests are non-specific. Hepatocellular damage is reflected by an elevated aspartate transaminase (AST) and, to a lesser degree, alanine aminotransferase (ALT). The AST is rarely elevated above 300 IU/l; if it is, another cause should be considered. Cholestasis is common. Alcoholic hepatitis may sometimes mimic obstructive jaundice with striking elevations of bilirubin, alkaline phosphatase and γ glutamyl transpeptidase. Such patients should never be subjected to laparotomy unless true obstruction has been unequivocally confirmed by ultrasound or endoscopic retrograde cholangiopancreatography (ERCP). Surgery in the face of alcoholic hepatitis carries an appalling mortality.

Treatment

Various forms of specific therapy have been advocated for acute alcoholic hepatitis but, with the exception of corticosteroids, none has withstood the rigor of repeated prospective, randomized, double blind trials. Therefore treatment for this condition is largely supportive. Abstinence is essential. Fluid and electrolyte balance should be assessed and corrected since disturbances are common. Alcohol suppresses antidiuretic hormone causing an obligatory diuresis. This, coupled with nausea and vomiting, frequently results in dehydration. Hypokalemia may be severe and is due in part to the renal tubular acidosis which is often encountered in alcoholics. Apart from the other risks associated with hypokalemia, it is also liable to induce or aggravate hepatic encephalopathy. Diuretics should only be used when absolutely necessary and then with caution. Patients with acute or acute on chronic hepatic decompensation tend to respond unpredictably and may develop electrolyte disturbances, renal dysfunction or hepatic encephalopathy in response to diuretics. Renal dysfunction is common; prerenal failure, acute tubular necrosis and functional renal failure should be prevented where possible and treated when present.

Infection is a common complication of alcoholic hepatitis and should be actively looked for and treated. Any fever or unexplained deterioration in the presence of ascites demands a diagnostic paracentesis with ascitic white cell count and culture because of the high and increasingly recognized risk of spontaneous bacterial peritonitis (Chapter 16).

Patients with alcoholic hepatitis are commonly malnourished and require nutritional support. Energy requirement is increased. Inadequate provision of calories results in protein being used as an energy source. Both energy and protein should be provided in adequate amounts (Chapter 25).

Vitamin supplementation with folate, thiamine, pyridoxine and, where appropriate, vitamin K is important. Trace metals such as zinc and magnesium may also be required.

Medication should be prescribed with caution. The patient admitted with alcoholic hepatitis often has induction of cytochrome P450. This may result in increased requirements for sedation in the face of early alcohol withdrawal. Administration of paracetamol – even in therapeutic doses – may result in liver cell necrosis because of an increased metabolism to toxic products. Conversely, as liver function deteriorates, drug tolerance diminishes markedly and standard doses of sedatives may result in oversedation and the precipitation of hepatic coma.

There is now considerable evidence that corticosteroids may improve the outcome in more severe cases. This has been shown for patients who develop encephalopathy in association with alcoholic hepatitis, and prednisone may be prescribed for such patients.

Orthotopic liver transplantation may be life-saving in fulminant hepatic failure due to alcohol and appears to be technically feasible. The debate as to whether it is justifiable in this setting revolves around ethical issues and is, as yet, unresolved.

Course

The toxic effects of alcohol may persist for 8 to 12 weeks after cessation of drinking. Thus the patient may continue to deteriorate even after admission to hospital. Apart from the degree of pre-existing and current liver damage, the outcome depends on the nutritional status of the patient, the presence of extrahepatic manifestations of alcohol such as delirium tremens and the response to possible infections. Encephalopathy, functional renal failure and severe coagulopathy are indicators of a poor prognosis.

Prognosis

The mortality in severe alcoholic hepatitis approaches 50%. Alcoholic hepatitis carries a risk of progression to cirrhosis of 40% where drinking continues. Even with abstinence, cirrhosis may ensue in up to 20% of patients. Following recovery, the most important principle of management is the encouragement of abstinence. Unfortunately, this is often unsuccessful, and many patients will suffer one or more relapses with a rapid deterioration hepatic reserve, cirrhosis and death.

CIRRHOSIS

Approximately 10–15% of alcoholics will develop cirrhosis. This appears to depend partly on the degree and duration of alcohol consumption and partly on as yet undefined genetic factors. As with alcoholic hepatitis, cirrhosis is, strictly speaking, a histological term which describes a liver showing characteristic features of fibrosis and hepatocyte regeneration, yet it is associated with a well-defined clinical syndrome which also allows its consideration as a clinical entity. Up to 40% of patients with cirrhosis are asymptomatic and here the diagnosis is often made by chance or post-mortem.

Clinical features

The classic physical findings associated with alcoholic cirrhosis; palmar erythema, Duypuytren's contractures, white nails, mild clubbing, spider angiomata, bruising, jaundice, enlarged parotid glands, ascites, dilated superficial abdominal wall veins, hepatosplenomegaly, gynecomastia and testicular atrophy are diagnostically useful but not invariably present in alcoholic cirrhosis. In contrast to many other forms of cirrhosis the liver is often enlarged in alcoholic cirrhosis as a result of fatty infiltration and inflammation. A large liver should also raise the question of hepatocellular carcinoma, the incidence of which is increased in alcoholic cirrhosis, particularly in association with concomitant hepatitis C infection. Malnutrition and extrahepatic manifestations of alcoholism such as peripheral neuropathy may be noted.

With the exception of liver biopsy, laboratory tests do not offer a definitive diagnosis of cirrhosis. In compensated cases, serum biochemistry is often normal, or may show mild elevation of transaminases and bilirubin. When abnormal the AST : ALT ratio is frequently higher than 2 (Chapter 2).

The most frequent findings on hematological examination are an increased mean corpuscular volume, thrombocytopenia and a prolonged prothrombin time (Chapter 3). Alcoholic cirrhosis is not uncommonly accompanied by hepatic iron overload. Ferritin concentration and transferrin concentration and saturation should be determined and may distinguish iron overload in alcoholic liver disease from hemochromatosis. A liver biopsy may provide a definitive diagnosis. Imaging techniques are becoming more useful as their resolution improves (Chapter 4) but currently provide only indirect evidence in support of the diagnosis such as changes in the size and homogeneity of the liver, hypertrophy of the caudate lobe, splenomegaly and evidence of portal hypertension.

Treatment

Abstinence

The first principle in the treatment of alcoholic cirrhosis is the encouragement of abstinence. Alcohol withdrawal is not without hazard; it may result in delirium tremens, the treatment of which is complicated by the varying sensitivity of cirrhotics to sedatives and the increased risk of encephalopathy.

Social intervention

Adequate social support is essential. Attempts to improve patients' understanding of their condition and to boost the chances of their abstaining are vital, as are those intended to encourage cooperation with their treatment regimen. The assistance of family, friends, employers and social agencies such is helpful.

Nutrition

Alcoholics are often malnourished. The causes of malnutrition are legion and include the substitution of alcohol calories for energy from more appropriate sources, an inadequate diet, the direct catabolic effects of alcohol and liver disease and the presence of other diseases such as tuberculosis. To this list must be added misguided restriction of the patient's protein intake by his or her doctor in the belief that this is *per se* an integral part of the management of cirrhosis.

Nutritional support is important and goes far beyond vitamin replacement alone. A healthy, balanced diet including carbohydrate, fat and protein supplements should be recommended. Protein should be freely given to all cirrhotic subjects except where encephalopathy is present (Chapter 13). Protein restriction is otherwise counterproductive; an intake of less than 50–60 g/day is incompatible with an adequate nitrogen balance in patients with chronic liver disease and should not be prescribed unless there is hepatic encephalopathy and then only for as short a period of time as possible.

Vitamin and trace element replenishment is important. Folate and the vitamin B complex, particularly thiamine, are frequently required as may vitamin C be where diet has been deficient. Vitamin K may be necessary in jaundiced patients. In cholestatic patients vitamin A and K deficiencies are frequent and require replacement treatment. Vitamin A has been found to be depleted in alcoholic liver disease. It is normally stored in the Ito cells, but as liver disease progresses these transform to fibroblastic cells and the vitamin A content of the liver falls. This may manifest in severe cases as night-blindness, but sub-clinical deficiency is common and is not thought to be detrimental. Supplementation must be performed only where decreased concentrations have been demonstrated and then cautiously since excessive amounts of vitamin A are hepatotoxic.

Trace metals such as magnesium and zinc may be depleted and should be supplemented. Electrolyte disturbances such as hyponatremia and hypokalemia are particu-

larly frequent in the presence of ascites. Their management is addressed in Chapter 16.

Therapy for specific complications

Major complications of cirrhosis include encephalopathy, ascites and variceal hemorrhage. Management of these is discussed in Chapters 13, 14 and 16. It is increasingly recognized that cirrhosis represents an immunocompromised state and infections should thus be actively sought and treated. Classic signs of infection may be absent, and infection may be heralded only by an unexplained deterioration in the patient's clinical state.

The increased incidence of hepatocellular carcinoma in alcoholic cirrhosis must also be borne in mind. It is always advisable to determine the serum alpha-fetoprotein level and perform an ultrasound examination of the liver when a patient with cirrhosis deteriorates unexpectedly.

Drug therapy

Various drugs have been suggested for the treatment of alcoholic cirrhosis, though none has shown a consistent benefit. This may, however, be due in part to the influence of continued drinking on the progression of the disease. Corticosteroids and anabolic steroids may be harmful in cirrhosis and should not be used. Colchicine, propylthiouracil, phospholipid supplements and silymarin are not yet generally accepted as conferring additional survival on patients with alcoholic cirrhosis.

ORTHOTOPIC LIVER TRANSPLANTATION

In most transplant centres there is a requirement of a period of proven abstinence of 6 months to a year. The subsequent survival of such patients is similar to those with other illnesses coming to transplant.

Prognosis

The prognosis of alcoholic hepatitis and cirrhosis is in large part determined by three factors: ongoing exposure to alcohol, the degree of hepatocellular dysfunction and the presence of major complications such as encephalopathy and ascites. Abstinence is the hallmark of treatment. However, it is a difficult goal. The 5-year survival of uncomplicated cirrhosis is approximately 90% in those who stop drinking and 70% in those who continue. It has been shown that abstinence improves the prognosis except where gastrointestinal bleeding has developed. The presence of jaundice, ascites or gastrointestinal tract bleeding denote a poor prognosis, with a 5-year survival of 60% in those who stop and only 35% in those who continue taking alcohol. Such a poor outlook is akin to that of many types of cancer.

RECOMMENDED READING

Gluud, C., Henriksen, J.H., Nielsen, G. and the Copenhagen Study Group for Liver Diseases (1988) Prognostic indicators in alcoholic cirrhotic men. *Hepatology*, **8**, 222–7.

Hayes, P.C. (ed.) (1993) Alcoholic liver disease. *Baillière's Clinical Gastroenterology*, **7**(3).

Kirsch, R.E. (1985) Alcoholic liver disease in South Africa, in *Alcoholic Liver Disease* (ed. P. Hall), Edward Arnold, London, pp. 184–92.

Lieber, C.S. (1988) Biochemical and molecular basis of alcohol-induced injury to liver and other tissues. *N Engl J Med*, **25**, 639–50.

Lieber, C.S. and Salaspuro, M.P. (1992) Alcoholic liver disease, in *Wright's Liver and Biliary Disease*, 3rd edn (eds G.H. Millward-Sadler, R. Wright and M.J.P. Arthur), WB Saunders, London.

Maddrey, W.C. (1988) Alcoholic hepatitis. *Semin Liver Dis*, **8**, 91–102.

8

Viral hepatitis

SIMON ROBSON, WENDY SPEARMAN and
GEOFFREY DUSHEIKO

INTRODUCTION

Viral hepatitis, an inflammatory and necrotic process in the liver, is a common infectious disease and a major public health problem worldwide. Acute viral hepatitis, although a generalized systemic infection, presents with clinical manifestations relating directly to inflammation of the liver with hepatocellular dysfunction and jaundice. The clinical severity of acute hepatitis is extremely varied. Most infections are asymptomatic, sub-clinical, or anicteric with mild gastrointestinal symptoms only. Less common are the typical episodes of acute illness characterized by jaundice and malaise. Rarely infection results in acute fulminant hepatitis associated with a high mortality.

Infection with hepatitis B (and associated D) or C may be associated with a persistent carrier state, chronic hepatitis or the more serious complications, cirrhosis and portal hypertension.

Worldwide, hepatitis viruses are responsible for the majority of all forms of chronic liver disease. The economic and human cost of these viruses is further exacerbated by their association with hepatocellular carcinoma – one of the 10 most common malignant tumors.

The hepatitis viruses identified by the late 1980s were the hepatitis A virus (HAV, infectious or epidemic hepatitis), the hepatitis B virus (HBV, previously termed serum hepatitis) and the hepatitis D virus (Delta agent or HDV).

The non-A, non-B viral hepatitis group (NANB), until quite recently, remained a diagnosis based on the exclusion of the above viruses and of other possible etiological agents such as alcohol, drugs and toxins. The heterogeneity of the NANB grouping was, however, quite apparent. Infection with these viruses resulted in a variety of epidemiological and clinical presentations. Both parenterally transmitted and sporadic community-acquired forms of infection were noted, and there was a variable tendency for infected individuals to develop chronic hepatitis and cirrhosis.

After extensive research into possible etiological agents of NANB hepatitis, two further hepatitis viruses have been identified and their genomes fully cloned. Diagnostic serological tests are now available. The hepatitis C virus (HCV) was the major etiological agent of transfusion-associated NANB hepatitis described prior to the advent of specific serological tests for HCV and accounts for the major proportion of sporadic community-acquired NANB hepatitis. The hepatitis E virus (HEV or E-NANB) causes enterally transmitted NANB hepatitis epidemics as well as sporadic disease in certain endemic communities. Other viruses that can cause acute hepatitis include the Epstein–Barr virus, cytomegalovirus (CMV) and the exotic hemorrhagic fever viruses such as yellow fever virus. The diseases caused by these latter viruses, however, are not generally included in the term viral hepatitis.

There is also increasing epidemiological evidence for a further hepatitis virus, the so-called hepatitis F virus (F-NANB), which appears to be transmitted in a sporadic community-acquired form. It may account for some cases of fulminant and sub-fulminant liver failure in NANB hepatitis infection. This virus, however, has not been identified, and there are no established serological tests for its detection.

HEPATITIS A VIRUS

EPIDEMIOLOGY

Hepatitis A is endemic in all parts of the world. Its exact incidence is difficult to estimate because of the high proportion of asymptomatic and anicteric infections, differences in surveillance and different patterns of the disease. In developing countries infection, as judged by the presence of antibodies, is almost universal by the end of the second decade of life. The vast majority of infections occur in childhood and most appear to be sub-clinical and anicteric. In industrialized countries, the prevalence of hepatitis A is much lower. Here, the minority of young adults have antibodies to HAV. In these communities localized outbreaks in crèches

and other institutions often spread to involve a significant number of adults, thus causing minor epidemics.

HAV is spread predominantly by the fecal–oral route, most commonly by person-to-person contact. Therefore infection is particularly common under conditions of poor sanitation and overcrowding. Common source outbreaks result most frequently from fecal contamination of drinking water and food, but water-borne transmission does not appear to be a major factor in industrialized urban communities. An increase in the number of food-borne outbreaks has also been reported in developed countries. The consumption of raw or inadequately cooked shellfish, cultivated in polluted water, has been associated with high risk of hepatitis A infection, particularly in South American countries and in Asia.

Hepatitis A infection is also common in male homosexuals. In general this virus is not transmitted parenterally by blood and blood products except under experimental conditions.

CLINICAL FEATURES

The incubation period of hepatitis A is 3–5 weeks with a mean of about 28 days. Although the disease has a low mortality, adult patients may be incapacitated for many weeks. Complications of HAV infection include fulminant hepatitis in a small proportion of patients. This is characterized in the early stages by protracted vomiting, dehydration, confusion and encephalopathy. These patients are also prone to hemorrhagic complications, cerebral edema, renal failure and hypoglycemia (Chapter 12). Further complications of HAV infection include a protracted cholestatic illness which may be precipitated or aggravated by a premature return to normal daily activities or to exercise. There is no evidence for persistence of HAV infection although early virological relapse has been described. Progression to chronic liver disease does not occur.

DIAGNOSIS

Specific serological tests for HAV antigen and antibodies include radioimmunoassay and enzyme-linked immunosorbent assays. Serological diagnosis of recent infection can be established by the demonstration of anti-HAV of the IgM class. HAV IgM is detectable in serum for 45–60 days after the onset of symptoms. Anti-HAV IgG is always demonstrable during the early phase of the illness and titers increase rapidly. The antibody usually persists for many years and its presence indicates immunity. The presence of HAV IgG alone indicates previous exposure, but not current infection.

MANAGEMENT

Control of infection is difficult since fecal shedding of the virus is highest during the late incubation and prodromal phases of the illness. Therefore strict isolation is not a useful control measure as the spread of HAV is maximal well before diagnosis of the disease. The spread of hepatitis A may be reduced by simple hygienic measures and by the sanitary disposal of excreta.

PASSIVE IMMUNIZATION

Normal pooled human immunoglobulin (containing titers of at least 100 IU/ml of anti-HAV) may be given intramuscularly before or soon after exposure to HAV in order to prevent or attenuate the clinical illness. The dose should be at least 2 IU of anti-HAV/kg body-weight. In pregnancy or in patients with liver disease, the dose should be doubled to ensure full protection. The immunoglobulin does not always prevent infection and excretion of HAV with non-apparent or sub-clinical hepatitis may develop.

Passive immunization is used for close personal contacts of patients with hepatitis A and for those exposed to contaminated food. This mode of control may also be used in limiting outbreaks in institutions. Prophylaxis with immunoglobulin is recommended for people without antibodies to hepatitis A virus about to visit endemic areas. The period of protection is about 6 months. Effective and safe hepatitis A vaccines are now entering clinical practice and are licensed in some countries. Adverse reactions are infrequent, and these vaccines induce high levels of protective antibody. In developed countries, the vaccine should be given to travelers to countries where HAV is endemic but may be extended to crèches and schools in certain countries.

HEPATITIS E

EPIDEMIOLOGY

Epidemic hepatitis, resembling hepatitis A but serologically distinct from it, has been reported from Mexico, India, Central and South East Asia, the Middle East, North and southern Africa. Hepatitis E is therefore observed in developing countries, both in local outbreaks and in a sporadic form. In Western industrialized countries, hepatitis E has not been documented apart from sporadic cases in persons returning from endemic areas. The illness is predominantly acute, self-limiting and appears to occur predominantly in young adults. The incubation period is 30–40 days. The hepatitis appears to be more severe in pregnancy, especially during the last trimester, where it is associated with a mortality rate of up to 20%. The infection is spread by the ingestion of contaminated water and probably food. The source of the infection is human fecal contamination of water. Few secondary cases are reported but when household contacts of the index case are examined, serial biochemical tests of liver function are abnormal in about 20% of these contacts.

Hepatitis E appears to be a non-enveloped RNA virus similar to the caliciviruses.

CLINICAL FEATURES AND DIAGNOSIS

The clinical and histopathological characteristics of the disease are similar to those of other forms of acute viral hepatitis. Hepatitis E-specific antigen (HEV-Ag), immunologically related to the virus-like particles of HAV, is expressed in the cytoplasm of hepatocytes during the early acute phase of infection and is also found to induce specific antibodies in infected primates. Specific anti-HEV antibodies are found in acute and convalescent sera from patients with hepatitis E in geographically isolated outbreaks. Sporadic community-acquired NANB hepatitis observed in Western countries appears serologically unrelated to hepatitis E observed in developing countries.

HEPATITIS B VIRUS

STRUCTURE

Hepatitis B virus (HBV, also called the Dane particle) is classified as a hepadna virus type I (Fig. 8.1). It has a diameter of 42 nm with a 27 nm inner core corresponding to the hepatitis B core antigen (HBcAg). Hepatitis B e antigen (HBeAg) is a soluble component of the core antigen and is detected in the blood of patients infected with hepatitis B virus. The virus also contains a unique circular DNA molecule which is partially double-stranded and is associated with a DNA polymerase. The entire DNA of HBV has been cloned in *E. coli*, in yeasts and in several mammalian cell lines. Three types of particle may be seen by electron microscopy in serum from

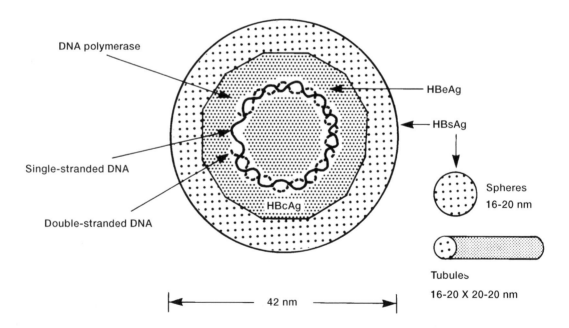

Figure 8.1 Structure of hepatitis B virus. Excess viral proteins are seen as spheres and tubules.

patients with acute or chronic hepatitis B infection. These are the large complex Dane particles, and the spheres and tubules which represent excess virally-coded proteins. The surface of all three particles displays the major protein known as hepatitis B surface antigen (HBsAg).

GEOGRAPHICAL DISTRIBUTION

An estimated 300 million people are carriers of HBV virus. The rate of antigen expression in patients varies from a low of 0.1–0.5% in Western Europe to a high of 8–15% in Africa and the Far East. The rate of chronic infection is greater in males. The prevalence of past and present HBV virus infection as determined by antibody to HBsAg is higher, ranging from 4–6% in the low-prevalence areas to 70–95% in Asia and Africa.

ACUTE HEPATITIS B

The clinical expression of acute HBV virus infection is extremely variable and ranges from a fulminant disease, which is rare, to sub-clinical infection, which is very common. Hepatocyte damage appears to be mediated by the host immune response, predominantly by cytotoxic T cells and natural killer cells. HBV, *per se*, is probably not cytopathic. Jaundice preceded by nausea, anorexia and vomiting appears in about 20–50% of patients, and a minor flu-like syndrome may occur, particularly in children. Clinical features which may point to hepatitis B virus include a long prodromal period, arthralgia and skin rashes. The diagnosis of HBV infection includes the use of laboratory tests which show increased serum aspartate aminotransferase (AST) and alanine aminotransferase (ALT) activity and must be confirmed in every case by demonstrating the appropriate hepatitis B serological markers.

The serological profile of a typical case of acute hepatitis B is shown in Figure 8.2. HBsAg is detectable for about 3 months in this patient. Following the disappearance of HBsAg, anti-HBs appears after a variable lag period of several weeks. Anti-HBc appears early on in the disease. Anti-HBs and anti-HBc persist for years after the patient has recovered and constitute the most lasting evidence of previous HBV infection. IgM anti-HBc disappears at or before 6 months, when the patient recovers from acute hepatitis B. Total and IgM anti-HBc are present during the 'window' period after HBsAg is lost but before anti-HBs antigen appears. Anti-HBe develops following the disappearance of HBeAg.

OUTCOME OF ACUTE HBV INFECTION

Most adults with acute HBV infection recover fully within 6 months. Approximately 5–10% progress to chronic HBV infection. In contrast, 30–40% of children and up to 90% of neonates with acute HBV infection become chronically infected.

Risk factors for chronicity of infection include the male gender, youth or age at the time of infection and immunocompromised states. Chronic carriers of hepatitis B virus may typically have a mild or asymptomatic initial episode of disease and therefore often do not give a history of previous acute hepatitis.

CHRONIC HEPATITIS B

By current definition patients with HBsAg persisting for longer than 6 months, and HBeAg persisting for longer than 3 months, are chronic carriers. Carriers may be symptomatic (fatigue, malaise) or may be considered asymptomatic or 'healthy'. In symptomatic carriers with chronic disease, HBsAg and HBeAg, and DNA from HBV are usually present in serum or liver. Healthy carriers usually produce HBsAg alone and do not have evidence of active or marked viral replication.

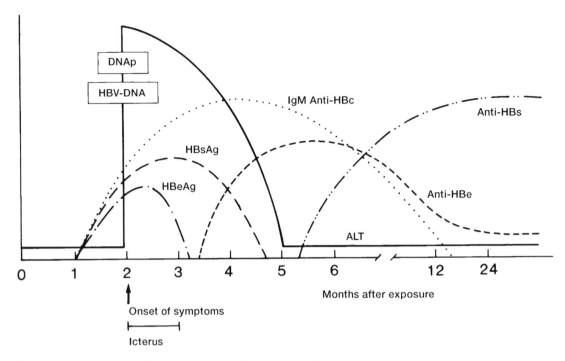

Figure 8.2 Serological profile of typical case of acute hepatitis B. ALT, alanine aminotransferase.

The serological profile of a typical case of symptomatic chronic hepatitis B is shown in Figure 8.3. In this patient markers of active viral replication, HBeAg and HBV DNA were present for almost 5 years. At about 5 years after the onset of disease seroconversion to the non-replicative state occurred. Sero-conversion is associated with disappearance of HBeAg and HBV DNA. The development of anti-HBe indicates the cessation of active viral replication although, as in this case, HBsAg may still be produced, signifying that the HBV has become integrated into the hepatocyte genome. Some patients may relapse clinically or biochemically and again develop markers of viral replication. Abortive seroconversions are also documented with transient flares of hepatitis unaccompanied by loss of HBeAg.

Polymerase chain reaction (PCR) amplification plus sequencing of HBV genomic DNA in infected liver tissue indicates that one or more nucleotide substitutions in the pre-C region of the genome account for the absent expression of HBeAg. A point mutation from guanine to adenine at nucleotide 896, creating an in-frame stop codon, is the most common finding.

OUTCOME OF CHRONIC HBV INFECTION

Chronic HBV infection may produce an asymptomatic carrier state (with an increased risk of hepatocellular carcinoma), chronic mild hepatitis or severe chronic hepatitis. Mild chronic hepatitis, which is most often a relatively benign condition, may occasionally progress to severe disease characterized histologically by mixed inflammatory changes in portal tracts and erosion of the marginal plates with piecemeal necrosis of the liver. Patients with mild chronic hepatitis have a good prognosis with less than 10% progressing to cirrhosis. In contrast, roughly 55% of patients with severe disease develop cirrhosis.

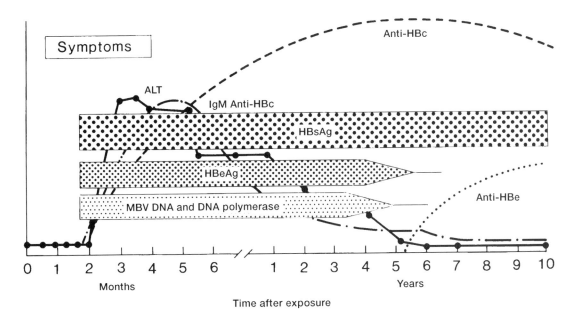

Figure 8.3 Serological profile of typical case of chronic hepatitis B infection. Seroconversion to anti-HBe noted at 5 years from disease onset (see the text for details). (Adapted from Hoofnagle and Schafer, 1986.)

Another potential complication of chronic HBV infection is primary liver carcinoma. Several studies have shown integration of HBV DNA into the genome of human hepatoma cells. The risk of developing liver cancer with chronic hepatitis B virus infection is of the order of 42 times greater than that of the general population in Western countries. In the East, the lifetime risk of developing liver cancer may be as high as up to 50% in selected patient groups with chronic hepatitis B virus infection.

A small percentage of patients with chronic HBV infection may develop extrahepatic manifestations such as polyarteritis nodosa, glomerulonephritis, peripheral neuropathy and marrow hypoplasia. These conditions are felt to be related to the formation of immune complexes.

EPIDEMIOLOGY

The incubation period of hepatitis B infection is 60–180 days. Laboratory tests for hepatitis B have confirmed the importance of parenteral transmission and the infectivity of blood products. However, hepatitis B is not spread exclusively by blood and blood products. There is also much evidence for the sexual transmission of hepatitis B. Here, male homosexuals and promiscuous individuals appear to be at very high risk. HBsAg has been found not only in blood, but also in saliva, menstrual and vaginal discharges, seminal fluid and serous exudates. These have been implicated in the spread of infection. Infection may result from accidental inoculation of minute amounts of blood or fluids contaminated with blood (such as may occur during medical, surgical and dental procedures), immunization with inadequately sterilized syringes and needles, intravenous and percutaneous drug abuse, tattooing, ear-piercing, nose-piercing, acupuncture, laboratory accidents and accidental inoculation with razors and toothbrushes.

In certain parts of the world, additional factors may play a role. These include traditional tattooing, scarification, ritual circumcision and perhaps repeated bites by blood-sucking insects, although this is unproven.

Hepatitis B may also be transferred from carrier mothers to their babies during the perinatal period. This vertical transmission appears to be important in South East Asia where the risk of infection may reach 50–60% or more. There is also a substantial risk of perinatal infection if the mother has acute hepatitis B in the second or third trimester of pregnancy or within 2 months of delivery. Although hepatitis B virus can affect the fetus *in utero*, this is uncommon and appears to occur in fewer than 5% of cases. In contrast to countries like Taiwan, the peak occurrence in southern Africa, Greece and Hong Kong is in children rather than in neonates. In this horizontal spread, infection in the first year of life is rare. In certain rural areas of South Africa large numbers of children are infected between 1 and 5 years of age. The same areas have an extremely high incidence of hepatocellular carcinoma with an average age at onset of 27 years. Thus immunization during the first year of life may have a major impact on subsequent morbidity and mortality in these regions.

IMMUNIZATION

Passive immunization

Hepatitis B immunoglobulin is prepared from pooled plasma which contains a high titer of anti-HBs. This preparation may confer temporary passive immunity and is useful for post-exposure prophylaxis in combination with active immunization. The major indication for the administration of this immunoglobulin is a single acute exposure to HBV such as where blood containing the virus is inoculated, ingested or splashed on to mucous membranes or the conjunctiva. Doses of 250–500 IU have been used effectively. The immunoglobulin should be administered as early as possible after exposure, preferably within 48 hours. There appears to be little benefit from the administration of the immunoglobulin more than 7 days after exposure to the virus. It is recommended that two doses of the immunoglobulin be given 30 days apart. The recommended adult dosage (of hepatitis B immunoglobulin) is about 3 ml and the dose in the newborn infant is 1–2 ml. The immunoglobulin is given by deep intramuscular injection. Passive immunoprophylaxis should be combined with active immunization which is essential for long-term protection.

Active immunization

Active immunization against hepatitis B is essential for groups who are at high risk and do not have serological evidence of past or present HBV infection. These include individuals requiring repeated transfusions of blood or blood products, prolonged in-patient treatment, frequent tissue penetration or repeated arterial or venous access, and patients with natural or acquired immunodeficiency. Viral hepatitis is an occupational hazard among health care personnel and staff of institutions for the mentally disabled. High rates of HBV infection also occur in narcotic drug addicts, drug abusers, homosexuals and commercial sex workers. Individuals working in high endemic areas are also at an increased risk. Young infants, children and susceptible adults living in poor socio-economic conditions in areas where the prevalence of hepatitis B is high should be immunized. The immune response to current hepatitis vaccines is good in the young but may be poor in immunocompromised patients and in elderly people.

The current indications for the use of hepatitis B vaccines in low prevalence areas are listed in Table 8.1.

Table 8.1 Indications for the use of hepatitis B vaccines

---

1. All health care personnel in frequent contact with blood and needles.

2. Patients who are likely to acquire a large number of blood transfusions at major elective surgery. Patients treated by maintenance hemodialysis, or those being admitted to residential institutions for the mentally disabled where there is a known high incidence of hepatitis B.

3. Spouses and sexual contacts of patients with acute or chronic hepatitis B. Other family members in close contact should also receive the vaccine.

4. Infants born to mothers who are persistent carriers of HbsAg or who are positive as a result of recent infection.

5. Individuals who frequently change sexual partners, particularly promiscuous male homosexuals and commercial sex workers. Narcotic and intravenous drug abusers. Long-term prisoners and prison staff, ambulance and rescue service staff and selected police personnel. Military personnel also require immunization in certain countries.

6. Immediate protection may be required under certain circumstances following potential and recent exposure to HBV. In this setting, active immunization with the vaccine is combined with simultaneous administration of hepatitis B immunoglobulin at a different site.

SPECIFIC ISSUES IN HBV VACCINATION

Vaccines currently available consist of plasma-derived or recombinant yeast-produced HBsAg. These vaccines are safe, immunogenic and effective. Vaccines are usually administered by intramuscular injection into the deltoid muscle (or thigh of newborn infants) at 0, 1 and 6 months. There is no risk of HIV or of other hepatitis virus transmission. In protective efficacy studies, the plasma-derived and yeast-derived vaccines appear to be equivalent. A variable proportion of healthy individuals may lose protective levels of anti-HBs at about 5 years after the first vaccine dose. Most, but not all of these individuals, appear to be protected against HBV infection. Booster doses are not currently recommended routinely but should be strongly considered for individuals who remain in high-risk categories. Hypo-responders, who may be identified by post-vaccination anti-HBs testing, may respond to attempts at re-vaccination.

Intradermal administration of one-tenth the usual dose of HBV vaccine induces anti-HBs in most recipients, but the peak response and duration of protection appear to be less than that achieved by intramuscular administration. Intradermal administration for booster inoculation remains to be evaluated. The rapid induction of anti-HBs with an accelerated HBV vaccination schedule may have potential for post-exposure prophylaxis. Several investigators have reported the detection of antibody escape mutants in children vaccinated against hepatitis B.

Other experimental HBV vaccines include polypeptides containing specific HBV antigenic determinants. Clinical trials of polypeptide vaccines are in progress but do not appear to be resulting in effective antibody titers. Hybrid virus vaccines utilizing recombinant vaccinia viruses have been constructed for HBV. These vaccines have certain theoretical advantages in that a single strain of vaccinia may be designed to present antigens characteristic of several viral diseases simultaneously. However, at present the use of vaccinia virus remains experimental and potentially hazardous. Other recombinant viruses being investigated as vectors for hepatitis vaccines include adenoviruses and polioviruses which may even be effective when given by mouth.

TREATMENT OF CHRONIC HBV INFECTION

The rationale for anti-viral treatment of chronic HBV infection is that even mild forms of liver injury may progress during episodes of reactivation or seroconversion, the increased risk of hepatocellular carcinoma and that untreated patients serve as a reservoir of infection. The goals of treatment therefore are to diminish infectivity of the host, to normalize liver inflammation and improve symptomatology. This effect may be predicted by the sustained disappearance of markers of HBV virus replication.

Of all the agents that have been used to treat chronic type B virus hepatitis, α interferon (IFN) as the single modality of therapy offers the most promise. IFN is usually well tolerated in clinically compensated patients with chronic hepatitis B. Its use is more difficult in patients with decompensated forms of the disease. 'Steroid priming' prior to IFN use should never be attempted in this group of patients because of the risk of further decompensation. Such variables as the pretreatment levels of circulating HBV DNA, aminotransferases, and degree of histological activity as well as the ethnic group, sexual lifestyle and HIV status of the patient influence the response to treatment.

Approximately 40% of patients seroconvert from HBeAg-positive to HBeAg-negative and anti-HBe-positive following standardized treatment regimens, compared with a spontaneous seroconversion rate of approximately 10% per annum. The long-term benefits of

this treatment are still being assessed but potential for 'cure' exists.

A high proportion (60–70%) of patients with anti-HBe may respond, but relapse rates are high in this group. Children with active disease or nephrotic syndrome associated with HBV may respond to IFN, or to steroid priming plus IFN. Studies also need to address whether early treatment of individuals with persistent viral replication 12 or more weeks after the onset of illness may prevent evolution to chronic infection.

HEPATITIS D VIRUS

STRUCTURE

The hepatitis delta virus (HDV) is a small defective RNA virus. This is the only known human viral pathogen that cannot infect cells or replicate on its own. HDV requires the hepatitis B virus as a 'helper' DNA virus for its survival. HDV has an outer coat composed of HBsAg, of HBV origin, its own delta antigen and small genome. HDV resembles the so-called satellite viruses of plants, which are also coated by capsid material of obligatory helper viruses. The virus appears to be directly cytopathic in contrast to hepatitis B where damage appears to be immune-mediated.

CLINICAL FEATURES

When acute delta hepatitis occurs in a chronic HBsAg carrier it is known as superinfection. Simultaneous acute delta and acute hepatitis B infection is called co-infection. Superinfection often leads to chronic delta infection with progressive hepatocellular dysfunction. Co-infection may be serious, leading to fulminant hepatitis but seldom results in chronic delta infection. Therefore delta hepatitis, although not as common as the other hepatitis viruses in southern Africa, is important because of its severity.

EPIDEMIOLOGY AND CONTROL

The geographic prevalence of hepatitis D virus in carriers of HBsAg suggests that this infection is important in the Middle East, parts of Africa and South America. Studies performed in southern Africa to date, suggest that delta agent is absent or very rare despite the large pool of HBsAg carriers. The mode of transmission of HDV is similar to that of HBV, that is predominantly parenteral, but non-parenteral spread also occurs. Immunization against hepatitis B protects against infection with the delta agent by depriving the HDV of its protective HBsAg coat.

TREATMENT

Established delta hepatitis is currently treated along the same lines as chronic hepatitis B infection, with interferon. There is presently no alternative treatment for this serious disease. Improvement may only occur in about 25% of patients and chronic HDV infection appears to require long-term treatment.

HEPATITIS C VIRUS

STRUCTURE

The hepatitis C virus (HCV) is an RNA virus with a lipid envelope about 18 nm in diameter which belongs to a unique family related to the toga and flavivirus group. Interestingly, both these families are arboviruses, a group of viruses usually transmitted by insect bites.

EPIDEMIOLOGY

HCV is a major cause of transfusion-associated non-A, non-B (NANB) hepatitis throughout the world but may also play a role in community-acquired NANB hepatitis. Approximately 75–85% of patients with chronic post-transfusion hepatitis (PTH) in the USA, Japan and Italy have been found to have markers of HCV infection. In addition, about 58% of community-acquired chronic NANB hepatitis cases with no identifiable source of parenteral exposure appear to be positive for anti-HCV.

Predominant modes of transmission for HCV virus include contact with blood or blood products, the sharing of contaminated needles or syringes and sexual or intimate contact with an HCV carrier. At highest risk are recipients of multiple units of blood and especially recipients of commercial Factor VIII concentrates. We have recently shown that 60% of hemophiliacs at Groote Schuur Hospital, Cape Town, have markers for hepatitis C virus. This is in agreement with the international literature.

CLINICAL FEATURES

Acute hepatitis C appears to run a mild anicteric course in about 75% of patients (Fig. 8.4). Because of the frequency of asymptomatic mild disease, many cases of hepatitis C remain undetected. Despite its relatively mild, often asymptomatic course, acute hepatitis secondary to HCV tends to progress to chronic liver disease in about 50% of patients. Fluctuating elevations in transaminase activity most often persist for some time, although the magnitude of ALT elevation decreases, as demonstrated in Figure 8.5. Despite mild or absent symptoms, hepatitis C may progress very rapidly with the early onset of chronic hepatitis and cirrhosis. There also appears to be a strong association with hepatocellular carcinoma.

DIAGNOSIS

Antibodies against HCV serve as markers for this infection. Although only 54% of acute phase sera test positive, this figure increases to

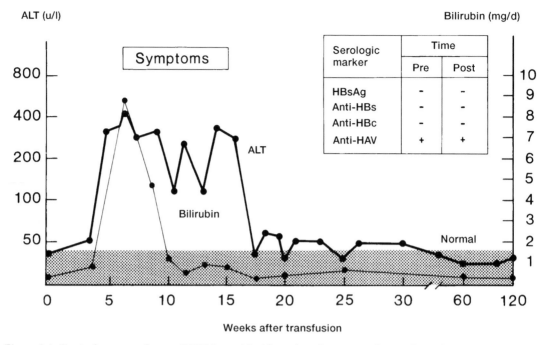

ALT (u/l)   Bilirubin (mg/d)

Serologic marker	Time	
	Pre	Post
HBsAg	-	-
Anti-HBs	-	-
Anti-HBc	-	-
Anti-HAV	+	+

Weeks after transfusion

Figure 8.4 Typical course of acute HCV hepatitis. Note that the patient has IgG markers for HAV. Anti-HCV antibodies were recorded as positive at 6 months. The shaded area represents normal ALT (alanine aminotransferase) levels.

67% in chronic phase sera taken 6–36 months from onset. Therefore in the acute setting, the diagnosis of HCV is still by exclusion. Additional data which aid in the diagnosis are epidemiological factors such as a history of exposure to blood or blood products, intravenous drug addiction and the episodic fluctuating ALT pattern (Fig. 8.5).

CONTROL

Testing for anti-HCV substantially improves the safety of transfusion of blood and blood products. In addition, steps taken to reduce the transmission of HIV have led to the exclusion of those donors most likely to carry HCV infection. Passive immunization against HCV has not been effective but conclusive investigations have still to be published. There are no vaccines for HCV at present.

TREATMENT

The treatment of chronic HCV infection remains a difficult problem. Because of the lack of markers until recently, many clinical studies have been performed on heterogeneous groups of patients with NANB hepatitis. The only recognized effective mode of treatment is α interferon doses of 3–5 million units three times weekly for 6 to 12 months. Approximately 15–25% of patients have a sustained response. Higher doses, longer treatment (>6 months) or interferon combined with other anti-viral agents appear to improve response rates. Liver transplantation for severe chronic hepatitis is followed by reactivation and infection of the graft in 79%.

HEPATITIS F VIRUS

Hepatitis F virus (HFV or F-NAB) is an epidemiological entity with no specific

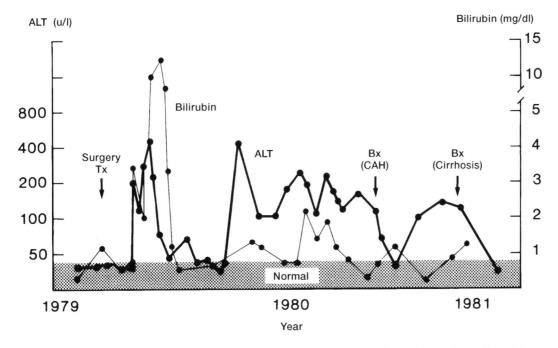

Figure 8.5 Typical case of post-transfusional chronic hepatitis C virus (HCV) infection. Note fluctuating alanine aminotransferase (ALT) values and rapid progression to cirrhosis. This patient developed anti-HCV antibodies at 6 months post-transfusion and was HCV RNA positive by RT–PCR (reverse transcriptase–polymerase chain reaction) (not shown in figure). The shaded area respresents normal ALT levels. Tx, transplantation; Bx, biopsy; CAH chronic active hepatitis.

serological markers. It may arise sporadically or in outbreaks, and results in fulminant and sub-fulminant hepatitis in a large proportion of patients. Patients usually develop encephalopathy up to 12 weeks after the onset of jaundice, and have a fluctuating clinical course characterized by periodic elevations of transaminase activities. The presence of jaundice, marked coagulation disturbances, renal impairment and an age of 40 years or more appear to indicate a poor prognosis with a mortality in excess of 90%. The only recognized treatment in this instance is liver transplantation.

Non-B, non-C post-transfusional hepatitis has also been termed HFV by several authors.

CONCLUSION

This clinical review has summarized current information on the hepatitis A, B and NANB viruses. The NANB hepatitis virus group, although heterogeneous, is now sub-classified with the advent of serological markers for the identification of the hepatitis C and hepatitis E viruses.

A major concern is to control hepatitis B virus and prevent the appalling sequelae of chronic infection with this virus. Universal vaccination of infants in high-risk areas is vital but will only be possible in those areas of greatest need once the costs of vaccine are reduced.

RECOMMENDED READING

Alter, H.J. (1989) Non-A, Non-B hepatitis: sorting through a diagnosis of exclusion. *Ann Intern Med*, **110**(8), 583–5.

Dienstag, J.L. and Alter, H.J. (1986) Non-A Non-B Hepatitis: Evolving epidemiologic and clinical perspectives. *Semin Liver Dis*, **6**, 67–81.

Esteban, R. (1993) Epidemiology of hepatitis C infection. *J Hepatol*, **17**, S67–71.

Ganem, D. and Varmus, H.E. (1987) The molecular biology of the hepatitis B virus. *Annu Rev Biochem*, **56**, 651–93.

Genesca, J., Esteban, J.I. and Alter, H.J. (1991) Blood-borne non-A non-B hepatitis: hepatitis C. *Semin Liver Dis*, **11**, 147–64.

Hoofnagle, J. (1989) Type D (Delta) Hepatitis. *JAMA*, **261**(9), 1321–5.

Hoofnagle, J.H. (1989) Towards universal vaccination against hepatitis B virus. *N Engl J Med*, **321**, 1333–4.

Hoofnagle, J.H. and Schafer, D.F. (1986) Serologic markers of hepatitis B virus infection. *Semin Liver Dis*, **6**, 1–10.

Hoofnagle, J.H., Peters, M., Mullen, K.D. *et al.* (1988) Randomized, controlled trial of recombinant human alpha interferon in patients with chronic type B hepatitis. *Gastroenterology*, **95**, 1318–25.

Kirsch, R.E. and Robson, S.C. (1989) Prevalence of Hepatitis B in Southern Africa (Editorial). *S Afr Med J*, **75**, 461.

Kuo, G., Choo, Q.-L., Alter, H.J. *et al.* (1989) An assay for circulating antibodies of a major etiologic virus of human non-A, non-B hepatitis. *Science*, **244**, 362–4.

Kuroki, T., Nishiguchi, S., Fukada, K. *et al.* (1993) Vertical transmission of hepatitis C virus detected by HCV-RNA analysis. *Gut*, **34**, S52–3.

Lemon, S.M. (1985) Type A viral hepatitis. *N Engl J Med*. **313**, 1059–67.

Margolis, H.S., Alter, M.J. and Hadler, S.C. (1991) Hepatitis B: evolving epidemiology and implications for control. *Semin Liver Dis*, **11**, 84–92.

Margolis, H.S., Alter, M.J. and Hadler, S.C. (1991) Hepatitis B: evolving epidemiology and implications for control. *Semin Liver Dis*, **11**, 84–92.

Perillo, R.P. (1993) Hepatitis B: transmission and natural history. *Gut*, **34**, S48–9.

Perillo, R.P., Schiff, E.R., Davis, G.L. *et al.* (1990) A randomized, controlled trial of interferon alfa-2b alone and after prednisone withdrawal for the treatment of chronic hepatitis B. The Hepatitis Interventional Therapy Group. *N Engl J Med*, **323**, 295–301.

Ramalingaswami, V. and Purcell, R.H. (1988) Waterborne non-A, non-B hepatitis. *Lancet*, **1**, 571–3.

Rizzetto, M. and Verme, G. (1985) Delta hepatitis – present status. *J Hepatol*, **1**, 187–93.

Robinson, W.S. (1990) Hepadnaviridae and their replication, in *Virology* (eds B.N. Fields and D.N. Knipe), Raven Press, New York, pp. 2137–69.

Roudot-Thoraval, F., Pawlotsky, J.M., Thiers, V. *et al.* (1993) Lack of mother to infant transmission of hepatitis C virus in human immunodeficiency virus negative women: a prospective study with hepatitis C virus RNA testing. *Hepatology*, **17**, 772–7.

Sarver, D. (1986) Hepatitis in clinical practice. *Postgrad Med*, **79**(4), 194–214.

Schoub, B.D., Johnson, S., McAnerny, J. *et al.* (1991) Exposure to hepatitis B virus among South African health care workers – Implications for pre-immunisation screening. *S Afr Med J*, **79**(1), 27–9.

Sutherland, S. (1986) Update on viral hepatitis. *The Practitioner*, **230**, 237–46.

Tiollais, P., Poursel, C. and Dejean, A. (1985) The hepatitis B virus. *Nature*, **317**, 489–95.

Zuckerman, A.J. (1989) The elusive Hepatitis C virus. *Br Med J*, **299**, 871–3.

9

Chronic hepatitis and autoimmune liver diseases

SIMON ROBSON and JAMES NEUBERGER

INTRODUCTION

Chronic active hepatitis, a syndrome due to many causes (Table 9.1), is characterized by clinical, laboratory and histological changes representing features of both chronic and active hepatitis. Histologically there is piecemeal necrosis with inflammatory infiltrates, consisting predominantly of mononuclear cells, eroding the marginal plate and extending into the adjacent liver lobule. The process may extend from portal areas to central veins. Bridging necrosis has a particularly bad prognosis and may progress rapidly to cirrhosis. Chronic persistent hepatitis is a 'benign' histological variant characterized by mononuclear cell infiltrates confined to the portal tracts. These histological classifications are often of little help in specific diagnosis and management. Currently the trend has been to describe the severity of the histological picture and to classify the condition of chronic hepatitis according to its presumed etiology.

A detailed description of chronic viral hepatitis B and C (HBV and HCV) is found in Chapter 8 and we will not deal with these except to stress that the presence of viral markers is of pivotal importance in prognosis and management of chronic liver disease. Patients with markers of HBV or HCV do not respond favorably to immunosuppressive therapy. In the case of HBV infection, steroids should only be used for the 'immune rebound'

Table 9.1 Causes of chronic hepatitis

Autoimmune
    Classic lupoid autoimmune hepatitis
    Liver and kidney microsomal (LKM) antibody-
      positive group
    Soluble liver antigen (SLA) group
    Smooth-muscle antibody (SMA)-positive group
    Overlap group

Viral
    Hepatitis viruses B and C

Drugs
    Alpha-methyldopa
    Nitrofurantoin

Alcohol

Wilson's disease

Hemochromatosis

Alpha-1 antitrypsin deficiency

effect following their withdrawal and then only in highly selected cases. In addition, steroids should not be used alone, but should always be followed by antiviral therapy such as alpha interferon.

It is important that patients with potentially reversible metabolic conditions such as hemochromatosis and Wilson's disease be recognized at an early stage. This possibility is greatly enhanced by a thorough clinical evaluation extending beyond the abdomen and encompassing a full family history and careful examination of the cardiovascular, endocrine and nervous systems. All young patients (age below 40 years) with unexplained liver disease should have a slit-lamp examination of the cornea for Kayser Fleischer rings to exclude Wilson's disease. A full drug history should be taken as some drugs may cause chronic hepatitis, which usually resolves after cessation of the causative agent.

Routine investigations should include a full blood count, coagulation profile, and serum chemistry. The alanine aminotransferase (ALT) and aspartate aminotransferase (AST) are particularly important in gauging the degree of liver inflammation. The serum globulins are usually increased with a polyclonal gammopathy. This is commonly associated with autoimmune lupoid hepatitis but is also seen in HCV and non-B, non-C chronic active hepatitis and in established cirrhosis from any cause.

Further investigations may include tests for autoantibodies and, where available, antibodies for soluble liver antigen. Serum iron, copper, ceruloplasmin, and the alpha-1 antitrypsin level and phenotype should be determined where indicated.

Imaging techniques will be utilized according to their indication. All patients should undergo ultrasound examination. If there is concern about underlying biliary disease or carcinoma, endoscopic retrograde cholangiopancreatography (ERCP), computed tomography (CT) scan or magnetic resonance imaging (MRI) will be indicated (Chapter 4).

AUTOIMMUNE CHRONIC HEPATITIS

IDENTIFICATION OF SUB-TYPES

This heterogeneous syndrome has been subdivided, by autoantibody analysis, into several sub-types (Table 9.1). The different antibody profiles may have pathogenetic significance. It is thought that K cells and antibody-dependent cellular cytotoxicity are important in the pathogenesis of liver damage in autoimmune chronic hepatitis.

Autoimmune reactions are, however, noted in a variety of liver diseases. These include alcoholic hepatitis and cirrhosis, alpha-1 antitrypsin deficiency, hemochromatosis and Wilson's disease. We will, however, concentrate our discussions initially on the conditions generally accepted as having a major autoimmune component and which can be classified as follows.

Classic lupoid autoimmune hepatitis

This is classically associated with serum antinuclear factors (ANF), high gamma-globulin levels, major histocompatability complex (MHC) or HLA B8 and DR3 or DR4. The DR4 haplotype is more common in older patients and in Japanese with chronic active hepatitis. This sub-type is predominantly seen in females and is the most common form of chronic active hepatitis. Fortunately, it responds very well to steroid therapy.

Liver and kidney microsomal (LKM) antibody-positive group

This is much less common than the classic ANF-positive group. Patients tend to be younger and respond to steroids. Some patients with LKM-1 antibody-associated chronic hepatitis have infection with hepatitis C virus, which may induce an autoimmune reaction. These patients are older, have lower serum transaminases and respond less well to steroids.

Soluble liver antigen (SLA) group

These antibodies are not detected by routine immunofluorescence tests and will therefore be missed unless measured by ELISA. This predominantly young female sub-set also responds to corticosteroids. The presence of SLA distinguishes this group from patients with HCV or presumed non-B, non-C chronic hepatitis who should not be given corticosteroids. The SLA group tend to be negative for anti-nuclear and liver and kidney microsomal antibodies which are markers for the above two autoimmune chronic hepatitis subgroups. A very marked serum hypergammaglobulinemia may be present and is often a useful clue for SLA autoimmune chronic active hepatitis (CAH).

Smooth-muscle antibody (SMA)-positive group

These patients have negative tests for other autoantibodies. There is some overlap with chronic viral hepatitis and this group does not appear to respond favorably to corticosteroids.

Overlap group

Here autoimmune reactions are directed at both biliary and hepatocyte constituents. Patients tend to present initially as fairly classic autoimmune chronic hepatitis. However, anti-mitochondrial antibodies may be detected and patients tend to evolve towards biliary cirrhosis. Long-term response to immunosuppressive therapy is therefore relatively poor.

CLINICAL FEATURES

Patients with autoimmune chronic hepatitis are predominantly female and are commonly of European or of mixed ancestry. There are two peak ages of presentation: during the teens and the peri-menopausal period. Elderly patients with established liver disease may also be seen. The symptoms and signs depend on the tempo and severity of the illness. Patients, particularly those in their teenage years, usually present with fatigue, malaise and jaundice. They frequently complain of acne and striae. Lymphadenopathy and fever are less frequent manifestations. Late signs include ascites, encephalopathy and variceal bleeding. These are less common and are usually seen in the older group of patients.

On examination patients often have florid stigmata of chronic liver disease. Hepatosplenomegaly is frequently found. Ascites and edema are late manifestations. Patients may also have features of other autoimmune conditions including thrombocytopenia, anemia (warm autoimmune variety), arthritis (usually non-deforming polyarthritis), thyroiditis and skin lesions, including vasculitis and pyoderma gangrenosum. Patients may also be found to have endocrine disorders, including hypothyroidism and hypopituitarism.

Following recognition, it is imperative that an absolutely firm clinical and histological diagnosis is made, both for prognosis and institution of appropriate therapy. Therefore all patients must undergo liver biopsy prior to introduction of immunosuppressive therapy. Under certain circumstances, if patients are very ill with bleeding disorders or severe ascites, a percutaneous liver biopsy may not be possible. If a trans-jugular biopsy cannot be obtained, these patients may be given a short trial of steroids but should have a future liver biopsy as soon as their general condition will allow this procedure.

TREATMENT

Patients with autoimmune chronic active hepatitis must be identified so that immunosuppressive therapy may be commenced. Left untreated there is a high morbidity and mortality, with rapid progression to cirrhosis, liver failure and death. Steroids are life-saving in the short term but are not without complications. Long-term management is further complicated in many cases by the slow, inexorable development of cirrhosis within 10–15 years of commencement of therapy.

The following indications for immunosuppressive therapy are suggested:

- florid hepatitis with transaminases in excess of 10 times normal;
- transaminases five times normal plus serum globulins twice normal;
- associated complications such as thrombocytopenia, warm autoimmune hemolytic anemia or inflammatory bowel disease;
- symptomatic patients with fatigue, malaise and jaundice;
- patients with transaminases elevated to twice normal but with significant inflammatory activity on biopsy.

Immunosuppressive therapy usually consists of prednisolone, prednisone or methylprednisolone at appropriate dosages (approximately 20 mg of prednisolone daily for the average adult). In teenagers the dosage may be modified to 0.5 mg/kg/day of prednisone. This should induce a rapid remission. This dosage is usually maintained until the patient is asymptomatic and until there is resolution of jaundice with decreasing transaminase levels. The dose is then slowly reduced.

Once in remission, most patients are given azathioprine (0.5–1 mg/kg/day). We never use doses higher than 50–75 mg of azathioprine/day as significant side effects such as infection and pancytopenia may result. Azathioprine may cause gastrointestinal upset and may rarely produce idiosyncratic liver damage. Once azathioprine therapy has been commenced steroid doses are slowly decreased to maintenance levels (usually <10 mg prednisone/day).

The major complications of steroid use include weight gain, hypertension, cataract formation, bone loss, increased risk of infection and adrenal suppression with long-term usage. All patients should receive a Medic-Alert token indicating that they have chronic hepatitis and are on prednisone and azathioprine therapy.

The aims of long-term management are to maintain remission and to avoid the development of long-term complications of autoimmune chronic active liver disease.

There is some debate about withdrawal of therapy. This should never be done in patients with established chronic liver disease or with significant histological changes on a recent liver biopsy. Where biochemical activity is still present, patients are usually monitored by annual or 18-monthly biopsies. It is occasionally possible to withdraw prednisone while continuing with azathioprine. Azathioprine alone will not induce remission but may maintain clinically quiescent disease. In some patients withdrawal of steroids is associated with arthralgia, necessitating reintroduction of low-dose prednisone for clinical comfort and symptomatic relief. Low-dose maintenance prednisone and azathioprine are utilized in the majority of our patients. In the very few patients unable to tolerate prednisone and azathioprine, cyclosporine is effective, although possibly more toxic. .

Withdrawal of all immunosuppressive therapy, if attempted, should be carried out after at least 18–24 months' therapy, in patients with clinically quiescent disease, normal transaminase levels and an inactive liver biopsy. Prednisone is slowly withdrawn, followed by azathioprine. If patients remain in clinical remission, a biopsy can be performed after 6 months. If this biopsy is normal the patient may safely be followed without immunosuppressive therapy until (or if) they relapse. We anticipate that up to 80% of patients relapse. Early relapses are invariable if there are features of established chronic disease, elevated transaminases or marked activity on liver biopsy.

COMPLICATIONS OF DISEASE

The complications of autoimmune chronic active liver disease include portal hypertension with variceal bleeding, which is managed along conventional lines. There may be a place for prophylactic propranolol in this group of patients if they have large varices (Chapter 14) but there is no place for prophylactic sclerotherapy. Following variceal bleeding, these patients should have long-term sclerotherapy or esophageal transsection. At this time, liver transplantation should be considered.

Further complications include ascites, hepatorenal failure, infection and bone disease. Encephalopathy may also develop at this point, necessitating lactulose therapy and the introduction of a low-protein diet (Chapter 13). Patients should be assessed for liver transplantation prior to this stage.

SPECIAL CIRCUMSTANCES

Pregnancy

Amenorrhea is a common manifestation of severe disease, but after institution of immunosuppressive therapy menses return and patients may become fertile, albeit at a reduced rate. There is increased fetal loss during the first trimester and some degree of growth retardation in those patients with full-term pregnancies. One is obviously concerned with the potential teratogenicity of both prednisone and azathioprine. However, it must be stressed that withdrawal of immunosuppressive therapy during pregnancy may be associated with severe clinical relapse and hepatitis. This is far more detrimental to the outcome of the pregnancy than the minor and often negligible effects of low-dose azathioprine and prednisone. Healthy babies with no increased incidence of congenital anomalies have been born to numerous patients with autoimmune chronic active liver disease maintained on low-dose prednisone and azathioprine.

In the intelligent patient who comes to a physician for preconception counseling, azathioprine may be withdrawn, provided that she is in clinical remission, is menstruating and has a normal liver biopsy. The patient should be maintained on prednisone. In the postpartum period, steroids may be increased as these patients may relapse during this time. The clinical course during pregnancy is, however, unpredictable and patients should be monitored more closely.

Geriatric patients

Elderly patients with autoimmune chronic hepatitis often present at a late stage of disease and are difficult to manage. The presence of ascites suggests that a poor response to corticosteroids and immunosuppressive therapy may be expected. However, this therapy should be embarked on, albeit at low doses and for a trial period.

Smooth-muscle antibody group

The atypical chronic hepatitis group includes those with only smooth-muscle antibodies. This group overlaps with chronic non-B, non-C or hepatitis C virus infections. Poor responses to steroids are usual. We recommend that if there is no clinical or biochemical improvement within 3 months of commencing steroids that this therapy be withdrawn. The risks of continued immunosuppression under

105

these circumstances are more hazardous than observing the patient and monitoring progress alone.

Overlap group

The last special instance is that of the overlap syndrome where patients may progress from a chronic active hepatitis syndrome to a predominantly cholestatic illness overlapping with primary biliary cirrhosis. These patients have an initial partial response to steroids. The progressive cholestasis is poorly responsive to any form of specific therapy, including bile salt replacement and immunosuppressive therapy.

HCV and autoimmune hepatitis

Finally, there are several recent reports of a high frequency of anti-HCV positivity in patients with autoimmune chronic hepatitis. This has been interpreted as either a causal relationship or simply representing coincidental HCV infection. High frequency of anti-HCV has also been noted in another condition associated with hypergamma-globulinemia, namely alcoholic cirrhosis. A further possibility is that these results represent a false-positive reaction in hypergamma-globulinemic disease. Support for false positivity comes from recent studies at King's College Hospital, London. All HCV tests should now be verified by neutralization tests, recombinant immunoblots or by polymerase chain reaction (PCR) for HCV RNA.

PRIMARY BILIARY CIRRHOSIS

Primary biliary cirrhosis (PBC), or chronic non-suppurative destructive cholangiohepatitis (Chapter 11), has been considered by many as a model autoimmune disease. While a wide variety of autoantibodies are found in patients with PBC, the characteristic antibodies are anti-mitochondrial antibodies (AMA). Indeed,

patients with the antibodies but normal liver function tests may have histological features of PBC on liver biopsy. Since 1987 there has been a vast improvement in the definition of the biochemical and molecular nature of the target auto-antigens. The major auto-antigen is the E2 sub-unit of pyruvate dehydrogenase (PDH-E2). Immunodominant sites on PDH-E2 have been mapped and have been shown to be the site of attachment of the functionally important lipoic acid prosthetic group. The cloning of cDNAs for mitochondrial antigens has led to the identification of three of the 2-oxo-acid dehydrogenase family as autoantibody targets.

Immunization of rodents and other experimental animals with mitochondrial antigens leads to the development of anti-mitochondrial antibodies without any biliary disease. Reproduction of biliary ductular lesions by transfer of peripheral blood lymphocytes purified from patients with PBC into nude or immunocompromised mice has been described. Some workers have suggested that rough forms of *E. coli* and recurrent bacterial infections may be implicated in the disease.

IMMUNOLOGY

PBC is classically associated with high IgM levels and abnormal T-suppressor cell function. Histological analysis of the mononuclear cells infiltrating the liver in PBC suggests that helper (CD3-, CD4-positive) T lymphocytes expressing the T-cell receptor β chain are the predominant cell type surrounding the portal triads. Cytotoxic T cells (CD3-, CD8-positive) are noted where there is significant piecemeal necrosis (often in the overlap syndrome between this condition and chronic active hepatitis). T lymphocytes are clearly the predominant cell type present in both infiltrates and necrotic areas in PBC. The newly recognized class of T cells bearing the γ/δ rather than the α/β T-cell receptor are also present in large numbers, particularly in early active granulomatous responses. These cells may have a special role in autoimmune reactions since they are present in abundance in rheumatoid synovium and in other areas of autoimmune reactions. These γ/δ T cells are thought to preferentially recognize heat shock and MHC class I proteins.

The actual cause of biliary ductular damage in PBC is unknown. Activated T cells may produce lymphokines which act locally to recruit non-specific T cells to the site of inflammation. 'Cholestatic' lymphokines are produced by T cells. Macrophages are also able to increase the expression of MHC class II proteins by biliary cells via specific mediators which include gamma interferons.

CLINICAL PRESENTATION

The clinical presentation of PBC depends on when the disease is diagnosed. This progression is impossible to predict but there appear to be two large groups. The one group with chiefly asymptomatic disease has a better prognosis. Indeed, apart from elevated alkaline phosphatases and anti-mitochondrial antibodies, there is little else to base the diagnosis on. Histology of these livers usually shows portal tract infiltration and later ductular injury. The other major group presents with symptomatic disease. Here increasing symptomatic cholestasis, florid signs of liver disease, elevated bilirubin and alkaline phosphatases are noted. All patients have large livers but splenomegaly may be a later manifestation. Patients classically present with pruritus, jaundice, fatigue, malaise and, at times, fever and lymphadenopathy. Later presentations include ascites, peripheral edema, encephalopathy and variceal bleeding. Patients have an increased tendency to develop sicca syndrome and scleroderma-like skin changes. Polyarthritis is also noted. There is an increased frequency of breast carcinoma, hepatocellular carcinoma and lymphoma.

Differential diagnosis

The histology of PBC may be fairly distinct, but at times may suggest a differential diagnosis ranging from sclerosing cholangitis to chronic active hepatitis. The early stages reflect ductular infiltrates with mononuclear cells. Ductular injury, fibrosis and scarring lead to the development of cirrhosis (Chapter 6). An ultrasound or ERCP is essential in all cases to document the absence of biliary obstruction (Chapter 4). A caveat to this is that gallstones are present in up to 30–40% of patients with PBC. The determination of 'symptomatic gallstones' may sometimes be difficult under these circumstances. Patients may also present with bone disease and 'hepatic osteodystrophy'. Steroids are not indicated in these patients as this treatment may accelerate their bone loss.

NATURAL HISTORY AND POTENTIAL THERAPIES

Although neither the initiation nor perpetuating mechanisms are well understood, immunologically mediated duct damage is felt to account for the progressive destruction of the biliary tract and the eventual development of biliary cirrhosis. Ideally, therapy should be aimed at turning off the initiation factors that lead to duct damage. Short of this, most therapies have been directed at arresting the inflammatory process and the progressive development of fibrosis which are prominent features. This is the rationale for the use of agents such as corticosteroids, colchicine, cyclosporine and methotrexate. The use of all these agents may be associated with short-term improvement in liver function tests.

The importance of secondary damage, postulated to be induced by bile salts and toxic factors, has received renewed support from early experience with ursodeoxycholic acid (UDCA). This alters bile acid composition with important decreases in the hydropho-bicity of the bile acid pool. However, all studies to date have utilized small numbers of patients followed up over a short period of time often in an uncontrolled manner. UDCA may improve liver biochemistry in the short term. However, there is currently no proof that this therapy prolongs life and prevents the progression of cirrhosis.

The early experiences with single thera-peutic agents suggested that combinations of anti-inflammatory and anti-cholestatic thera-pies may provide even better potential for the management of this condition. However, there is a need for continuing, controlled clin-ical trials.

Certain drugs are toxic (including penicil-lamine and chlorambucil) and should not be utilized under any circumstances. Steroids remain contraindicated outside of random-ized clinical studies. Steroids have detri-mental effects on bone density despite minor improvements in histology and liver biochemistry. Cyclosporine may also aggra-vate bone disease and has the additional complications of nephrotoxicity and hyper-tension with a potential increased risk of lymphoma. UDCA and colchicine appear to be relatively safe but proof of their long-term benefit is still awaited. Methotrexate is a hepatotoxic drug and there does not appear to be any rational reason for the general use of this agent in chronic cholestatic liver disease, although some isolated patients with PBC may show improvement. Azathioprine is associated with increased risks of infection but some studies have claimed an improved quality of life with this agent.

Symptomatic therapy is essential in the management of these patients. Therapy should be directed at the pruritis, with the use of cholestyramine, a bile acid-binding resin. If cholestyramine alone is not effective, further modalities of therapy including anti-histamines, cimetidine, rifampin and anabolic

steroids may be tried. UDCA has some effect on pruritus, as does cyclosporine at initiation of therapy.

Careful attention to nutrition including supplementation of the diet with medium-chain triglycerides and a low neutral fat diet in patients with steatorrhea is useful. We recom-mend that patients take additional calcium with skimmed or defatted milk and calcium supplements. Intramuscular vitamins are administered every month (vitamin A, 100 000 units; vitamin D, 100 000 units; vitamin K, 10 mg). Alternatively, vitamin A and D supple-ments may be administered orally on a daily basis. Vitamin E, where thought to be defi-cient, may be supplemented by injection. Patients are advised to expose themselves to sunlight for a short period of time every day. There may be an association with celiac disease and duodenal biopsies should be taken in those patients with significant malabsorption.

TRANSPLANTATION

The only therapy that has been shown to prolong the life of patients with PBC and to give excellent symptomatic results is liver transplantation (Chapter 27). The timing of transplantation still requires careful clinical judgment. The use of statistical survival modeling has given a degree of objectivity to this decision-making process. However, current models are not perfect and they only take into account time-dependent factors. These models are estimates of the probability of survival. None of these models takes into account the patient's quality of life and cata-strophic, life-threatening events such as variceal bleeding. Furthermore, the confi-dence limits, when applied to individual patients, are wide. On a more practical basis, when the serum bilirubin approaches 180 μmol/l, the life expectancy is about 18 months. Therefore when patients with PBC become progressively jaundiced, they are at high risk of death and should be referred for urgent transplantation. In moderately jaundiced patients who develop increasing symptomatology, an opinion should be sought at a liver transplant center.

Patients with end-stage liver disease have significantly more torrid peri-transplant courses, require more blood transfusions and spend more days in the intensive care unit and in hospital after transplantation. Transplantation in PBC at earlier advanced stages of disease may not only increase long-term survival but diminishes morbidity and the costs of liver transplantation.

PRIMARY SCLEROSING CHOLANGITIS

Primary sclerosing cholangitis is dealt with in detail in Chapter 11 and will not be discussed here.

ALCOHOLIC LIVER DISEASE

Chronic alcohol abuse may lead to the development of liver injury even when the diet contains all the required nutrients in the recommended amounts (Chapter 7). However, malnutrition is common in alcoholics. Alcohol may displace other nutrients from the diet and has toxic effects on the gastrointestinal tract. Ethanol may also interfere with vitamin and other nutrient activation or accelerate their breakdown. Alcohol's effects on the liver are as follows:

● metabolic changes directly related to the oxidation of alcohol;
● adaptive changes involving primarily increased microsomal functions;
● injurious effects, including marked structural and functional changes in mitochondria.

Many effects linked to the consumption of alcohol are secondary to the oxidation of alcohol to acetaldehyde via the alcohol dehydrogenase pathway and activation of the xenobiotics by the ethanol-inducible cytochrome P450 IIE1.

AUTOIMMUNITY

There are many unanswered questions in the possibility of an autoimmune pathogenesis for both alcoholic hepatitis and alcoholic cirrhosis. It is apparent that a minority of patients who abuse alcohol develop alcoholic hepatitis and cirrhosis. There are obviously both genetic and environmental factors which make patients susceptible to the development of alcoholism and alcoholic liver disease.

It is known that alcoholism runs in families and that there is a genetic predisposition to end-organ damage. The different familial types associated with alcoholism include the 'milieu limited', the 'male limited' and the 'anti-social behavior' groups.

The immunology of alcoholic liver disease is characterized by a combination of both immunodeficiency and enhanced specific and non-specific responses to altered tissue components. Immunoreactivity appears to be directed at acetaldehyde-induced epitopes, particularly on adducts of tissue proteins. Lipoproteins (LDL) are highly sensitive to such interactions by virtue of lysine residues. Mallory's hyaline (altered cytokeratin) is a highly immunogenic protein. Both T and B lymphocyte responses are implicated in the development of tissue damage secondary to alcohol exposure. There is an increase in intrahepatic T cells, which occur in the portal areas of patients with alcoholic hepatitis. Cytotoxic T cells extend into the liver lobule. Chemotactic factors secreted in response to alcoholic hyaline may cause accumulation of polymorpholeukocytes. There are increased levels of tumor necrosis factor, IL-6 and circulating adhesion molecules. Sinusoidal deposition of IgA is common in alcoholic liver disease. Circulating immune complexes do not appear to play a role in the pathogenesis of alcoholic liver injury but may contribute to renal injury.

Impaired delayed hypersensitivity *in vivo* may occur in advanced alcoholic liver disease. Alcohol or acetaldehyde added to cultures of peripheral mononuclear cells *in vitro* may induce lymphocyte transformation when these cells are purified from patients with alcoholic hepatitis. Similarly, homogenates of livers obtained from patients with alcoholic hepatitis will cause cell-mediated reactivity of autologous lymphocytes *in vitro*. Isolated alcoholic hyaline will also induce reactivity of peripheral blood lymphocytes *in vitro*. Circulating antibodies to acetaldehyde protein adducts are observed in patients with alcoholic liver disease. All of these mechanisms may be secondary phenomena but may require further evaluation in the future.

OTHER DRUGS

A variety of other drugs may induce an immune-mediated reaction that damages the liver. The disease may present as an acute hepatitis, such as with halothane, or as a chronic hepatitis. A classical form of chronic hepatitis was described with the now unavailable laxative, oxyphenisatin. Drugs such as methyldopa may be associated with a chronic hepatitis which usually regresses on withdrawal of the drug. In some cases, there are circulating autoantibodies which react with the cytochrome metabolizing the drug; the best example is the association of tienilic acid hepatotoxicity and the liver kidney microsomal antibody (LKM-2). Other than withdrawal and supportive therapy, no specific treatment is indicated (Chapter 10).

RECOMMENDED READING

Baggenstoss, A.H., Soloway, R.D., Summerskill, W.H.J. *et al.* (1972) Chronic active liver disease. The range of histologic lesions, their response to treatment and evolution. *Hum Pathol*, **3**, 183–98.

Bonsel, G.J., Klopmaker, J.J., Van't Veer, F. *et al.* (1990) Use of prognostic models for assessment of value of liver transplantation in primary biliary cirrhosis. *Lancet*, **335**, 493–7.

Chapman, R.W.G., Marborgh, B.A., Rhodes, J.M. *et al.* (1980) Primary sclerosing cholangitis: a review of its clinical features, cholangiography and hepatic histology. *Gut*, **21**, 870–7.

Combes, B. (1989) Prednisolone for primary biliary cirrhosis – good news, bad news. (Editorial) *Hepatology*, **10**, 511–13.

Dickson, E.P., Grambsch, P.M., Fleming, T.R., *et al.* (1989) Prognosis in primary biliary cirrhosis: model for decision making. *Hepatology*, **10**, 1–7.

Diehl, A.M., Goodman, Z.D. and Ishak, K.G. (1988) Alcohol-like liver disease in non-alcoholics. Comparison with alcohol-induced liver injury. *Gastroenterology*, **95**, 1056–62.

Hay, J.E., Czaja, A.J., Rakela, J. and Ludwig, J. (1989) The nature of unexplained aminotransferase elevations of a mild to moderate degree in asymptomatic patients. *Hepatology*, **9**, 193–7.

Homberg, J.-C., Abuaf, N., Bernard, O. *et al.* (1987) Chronic active hepatitis associated with antiliver/kidney microsome antibody type I: a second type of 'autoimmune' hepatitis. *Hepatology*, **7**, 1333-9.

Israel, Y., Hurwitz, E., Niemela, O. *et al.* (1986) Monoclonal and polyclonal antibodies against acetaldehyde-containing epitopes in acetaldehyde protein adducts. *Proc Natl Acad Sci USA*, **83**, 7923–7.

Kaplan, M.M. (1987) Primary biliary cirrhosis. *N Engl J Med*, **316**, 521–8.

Kaplan, M.M. (1989) Medical treatment of primary biliary cirrhosis. *Semin Liver Dis*, **9**, 138–43.

Lindor, K.D., LaRusso, N.F. and Wiesner, R.H. (1989) Prednisone and colchicine are not of benefit after two years in patients with primary sclerosing cholangitis. (Abstract) *Hepatology*, **10**, 638.

Long, R.G., Scheuer, P.J. and Sherlock, S. (1977) Presentation and cause of asymptomatic primary biliary cirrhosis. *Gastroenterology*, **72**, 1204–7.

MacFarlane, I.G. and Eddleston, A.L.W.F. (1989) Chronic active hepatitis, in *Immunology and immunopathology of the liver and gastrointestinal tract* (eds F. Targan and S. Shanohan), Igaken-Shoin, New York.

Maddrey, W.C. (1987) Subdivisions of idiopathic chronic active hepatitis. *Hepatology*, **7**, 1372–5.

Markus, B.H., Dickson, E.R., Grambsch, P.M. *et al.* (1989) Efficacy of liver transplantation in patients with primary biliary cirrhosis. *N Engl J Med*, *320*, 1709–13.

Matsuzaki, Y., Tanaka, N., Osuga, T. *et al.* (1990) Improvement of biliary enzyme levels and itching as a result of long-term administration of ursodeoxycholic acid in primary biliary cirrhosis. *Am J Gastroenterol*, **85**, 15–23.

Scheuer, P.J. (1986) Changing views on chronic hepatitis. *Histopathology*, **10**, 1–4.

Seeff, L.B. (1982) Drug-induced chronic liver disease, with emphasis on chronic active hepatitis. *Semin Liver Dis*, **1**, 104–15.

Sherlock, S. and Scheuer, P.J. (1973) The presentation and diagnosis of 100 patients with primary biliary cirrhosis. *N Engl J Med*, **289**, 674–8.

Starzl, T.E., Demetris, A.J. and Van Thiel, D.H. (1989) Liver transplantation. *N Engl J Med*, **321**, 1014–22, 1092–9.

Stiehl, A., Raedsch, R., Rudolph, G. *et al.* (1989) Treatment of primary sclerosing cholangitis with ursodeoxycholic acid: first results of a controlled trial. (Abstract) *Hepatology*, **10**, 602.

Van Ness, M. and Diehl, A.M. (1989) Is liver biopsy useful in the evaluation of patients with chronically elevated liver enzymes? *Ann Intern Med*, **111**, 473–8.

Zetterman, R.K. and Sorrell, M.F. (1981) Immunologic aspects of alcoholic liver disease. *Gastroenterology*, **81**, 616–24.

10

Drug-induced liver disease

RICHARD HIFT, RALPH KIRSCH and NATHAN BASS

INTRODUCTION

Adverse drug reactions are a common cause of liver damage. The possibility of drug-induced disease must be considered in the differential diagnosis of nearly every patient presenting with liver disease, be it with hepatitis, acute liver failure, cholestasis, fatty liver or cirrhosis. This is particularly important because, although drug-induced hepatotoxicity is potentially reversible, failure to recognize and withdraw the offending agent may result in death of the patient.

More than 600 drugs have been shown to have the potential to induce liver disease. This chapter aims to explain the mechanisms, prevention and treatment of drug-induced liver disease and to give important examples.

The relative contributions of specific drugs to the overall incidence of drug-induced liver disease in a particular population will reflect current prescribing practices in that population. Thus, anti-tuberculous drugs have been shown to account for approximately half of the severe drug-induced liver injury seen in southern Africa, but are a far less prevalent cause of acute liver disease in North America.

MECHANISMS OF DRUG-INDUCED LIVER DAMAGE

INTRINSIC TOXICITY AND IDIOSYNCRATIC REACTIONS

Drug-induced liver damage may occur as a result of intrinsic toxicity on the part of the agent, or as a consequence of an idiosyncratic and unpredictable response to it by the patient. Intrinsic toxicity is predictable in that liver disease will invariably follow exposure to a large enough dose (and is thus dose-dependent). It is also often reproducible in animal models. Paracetamol (acetaminophen) overdose is a well-studied, clinically important example.

Most drugs causing hepatotoxicity, however, appear to operate by idiosyncratic mechanisms. These reactions will not occur in all subjects (and often only in a very small proportion), are often dose-independent and unpredictable, and are difficult to reproduce experimentally. There may be a long and variable period of latency between initiation of therapy and onset of the liver disease. These reactions are frequently not recognized as a problem until a drug has been in use for

Table 10.1 Two types of hepatic drug reaction

	Intrinsic toxicity (e.g. paracetamol [acetaminophen])	Idiosyncratic reactions (e.g. isoniazid)
Predictable	Yes	No
Host-dependent	No	Yes
Dose-related	Yes	No
Temporal relationship	Yes	No
Reproducible in animals	Yes	No

several years. The differences between these two types of hepatic drug reaction are summarized in Table 10.1.

In most cases it is not the parent compound that induces liver damage, but products of its metabolism, particularly chemically reactive metabolites, electrophiles, drug free radicals and oxygen free radicals. These may directly modify cellular components by processes such as covalent binding, lipid peroxidation or protein thiol oxidation. This may impair cellular metabolism and result in cell death or induce secondary immune responses which then mediate toxicity. Genetic and environmental factors may determine the balance between the production of these toxic and reactive intermediates and their detoxification. A knowledge of these processes is helpful for the understanding of drug toxicity.

PRINCIPLES OF DRUG METABOLISM

Most drugs are lipophilic and circulate in blood bound to plasma proteins. The liver is the major site of drug biotransformation and is uniquely adapted for this purpose. Drugs are released from plasma proteins in the space of Disse and are subsequently taken up by the hepatocytes. Within the hepatocyte, they are converted to soluble metabolites by two principal types of reaction.

In so-called 'phase I' reactions, drugs are oxidized or hydroxylated to reactive intermediates, which can be covalently attached to a polar ligand such as glutathione, sulfate or glucuronic acid. This is the 'phase II' or conjugation reaction, and results in the formation of a water-soluble compound which may be excreted. Phase I reactions tend to lead to the production of reactive, and hence toxic, metabolites, while phase II reactions tend to produce less-reactive hydrophilic compounds which may be excreted.

Some drugs possess chemical groups suitable for conjugation and will proceed directly to a phase II reaction. Other drugs will require a phase I reaction to prepare them chemically for conjugation.

The microsomes of hepatocytes have been shown to contain enzymes responsible for phase I activity. These cytochromes absorb light with a wavelength of 450 nm and are thus termed 'cytochrome P450'. Over 20 different forms of P450 have been identified in human liver and as many as 50–100 distinct P450 proteins are thought to exist. This multiplicity accounts for the ability of hepatocytes to metabolize a wide variety of endogenous and exogenous compounds.

THE METABOLIC BASIS OF DIRECT HEPATOTOXICITY: THE PARACETAMOL AND CARBON TETRACHLORIDE MODELS

Paracetamol (acetaminophen) is metabolized by several routes, some of which are detoxifying while others lead to the production of toxic intermediates (Fig. 10.1). About 70–80% of the parent drug is conjugated to form nontoxic sulfates and glucuronides. Up to 20% is oxidized by hepatic cytochrome P450 (a phase I reaction) to produce the reactive intermediate

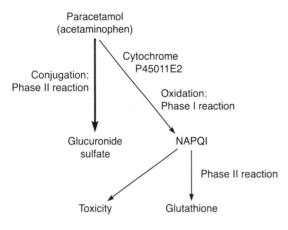

Figure 10.1 The metabolism of paracetamol (acetaminophen).

N-acetyl-*p*-benzoquinone imine (NAPQI). This toxic metabolite is largely inactivated by phase II conjugation with glutathione. However, in acute overdose, large amounts of NAPQI are formed, glutathione stores are depleted and NAPQI may then arylate or oxidize sulfydryl groups on critical cellular enzymes with resultant injury.

Carbon tetrachloride is another well-studied model of predictable hepatotoxicity. As with paracetamol, a phase I reaction catalysed by cytochrome P450 produces a hepatotoxic metabolite. This is the free radical $CCl_3 \bullet$. Some protection against the damaging effect of this free radical is afforded by glutathione and by free radical scavengers such as vitamin E. These defenses are readily overwhelmed by higher doses. The metabolic fate of carbon tetrachloride is critically dependent on the prevailing oxygen tension. Reduction to $CCl_3 \bullet$ is strongly inhibited by oxygen. Hence, CCl_4 toxicity is enhanced in the centrilobular area where oxygen tension is low. Necrosis induced by carbon tetrachloride is therefore characteristically centrilobular in distribution.

The liver is exquisitely vulnerable to drug-induced injury since it is the major site for drug clearance and biotransformation. The precise mechanisms of cellular injury are imperfectly understood. Drug free radicals may generate oxygen free radicals by redox cycling. This may result in lipid peroxidation with damage to the membranes of cells and organelles. There may also be direct interference with proteins resulting in functional and structural cellular alterations, including sustained increases in cytosolic calcium with activation of phospholipases and proteases.

FACTORS ACCOUNTING FOR VARIABILITY IN SENSITIVITY TO DIRECT DRUG TOXICITY

Several factors account for some degree of variability in an individual's susceptibility to direct hepatotoxins, which will translate clinically into differences in the threshold required for toxicity to become evident. These include the speed and extent of drug absorption and, more importantly, the rapidity with which the drug is metabolized to its toxic products. Genetically determined factors may play a role, while interactions with other drugs are clearly important. Cytochrome P450 is readily induced by exposure to alcohol or other enzyme inducers such as the anticonvulsants phenobarbitone and phenytoin. This enzyme induction is an important determinant of paracetamol (acetaminophen) toxicity. Thus, paracetamol will be more rapidly metabolized to its toxic intermediates in people who drink heavily or who are being treated with anti-convulsants. Toxicity even with therapeutic doses of paracetamol is now well recognized in chronic alcoholics.

CLINICAL FEATURES

Characteristically the onset of liver damage is rapid. About 48 hours after ingestion of paracetamol, an acute hepatitis develops, marked by vomiting, jaundice and tender hepatomegaly. The transaminases are elevated, often to extremely high levels. More severe cases rapidly develop signs of acute liver failure such as encephalopathy and a prolonged prothrombin time. Renal failure secondary to acute tubular necrosis is common.

MANAGEMENT OF PARACETAMOL POISONING

A rational approach to the therapy of paracetamol (acetaminophen) poisoning is based on an understanding of the biochemical mechanisms. N-Acetylcysteine (Parvolex®) is the antidote of choice. This is a sulfydryl donor which counteracts paracetamol by replenishing glutathione stores, thus allowing the formation of non-toxic glutathione adducts. Theoretically the risk of hepatotoxicity following paracetamol overdose should correlate with the serum paracetamol level. However, in practice this does not always hold true because of uncertainty about the timing of the overdose and individual variation in sensitivity, etc., and decisions on whether to treat should not be based on serum levels alone.

Initial therapy

Prompt treatment is essential. Any person who has ingested significant amounts of paracetamol should be immediately referred to hospital for definitive management. Where treatment is only commenced once liver disease has become clinically apparent, the outlook is very much poorer. Induced emesis or gastric lavage followed by administration of activated charcoal will reduce the absorption of paracetamol for a few hours after ingestion.

Specific therapy

Our current regimen comprises intravenous N-acetylcysteine in a dose of 300 mg/kg over 24 hours in step-wise fashion. N-Acetylcysteine is relatively safe, but up to 5% of patients develop allergic reactions and bronchospasm. While these are usually mild, facilities for management should be available. Since the efficacy of N-acetylcysteine decreases with time, therapy should be started as soon as possible whenever a significant amount of paracetamol is thought to have been ingested. However, even delayed administration of intravenous N-acetylcysteine may be more effective than was initially believed. There is evidence that mortality may be reduced and that fewer patients will develop advanced degrees of coma even where it is given between 10 and 36 hours, and perhaps even as long as 96 hours, after paracetamol ingestion.

Paracetamol blood levels are easily determined and have been used to define limits above which the likelihood of hepatotoxicity is high and treatment definitely indicated. We believe that decisions on treatment should not be based on serum paracetamol levels alone. These will vary with the rapidity of absorption of paracetamol from the stomach, the time since the ingestion (which may not be accurately reported to the doctor) and the speed with which paracetamol is metabolized. We recommend that treatment with N-acetylcysteine should be started immediately, and should continue wherever significant amounts appear to have been ingested or appreciably elevated paracetamol levels are demonstrated in the blood. It is important to recognize that in chronic alcoholics, normal therapeutic doses of paracetamol may result in severe liver damage. In such instances blood levels of paracetamol may be undetectable at the time of diagnosis of the liver injury.

Supportive care

General supportive measures are necessary following paracetamol poisoning. Hepatic and renal function must be monitored for up to 72 hours following ingestion as the onset of both renal and hepatic failure are typically delayed. Liver transplantation may be indicated in the rare patient who develops severe fulminant liver failure.

IDIOSYNCRATIC DRUG-INDUCED LIVER DAMAGE

Idiosyncratic reactions may be divided into two groups. A form akin to toxic hepatitis may follow variant metabolism of a drug as a result of environmental and host factors favoring the increased production of toxic intermediates, as described earlier. A second class consists of reactions that are thought to be immunologically mediated.

Where drug toxicity follows an idiosyncratic metabolic aberration, the duration of drug exposure varies from 1 week to 12 months or more. There are few, if any, clinical features of hypersensitivity such as rash, fever and eosinophilia, and there is often a delayed response to a drug challenge. Idiosyncratic responses secondary to immunoallergic or hypersensitivity responses tend to follow a shorter duration of exposure (usually less than 2 months); clinical features of hypersensitivity may be noted and the response to a challenge is often prompt. However, the distinction between reactions mediated by hypersensitivity and those resulting from a variation in metabolic handling of a drug is not absolute. In practice an educated guess as to the most likely mechanism, based on clinical features, must often be made since laboratory investigations are of little discriminatory value.

VARIANT DRUG METABOLISM

There are at least 10 distinct families of genes coding for cytochrome P450. Gene families 1, 2 and 3 in particular appear to determine the activity of those playing an important part in drug metabolism. These groups of P450 are differentially induced by various drugs and are subjected to genetic variability as a result of polymorphisms at the DNA level. Variant forms of P450 may predispose to hepatotoxicity if they increase the rate of production of reactive metabolites or are less able to detoxify or eliminate a toxic compound. This effect of genetic variability on the activity of cytochrome P450 is one mechanism thought to account for individual variation in susceptibility to drug-induced liver damage. Some of the more important polymorphisms that have been studied include the debrisoquine-type P450IID6, the mephenytoin-type involving cytochrome P450IIC and the N-acetyltransferases. Mutant alleles of the N-acetyltransferases for instance result in slow drug acetylation which may be linked to abnormal drug biotransformation. Acetylation is one of the mechanisms by which isoniazid is metabolized. It was at one stage believed that people with a slow acetylation status were more prone to isoniazid-induced hepatitis, though it appears more recently that this may not be so.

DRUG-INDUCED IMMUNOALLERGIC HEPATITIS

Before biotransformation, most drugs are poorly immunogenic. Most are small organic molecules which need to form stable bonds with circulating or tissue proteins to be immunogenic, i.e. they must form hapten–macromolecular complexes. Parent drugs are largely inert and their metabolites are more likely to be reactive and thus able to form complexes with proteins. Such reactive metabolites have tentatively been identified in a few allergic hepatotoxic drug reactions. For most, however, the formation of these reactive metabolites and their conjugation to cell proteins can only be inferred. Cellular proteins which have been altered as a result of infection, tissue damage or cell death may result in increased immunogenicity when complexed with drugs. This may explain why drug reactions appear to be more frequent in patients with pre-existing liver disease or chronic infection, as is seen for instance in alcoholics receiving anti-tuberculous drug therapy.

The varying susceptibility of individuals to immunoallergic hepatitis may be explained by two mechanisms, both of which, in the final analysis, are likely to be at least in part genetically determined. Thus, idiosyncratic pathways of metabolism may preferentially produce metabolites capable of eliciting an immune response in association with carrier proteins. Secondly, variations in immune responsiveness may make a person more or less liable to mount an immune response to such a hapten–carrier complex. It is not only the drug and its metabolites that can function as haptens or immunogens. Reactive drug metabolites may alter endogenous macromolecules by covalent interactions, oxidative modifications or the formation of abnormal disulfide linkages. These resulting macromolecules may themselves be immunogenic and elicit specific humoral and cellular responses. In general, immune responses may be directed against three classes of determinant: a covalently bound drug–protein conjugate (haptenic epitopes), novel epitopes of a carrier protein resulting from its covalent modification (neoantigenic determinants) and native epitopes, ordinarily seen as self where tolerance is bypassed as a consequence of the hapten–protein configuration (auto-antigenic determinants). Finally, some drugs such as procainamide and methyldopa may induce a systemic immune response to cytoplasmic antigens or nuclear components resulting in a form of autoimmune disease which may or may not be organ specific.

Drug-induced neoantigens are usually formed within the hepatocyte, but must be exposed to the extracellular environment to stimulate an immune response. This may occur when hepatocytes are damaged, either by the toxic effects of the drug or by hypoxia. Hapten conjugates may then come into contact with immunocompetent cells and induce primary immune responses. Subsequent exposure to the drug may result in secondary responses such as the formation of immune complexes, activation of complement, and localized inflammation. Neoantigens which are normally expressed on the hepatocyte plasma membrane are also accessible to immunocompetent cells. In halothane hepatitis, for example, proteins covalently altered by a trifluoroacyl hapten (the initiator of the immune response) appear to concentrate within the lumen of the endoplasmic reticulum, from where proteins are sorted for secretion or for incorporation into the plasma membrane. Once in the membrane, the protein–hapten complex may stimulate an immune response. Expression of class I or class II major histocompatibility complex antigens along with the neoantigen is necessary to evoke the immune response.

Immunological responses to drugs are not necessarily associated with typical clinical manifestations of hypersensitivity. Immune responses to drugs are diverse, attendant reactions are usually complex and these mechanisms are often difficult to evaluate experimentally.

CLINICAL FEATURES OF IMMUNOALLERGIC HEPATITIS

Drug-induced allergic hepatitis is independent of dose and often occurs after repeated exposure. This is for instance true of halothane hepatitis, where patients have typically been exposed to multiple halothane anesthetics over a period of weeks or months prior to the onset of the disease. Features of hypersensitivity such as fever and eosinophilia may be recognized and a re-challenge will frequently result in a recurrence. However, as this may be fatal, re-challenge should never be employed diagnostically.

In most cases, symptoms subside once the drug is discontinued. The time course after exposure to a drug is variable. Profound systemic immunoallergic phenomena may accompany hepatotoxicity within weeks of drug therapy, as is seen with phenytoin and nitrofurantoin. Yet others may cause delayed, slowly progressive liver disease with minimal accompanying systemic allergic features. This is typical of isoniazid-induced hepatitis which may represent an example of drug hepatoxicity that results predominantly from idiosyncratic metabolism.

DIAGNOSIS OF IDIOSYNCRATIC DRUG-INDUCED LIVER DISEASE

Approach to the diagnosis of drug-induced hepatotoxicity

The diagnosis of drug-induced liver disease is often missed. The combination of fever, jaundice, rash, adenopathy, tender liver, eosinophilia and raised transaminases associated with the recent introduction of a single therapeutic agent represents a caricature which is rarely seen in practice. In contrast, the more usual clinical problem is the wasted, often alcoholic, patient with systemic disease, receiving multiple drug therapy, including several agents known to cause liver disease, who gradually slips into liver failure. The clinical and biochemical data in these patients are often unhelpful. Features strengthening the diagnosis are a satisfactory response to withdrawal of the agent, negative serology for hepatitis viruses, and the presence of typical clinical features such as fever, nausea, jaundice and right upper quadrant pain.

Inadvertent re-challenge may be diagnostic but deliberate re-exposure of a patient to medication suspected of being hepatotoxic is dangerous and has resulted in deaths.

EXAMPLES OF IMMUNOALLERGIC HEPATITIS

Three examples will serve to demonstrate the variety of immunological mechanisms which may underline drug-induced immunoallergic hepatitis. Tienilic acid (a uricosuric diuretic) was associated with significant drug-induced liver injury in the USA and was consequently withdrawn. Patients who developed hepatitis with this drug were found to demonstrate a specific class of autoantibody which reacted with liver and kidney microsomes (LKM). These anti-LKM antibodies behaved slightly differently from the anti-LKM antibodies seen in some patients with autoimmune chronic active hepatitis, and were labeled anti-LKM2. It was shown that the anti-LKM2 antibodies were directed against a class of cytochrome P450 responsible for the metabolism of tienilic acid, and were themselves capable of inhibiting the metabolism of the drug by human liver microsomes. It appears that the drug bound to cytochrome P450, and that the resulting complex was immunogenic and gave rise to antibodies that were subsequently directed against conformational drug epitopes.

Alcohol is believed in part to produce liver damage through immunological reactions. The first metabolite of ethanol oxidation, acetaldehyde, has been shown to react with a variety of proteins including hepatic microsomal proteins, albumin and plasma proteins with which it forms both stable and unstable adducts. These acetaldehyde–protein adducts are able to induce humoral and cellular immune responses.

Halothane is oxidized by cytochrome P450 to a reactive intermediate which gives rise to trifluoroacyl (TFA) haptens which appear to bind to a variety of liver proteins giving rise to neoantigens in the liver. Though assays for the detection of antibodies against these TFA neoantigens are available as research tools, they are not yet in clinical use. Such a practical test would be of considerable value, as it could demonstrate sensitization to halothane and might predict hypersensitivity reactions after exposure to similar volatile anesthetics such as enflurane or isoflurane.

MANAGEMENT OF IDIOSYNCRATIC DRUG-INDUCED HEPATOTOXICITY

Early recognition of a drug-induced liver injury followed by removal of the drug is essential. There are few data supporting a beneficial effect of steroids in drug-induced liver injury, although they are frequently given, often in desperation because of the lack of definitive therapeutic alternatives. They may, however, have a place in those forms of immunoallergic hepatitis in which the immunological component is particularly prominent, as is seen with phenytoin.

As a general rule, patients should never be re-challenged with the drugs suspected to have induced the hepatitis. In some cases, such as tuberculosis, this may have to be modified since only one of several drugs may be implicated, and alternative regimens to rifampicin, isoniazid and pyrazinamide are less effective and prohibitively expensive. Here it is recommended that the need for treatment be re-assessed; and that the most dangerous agents (perhaps pyrazinamide, and the rifampicin–isoniazid combination) be avoided. While safe agents such as strepto-mycin and ethambutol are continued, isoni-azid may be cautiously re-introduced, in hospital, with frequent monitoring of the liver enzymes. Only when the patient is clearly tolerating this therapy should the addition of another agent, such as rifampicin, be considered.

The outcome of a severe hepatitis will be influenced by the standard of supportive care which the patient receives. This care, appro-priate to the management of acute liver failure, is discussed fully in Chapter 12. Liver transplantation may offer the only hope for patients with drug-induced fulminant liver failure and should be considered in the inex-orably deteriorating patient.

DRUG-INDUCED CHOLESTASIS

Cholestasis is the predominant clinical mani-festation of a number of drugs that are capable of disrupting the process of bile formation and secretion. These usually idiosyncratic reac-tions are important to recognize, particularly as they may mimic obstructive biliary disease.

The formation and secretion of bile are energy-dependent processes whereby solutes, bile acids and water from sinusoidal blood pass through the cytosol of the hepatocyte to the bile canalicular lumen. The energy for the uptake and secretion of bile acids is provided by the $Na^+ K^+$ pump in the hepatocyte while specific protein carriers in both the sinusoidal and canalicular membranes are involved in bile acid transport from plasma to bile. Bile flow itself is dependent upon several mecha-nisms, including the osmotic effects of bile acid molecules, passive diffusion and solvent drag. Bile acid-independent bile flow follows the secretion of inorganic ions and is also energy-dependent. Interference with any of these mechanisms will result in cessation of bile flow or cholestasis.

SYNDROMES OF DRUG-INDUCED CHOLESTASIS

Drugs may induce varying forms of cholestasis in susceptible patients. Cholestasis may occur after a single dose of the respon-sible medication or after many years of uncomplicated and continuous use. The severity may vary from symptoms of itch and jaundice to profound anorexia, vomiting, abdominal discomfort and fever. Clinically obvious jaundice is usual. Serum biochemistry suggests cholestasis with elevated alkaline phosphatase levels and bilirubin and, at most, moderately elevated transaminase levels.

Three forms of cholestatic drug reaction are recognized. Non-inflammatory or 'bland' isolated intrahepatic cholestasis, as seen with the C-17 alkylated steroids, is manifested by the centrilobular accumulation of bile within hepatocytes and bile canaliculi. Cholestatic hepatitis is typified by a combination of cholestasis and features of inflammation such as hepatocellular degeneration and a mixed mononuclear cell and eosinophilic infiltrate in portal tracts and the lobular parenchyma. This is typical of chlorpromazine and erythromycin. Bile duct damage (ductal or cholangiodestructive injury) represents the third type of cholestatic drug reaction and is seen following phenothiazine, haloperidol and allopurinol exposure. Here the clinical, laboratory and histological features may resemble those of primary biliary cirrhosis.

There are many reports of a chronic primary biliary cirrhosis-type syndrome (drug-induced chronic cholestasis), induced by psychotropic agents such as chlorpromazine, amitriptyline and carbamazepine, as well as some other drugs such as thiabendazole and piperazine. Their metabolism is thought to be influenced by genetic polymorphisms determining pathways of oxidation, sulfoxidation and hydroxylation. These aberrations in drug metabolism may lead to generation of toxic metabolites which trigger an autoimmune reaction that results in chronic bile duct injury.

DIAGNOSIS

Drug-induced cholestasis is a diagnosis of exclusion. Even in the presence of strong circumstantial evidence of a drug reaction, imaging studies and sometimes liver biopsy are necessary to exclude obstructive jaundice and other causes of liver disease, and the diagnosis often rests on the circumstantial evidence of the administration of a drug with the potential for inducing cholestasis.

EXAMPLES

17-Alkylated steroids such as ethinylestradiol and methyltestosterone decrease hepatocyte membrane fluidity and impair the function of membrane-bound enzymes. They reduce the hepatocellular uptake of substrates and alter the association of bile acids with intracellular organelles. Estrogens are thought to act principally at the hepatocyte basolateral membrane to produce cholestasis. Itching and jaundice are the major symptoms, and usually develop within 2–5 months of the initiation of therapy; symptoms may persist for a month after the cessation of drug therapy. The reactions are often idiosyncratic, but do not appear to be immune-mediated. Patients with a history of cholestasis during pregnancy appear to be at higher risk of developing estrogen-induced cholestasis.

Chlorpromazine and other phenothiazines induce a cholestatic hepatitis in 1–2% of patients. Chlorpromazine is thought to inhibit Na^+, K^+-ATPase activity, and its metabolites inhibit actin polymerization *in vitro*, suggesting that they may interfere with microfilament function *in vivo*. Chlorpromazine metabolism is complex and variable. The toxic effects are apparently related to hydroxylation of the drug with production of toxic free radicals. There may therefore be a metabolic basis for individual susceptibility to chlorpromazine-induced cholestasis. Recovery may take up to a year following withdrawal of the drug. Occasional patients appear to develop chronic, progressive cholestatic disease.

Tricyclic antidepressants may induce hepatocellular injury but at times a predominantly cholestatic pattern is observed. The features of drug-induced hepatitis are similar to those seen after phenothiazine use.

Erythromycin derivates, particularly the

estolate, may result in cholestasis and focal necrosis. Abdominal pain is often prominent. This drug appears to decrease bile acid secretion and bile flow in a dose-dependent manner. A mild inflammatory reaction induced by oxidized erythromycin metabolites may facilitate immune-mediated cholestasis.

MANAGEMENT

Drug-induced cholestasis usually improves following withdrawal of the responsible agent. This response may be delayed, even by 1 or 2 years. In such cases, supportive management of pruritus and fat-soluble vitamin malabsorption may be necessary. In rare instances cholangiodestructive processes may progress to chronic liver disease.

RARER FORMS OF DRUG-INDUCED LIVER DISEASE

VENO-OCCLUSIVE DISEASE AND VASCULAR INJURY

The central veins, hepatic veins and sinusoids may be damaged by drugs. Cytotoxic therapy, particularly with cyclophosphamide and busulphan, is associated with veno-occlusive disease, which is characterized by painful hepatomegaly and ascites. Oral contraceptives may cause thrombosis of large hepatic veins and the Budd–Chiari syndrome. Peliosis hepatitis may occur following administration of androgens, anabolic steroids and tamoxifen. This is characterized by the development of large blood-filled cavities distributed randomly through the liver parenchyma. The endothelial barrier is incompetent, and may even be traversed by erythrocytes. Perisinusoidal fibrosis may follow.

GRANULOMATOUS HEPATITIS

Non-caseating granulomas may develop in response to certain drugs, particularly quini-dine, allopurinol and phenylbutazone (buta-zolidin). They may be located either in the lobules of the parenchyma or in the portal tracts. The clinical presentation is that of hepatitis with elevated transaminases. Fever and other systemic symptoms such as skin rash may be prominent.

STEATOSIS

Drugs may impair hepatic lipid metabolism and lead to accumulation of fat vacuoles. The macrovesicular variety, accompanied by the presence of large fat droplets, is seen following exposure to corticosteroids, methotrexate and a few other agents. This type of injury usually follows a benign clinical course. The micro-vesicular variety may follow exposure to tetracyclines, sodium valproate and salicylates. It presents clinically with hepatomegaly, deranged liver function and, occasionally, fulminant liver failure. An unusual form of liver phospholipid accumulation (phospholipidosis) is caused by amiodarone, which less commonly may induce liver injury histologically similar to alcoholic hepatitis.

CONCLUSIONS

Drug-induced injury is a common cause of acquired liver disease. Such diseases take several forms and may vary greatly in severity. Severe drug-induced liver disease of any form should always be regarded as being potentially fatal. Indeed, in a study performed in Cape Town, the overall hospital mortality rate of drug-related liver disease was 24%. However, 40% of those in whom hepatitis was secondary to anti-tuberculous therapy died. This high mortality emphasizes the importance of withdrawing any drug capable of producing liver damage at an early stage and of not re-challenging apart from under the most exceptional circumstances.

RECOMMENDED READING

Bass, N. and Ockner, R.K. (1990) Drug-induced liver disease, in *Hepatology: A Textbook of Liver Disease* (eds D. Zakim and T. Boyer), WB Saunders, London, pp. 754–91.

Lee, W.M. (1993) Drug-induced hepatotoxicity. *Aliment Pharmacol Therapeut*, **7**, 477–85.

Parrish, A.G., Robson, S.C., Trey, C. and Kirsch, R.E. (1990) Retrospective survey of drug-induced liver disease at Groote Schuur Hospital, Cape Town – 1983–1987. *S Afr Med J*, **77**, 199–202.

Perry, M.C. (1992) Chemotherapeutic agents and hepatotoxicity. *Semin Oncol*, **19**, 551–65.

Thomas, S.H.L. (1993) Paracetamol (acetaminophen) poisoning. *Pharmacol Ther*, **60**, 91–120.

Watkins, P.B. (1990) Role of cytochrome P450 in drug metabolism and hepatotoxicity. *Semin Liver Dis*, **10**, 235–50.

Zimmerman, H.J. (1990) Update of hepatoxicity due to classes of drugs in common clinical use: non-steroidal drugs, anti-inflammatory drugs, antibiotics, antihypertensives, and cardiac and psychotropic agents. *Semin Liver Dis*, **10**, 322–38.

11

Cholestatic syndromes

ERIC LEMMER, SIMON ROBSON and TOM BOYER

INTRODUCTION

Intrahepatic cholestasis may be defined as the impairment of bile formation and/or secretion, and must be distinguished from extrahepatic obstructive jaundice. There has been renewed interest in the chronic cholestatic disorders following the advent of successful orthotopic liver transplantation.

MECHANISMS OF BILE FORMATION AND SECRETION

Bile formation and secretion are energy-dependent processes whereby solutes, bile acids, conjugated bilirubin and water from sinusoidal blood pass through the cytosol of the hepatocyte to the canalicular lumen. Energy for the uptake and secretion of bile acids is provided by the sodium pump. Bile flow itself is dependent upon several mechanisms, including the osmotic effect of bile acid molecules, passive diffusion and solvent drag. Canaliculi join to form ductules, interlobar and septal ducts which eventually drain via the common bile duct into the intestine.

CLINICAL FEATURES OF CHOLESTASIS

Early cholestasis may be asymptomatic. Raised serum alkaline phosphatase (ALP) and gamma-glutamyltransferase (GGT) activities are often the only signs. Generalized pruritus, usually worse in the evening and after a hot bath, is suggestive of cholestasis. The cause of the pruritus is not known. Elevated levels or altered ratios of serum bile acids are the most likely cause, but this is unproven. Many patients never become jaundiced; others, however, will develop dark urine, light stools and become icteric.

Examination of a severe long-standing case typically reveals intense jaundice, increased pigmentation of skin, scratch marks, xanthelasma and xanthomata. A firm hepatomegaly may be found. Splenomegaly signifies the development of portal hypertension. Sinus bradycardia may occur possibly due to the direct action of bile acids on the sino-atrial node. Clubbing is rare but when present is thought to reflect intrapulmonary shunting.

Malabsorption of fat and vitamins A, D, E and K result from lack of bile acids in the gut. Patients develop steatorrhea, easy bruising, hepatic osteodystrophy (osteoporosis more

commonly than osteomalacea), night blindness and neurological disturbances. Bleeding
varices, ascites and encephalopathy signify
end-stage biliary cirrhosis.

INVESTIGATION OF THE PATIENT WITH CHOLESTASIS

LABORATORY TESTS

Because symptoms are often absent during
anicteric cholestasis, recognition depends on
biochemical tests. A raised serum ALP
together with a raised GGT or 5′ nucleotidase
activity is most useful. An increased GGT
activity in the serum with a normal ALP
activity does not, however, necessarily indicate a cholestatic process. If jaundice
develops, the serum conjugated bilirubin
progressively rises and often plateaus at a
level of 250–400 μmol/l. The prothrombin
time, if prolonged, is correctable with
parenteral vitamin K. Serum albumin levels
remain normal unless cirrhosis has developed. Serum cholesterol levels are often
markedly raised and lipoprotein-X may be
present in the serum. Accelerated atherosclerosis appears not to be a major clinical
problem in patients with chronic cholestasis.

An anti-mitochondrial antibody (AMA) test
is positive in 95% of patients with primary
biliary cirrhosis, and makes this diagnosis
likely. AMA are a family of antibodies that
react with different antigens within the mitochondria. Anti-M_2, which is found most
commonly, recognizes a 70-kDa epitope of
the inner mitochondrial membrane enzyme
pyruvate dehydrogenase E2.

IMAGING STUDIES

The differentiation of intrahepatic cholestasis
from extrahepatic biliary obstruction is crucial
for patient management. Ultrasound is the
least expensive screening test, but cholangiog-

raphy is usually required to rule out mechanical biliary obstruction. Endoscopic retrograde
cholangiography (ERC) is the procedure of
choice, even when the intrahepatic ducts are
dilated. Percutaneous transhepatic cholangiography (PTC) is used in patients who have
a failed ERC, but this carries a risk of bleeding
or bile leakage. Typically, the cholangio-
graphic picture of sclerosing cholangitis is
that of multiple strictures of both intra- and
extrahepatic ducts with intervening dilated
segments giving a so-called 'beaded appearance' (Fig. 11.1) (Chapter 4).

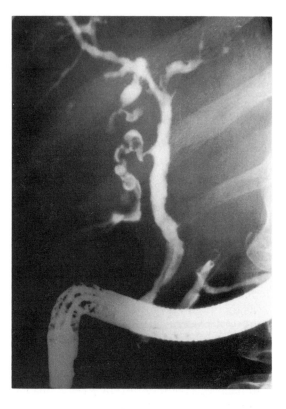

Figure 11.1 Endoscopic retrograde cholangiography (ERC) in a patient with primary sclerosing
cholangitis showing multiple strictures involving
intra- and extrahepatic bile ducts with intervening
dilated segments.

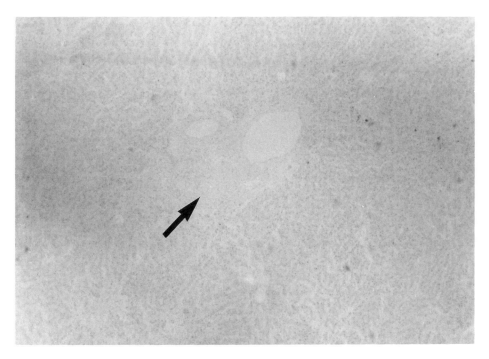

Figure 11.2 Liver biopsy specimen in a patient with primary sclerosing cholangitis showing a portal tract with dense periductal fibrosis which has resulted in disappearance of the portal bile duct (arrow). Fibrosis has extended beyond the portal tract to involve the hepatic parenchyma.

HISTOLOGY

Liver biopsy is frequently required, especially if the ERC is normal. Cholestasis is identified histologically by the presence of bile pigment in the liver. Ductular proliferation (possibly due to the mitogenic effect of the bile acids) and ductopenia ('vanishing bile ducts') may be present. Primary biliary cirrhosis is characterized by non-suppurative destructive cholangitis, and occasionally granulomas may be seen. The typical lesion in primary sclerosing cholangitis is a dense 'onion skin' periductal fibrosis (Fig. 11.2). The stage of the liver disease, as determined by liver histology, is used to judge prognosis.

CHOLESTATIC SYNDROMES

Causes of cholestasis and cholestatic syndromes are listed in Table 11.1

CHOLESTATIC VIRAL AND ALCOHOLIC HEPATITIS

Acute viral hepatitis A may rarely present as a prolonged cholestatic illness. Features include pruritus, fever, diarrhea and weight loss with unusually high serum bilirubin levels and a clinical course lasting 12 weeks or longer. The outcome is invariably favorable (Chapter 8). Alcoholic hepatitis is often associated with marked cholestasis, and its presentation may closely resemble that of acute calculous cholecystitis. Laparotomy on patients with unsuspected viral or alcoholic hepatitis carries a high morbidity, and it is thus important to be aware of these conditions (Chapter 7).

DRUG-INDUCED CHOLESTASIS

There is a wide spectrum of clinical manifestations associated with drug-induced cholestatic

Table 11.1 Causes of cholestasis

Viral and alcoholic hepatitis

Drugs

Benign recurrent cholestasis

Pregnancy

Sclerosing cholangitis

Primary biliary cirrhosis

Idiopathic adulthood ductopenia

Severe systemic illness ('cholangitis lenta')

'Postoperative jaundice'

---

injury. These may occur after a single dose of the responsible medication, or after many years of therapy (Chapter 10). Three forms of cholestatic drug reaction are seen. Isolated intrahepatic cholestasis ('bland cholestasis') is seen with 17-alkylated steroids such as estrogen and methyltestosterone. Cholestatic hepatitis may be caused by chlorpromazine or erythromycin estolate. Finally, there have been numerous reports of drugs causing cholangiodestructive injury similar to that seen in primary biliary cirrhosis. Drug-induced cholestasis is a 'diagnosis of exclusion'; there may only be circumstantial evidence of the administration of a drug with the potential for inducing cholestasis.

INTRAHEPATIC CHOLESTASIS OF PREGNANCY (ICP)

ICP represents a spectrum of cholestatic disease with an incidence of 1 in 1000 to 1 in 10 000 pregnancies (Chapter 23). Prominent pruritus during the third trimester is the initial symptom; 3–7 weeks later the patient may develop dark urine, and occasionally light stools with jaundice. Symptoms always resolve rapidly after delivery, but cholestasis may recur during subsequent pregnancies. Liver biopsy reveals mild cholestasis with intracellular bile pigment and canalicular bile plugs, without hepatocellular necrosis. The syndrome appears to be related to estrogenic hormones, and patients may develop cholestasis during use of the oral contraceptive pill. It has been postulated that changes in the permeability of the canaliculi, a decrease in the activity of the hepatocyte sodium pump or a change in membrane fluidity may all contribute to ICP. The course is not always benign. There may be an increased incidence of fetal distress, stillbirths and prematurity.

PRIMARY SCLEROSING CHOLANGITIS (PSC)

This is a syndrome of unknown etiology characterized by chronic fibrosing inflammation of both intra- and extrahepatic bile ducts. Approximately 70% of patients with PSC are males, usually under the age of 45 years. There is a strong association with inflammatory bowel disease, especially ulcerative colitis (UC). Presentation is usually with insidious cholestasis. Less commonly recurrent cholangitis occurs. Following an increased awareness of the condition, more cases are being detected after investigation of a raised serum ALP in otherwise asymptomatic patients with UC. Diagnosis rests on typical ERC findings and exclusion of secondary causes, most commonly choledocholithiasis or previous biliary tract surgery.

PSC is considered to be autoimmune in origin, and is probably caused by a disturbance in cell-mediated immunity. PSC is closely associated with HLA-B8, DR3 and particularly DRw52a haplotype. These findings indicate a strong genetic predisposition. Any hypothesis regarding the pathogenesis of PSC must explain the clinical associations with UC.

The course of patients with PSC is variable but usually progressive with the development of cirrhosis and liver failure. Both PSC and UC are associated with the development of cholangiocarcinoma.

Rare secondary causes of sclerosing cholangitis include AIDS (possibly related to biliary cryptosporidiosis), chronic liver graft rejection, intra-arterial chemotherapy and histiocytosis X (Chapter 9).

PRIMARY BILIARY CIRRHOSIS (PBC)

This is a chronic cholestatic disease of unknown origin characterized by progressive destruction of intrahepatic bile ducts. Ultimately scarring and cirrhosis occurs with the development of liver failure. The condition is uncommon with a world-wide prevalence of 5.7–14.4 per 100 000 and an annual incidence of 5.8–15 per 1 million. The typical patient is a middle-aged female (aged 30–66 years) who presents with fatigue and pruritus. Patients may also be asymptomatic. Here, the diagnosis is made during the investigation of unexplained hepatomegaly or raised serum ALP. Associated autoimmune disorders include scleroderma, Sjögrens syndrome, arthropathy, hypothyroidism and renal tubular acidosis. The diagnosis is confirmed by a positive AMA test and a compatible liver histology. Atypical cases should undergo ERC to exclude biliary obstruction or sclerosing cholangitis.

Immune mechanisms are likely in the pathogenesis of PBC. The anti-M_2 fraction of AMA cross-reacts with epitopes of the pyruvate dehydrogenase complex and intestinal microbes. Conceivably molecular mimicry between auto-epitopes and microorganisms may be involved in the pathogenesis of PBC.

The natural history of PBC is that of slow progression, and asymptomatic patients may have a near normal life expectancy (Chapter 9).

IDIOPATHIC ADULTHOOD DUCTOPENIA

This represents a newly defined entity, the nature of which remains unclear. Patients develop chronic cholestasis during adulthood and liver biopsy reveals a paucity of intralobular bile ducts. The histological picture resembles that of non-syndromic paucity of intrahepatic bile ducts, well described in infants and children. Idiopathic adulthood ductopenia may progress rapidly to end-stage liver disease, necessitating liver transplantation (Chapter 6).

CHOLESTASIS ASSOCIATED WITH SYSTEMIC ILLNESS

Severe septicemia may cause cholestatic jaundice in adults. Biochemical abnormalities include an increased concentration of conjugated bilirubin in the serum with only a modest increase in ALP levels. This suggests a selective defect in the excretion of conjugated bilirubin rather than true cholestasis. As the mortality is high an awareness of this entity allows attention to be correctly focused on sepsis originating outside the liver as the cause of cholestasis.

Patients with Hodgkin's disease may rarely present with an intense idiopathic cholestatic jaundice in the absence of any hepatic involvement by the malignancy. This presentation is presumably a paraneoplastic syndrome of unknown mechanism. A similar syndrome may occur in patients with advanced prostatic and ovarian carcinoma.

Cholestasis may be a relatively late complication of total parenteral nutrition, manifesting 3 weeks or more after the initiation of therapy. The pathogenesis is almost certainly multifactorial; biliary stasis followed by deposition of biliary sludge may be an important contributing factor. This entity is more common in children, and may rarely progress to cirrhosis.

MANAGEMENT OF THE PATIENT WITH CHOLESTASIS

GENERAL MEASURES

Nutrition of patients with chronic cholestasis requires close attention, particularly if transplantation is anticipated. Fat malabsorption due to lack of bile acids in the gut may be aggravated by concurrent therapy with cholestyramine. Patients should be on a low saturated fat diet, with adequate protein and calories (Chapter 25). A 40 g fat diet and supplementation with medium-chain triglycerides (MCT) is recommended if steatorrhea is present. Prophylactic therapy with a vitamin supplement containing A, D E and K should be considered in all patients. Regular exposure to sunlight and calcium supplementation (e.g. calcium gluconate 30 g/day) may retard progression of metabolic bone disease. In chronic cholestasis, bile acid sequestrant therapy is of value in the treatment of pruritus. Because the amount of bile acid in the gallbladder is greatest after an overnight fast, trapping this pool as it leaves the gallbladder after the morning meal is the best strategy. Cholestyramine should be administered as a sachet before and after breakfast (dosage 12 g/day). Resistant cases of pruritus may respond to treatment with rifampin or plasmapheresis. Very severe pruritus may be an indication for liver transplantation.

SPECIFIC THERAPY

Obviously relief of mechanical biliary obstruction is curative; however, this is frequently not possible in patients with sclerosing cholangitis. Recurrent bouts of bacterial cholangitis related to partial biliary obstruc-

tion should be treated with antibiotics (e.g. ampicillin and gentamicin, or ceftriaxone). In patients with prolonged cholestasis due to hepatitis A viral infection, corticosteroids may lower the serum bilirubin and afford symptomatic relief, but the clinical course is probably not affected. Steroids generally should not be used in chronic cholestatic disorders as they have not been shown to be beneficial and may accelerate the progression of bone disease.

There is no specific therapy for PBC or PSC. Ursodeoxycholic acid (UDCA), a non-toxic bile acid, appears to be beneficial in patients with PBC. The mechanism of action of UDCA is unclear, but may be due in part to a decrease in toxic hydrophobic bile acids by the hydrophilic UDCA. UDCA may also lead to a lowered immune-mediated injury of bile duct cells by a decrease in HLA expression by these cells. Methotrexate and other immunosuppressive agents have been tried in the treatment of both conditions. The use of these agents outside controlled clinical trials cannot be recommended at present.

LIVER TRANSPLANTATION

End-stage liver failure due to chronic cholestatic liver disease is one of the most common indications for orthotopic liver transplantation. Several centers have reported survival rates of greater than 90% at 1 year and 80% at 5 years following transplantation for PBC. Timing of liver transplantation is critical as the outcome is related to the general condition of the patient. Early referral to a specialist liver center is thus essential. In patients with PSC the decision is further complicated by the unpredictable occurrence of cholangiocarcinoma and previous biliary drainage procedures. Drainage procedures are best avoided in this condition, particularly if histological cirrhosis or late liver disease is present.

CONCLUSIONS

Cholestasis in the absence of mechanical bile duct obstruction is common and usually transient, reflecting resolving liver injury. Severe progressive chronic cholestasis, although less common, is an important cause of end-stage liver disease. Symptomatic therapy and prevention of malnutrition are essential in these patients, particularly if liver transplantation is considered.

RECOMMENDED READING

Blendis, L.M. (1989) Jaundice in systemic disease, in *Baillière's Clinical Gastroenterology* (ed. I.A.D. Bouchier), Ballière Tindall, London, vol. 3, pp. 431–46.

De Groote, J. and Fevery, J. (1991) Cholestatic liver disease. *Curr Opin Gastroenterol*, **7**, 388–95.

Desmet, V.J. (1990) Destructive intrahepatic bile duct diseases. *Recent Prog Med*, **81**, 392–8.

Gordon, S.C., Reddy, K.R., Schiff, L. *et al.* (1984) Prolonged intrahepatic cholestasis secondary to acute hepatitis A. *Ann Intern Med*, **101**, 635–7.

Javitt, W.B. (1989) Cholestatic liver disease and its management, in *Baillière's Clinical Gastroenterology* (ed. I.A.D. Bouchier), Baillière Tindall, London, vol. 3, pp. 423–30.

Kaplan, M.M. (1987) Primary biliary cirrhosis. *N Engl J Med*, **316**, 521–8.

Ludwig, J., La Russo, N. and Wiesner, R. (1990) The syndrome of primary sclerosing cholangitis, in *Progress in Liver Disease* (eds H. Popper and F. Schaffner), WB Saunders, Philadelphia, pp. 555–65.

Miller, D.J., Keeton, G.R., Webber, B.L. *et al.* (1976) Jaundice in severe bacterial infection. *Gastroenterology*, **71**, 94–7.

Quigley, E.M., Marsh, M.N., Shaffer, J.L. and Markin, R.S. (1993) Hepatobiliary complications of total parenteral nutrition. *Gastroenterology*, **104**, 286–301.

Reyes, H. (1992) The spectrum of liver and gastrointestinal disease seen in cholestasis of pregnancy. *Gastroenterol Clin North Am*, **21**, 905–21.

Seidel, D. (1987) Lipoproteins in liver disease. *J Clin Chem Clin Biochem*, **25**, 541–51.

12

Acute liver failure

MICHAEL VOIGT and ROGER WILLIAMS

INTRODUCTION

Acute liver failure (ALF) is a syndrome of severe hepatic dysfunction causing hepatic encephalopathy, which occurs within 3 months of the onset of the first symptoms of liver disease. It is associated with an extremely high mortality, but survivors generally return to completely normal function. Management in units where specialized multidisciplinary intensive care and facilities for liver transplantation are available, is crucial for optimal management of these extremely ill patients.

DEFINITION AND CLASSIFICATION

Acute liver failure is classified into sub-groups, according to the timing of the onset of hepatic encephalopathy (or coagulopathy) after the first symptom of liver disease or of jaundice. Such classification is required for comparison between therapeutic studies and in an attempt to identify more accurately patients requiring urgent admission for management of complications such as cerebral edema (e.g. hyperacute liver failure), and those with a poor prognosis (acute and sub-

acute/sub-fulminant) who should be placed on the urgent transplantation list, as sub-groups differ in their rate of complications and prognoses. A recent classification is given in Table 12.1. Sub-groups with different manifestations and prognoses may be defined according to the interval between the onset of jaundice and encephalopathy.

EETIOLOGY AND DIAGNOSIS

The epidemiology of ALF varies geographically and with time. Generally viral, drug-induced and toxic hepatitis account for the majority of cases.

VIRAL

Acute liver failure occurs in approximately 0.1–0.35% of hospitalized cases of hepatitis A virus (HAV) infection but this may account for up to 20% of cases of acute liver failure in some northern European countries. The risk of developing ALF-A increases with age particularly when contracted over the age of 40. High-titer IgM anti-HAV antibodies reliably diagnose HAV infection. HAV may persist in ALF-A and if patients undergo

Table 12.1 Classification of acute liver failure. (Adapted from O'Grady, Schalm and Williams, 1993.)

	Interval between onset of jaundice and encephalopathy	Complications	Mortality
Hyperacute liver failure	7 days	Cerebral edema 70–80%	Higher percentage survive with medical management
Acute liver failure	8 to 28 days after onset of jaundice	Cerebral edema 60–70%	Poor prognosis without transplantation
Sub-acute liver failure (late onset hepatic failure)	5 to 12 weeks (LOHF 8 to 24 weeks)	Cerebral edema 10–15%	Poor prognosis

LOHF, late onset hepatic failure.

orthotopic liver transplantation, reinfection of the graft may occur. In general, the prognosis for ALF-A is better than for other viral causes of ALF.

Hepatitis B accounts for up to 74% of cases of ALF in some countries. The most reliable diagnostic marker is a high-titer IgM-anti-HBc. HBsAg, HBeAg and HBV DNA are usually negative and anti-HBs and anti HBe may not be found at the time of presentation with ALF.

ALF-B may also be caused by mutant forms of the virus. A mutation at position 1896 of the precore region resulting in a stop-codon, preventing secretion of HBeAg, is associated with ALF-B. In addition, reactivation of precore mutant hepatitis B virus may lead to fulminant liver failure in chronic HBV carriers.

Hepatitis B may also be a common cause of acute liver failure in cases thought to have non-A, non-B hepatitis as diagnosed by the absence of serological HBV markers. Evidence of hepatitis B was found in the livers of seven out of 17 patients undergoing liver transplantation for apparent non-A, non-B hepatitis.

Co-infection of HBV and the delta hepatitis virus (HDV), an incomplete RNA virus that can only propagate in the presence of hepatitis B virus, accounts for a high proportion of cases of HBV related ALF in some countries.

Hepatitis C virus (HCV) usually causes a mild initial disease. Although seroconversion occurs late in the disease (mean interval from onset of hepatitis to seroconversion 15 weeks, range 4–32 weeks), which makes it difficult to exclude HCV as the cause of ALF, all indications are that this virus is not a common cause of ALF.

Hepatitis E virus infection (HEV), previously termed enteric non-A, non-B hepatitis (NANB), is an important cause of fulminant liver failure. The disease appears to be particularly severe in pregnant women. While it was originally described in third world countries such as the Indian sub-continent, Mexico and North Africa, HEV-ALF has recently been shown to be responsible for up to 10% of cases of viral ALF in developed countries such as the UK and USA.

Hepatitis 'G' has been used to refer to a syncitial giant cell hepatitis, thought to be caused by a paramyxovirus, and believed to cause late onset hepatic failure. However, the histological picture of syncitial giant cell

131

hepatitis is not specific as it has been shown in a number of different conditions including autoimmune chronic active and CMV hepatitis. The prognosis varies with the etiology and is not always ominous.

Herpes simplex virus, cytomegalovirus, varicella zoster and the Epstein–Barr virus may occasionally cause fulminant liver failure. Patients with herpes simplex ALF usually have disseminated herpes and may not be jaundiced.

Acute liver failure which develops in the absence of any discernible cause and in the absence of all viral markers, i.e. non-A, non-B, non-C, non-D, non-E hepatitis, accounts for 15–30% of all cases of ALF in some series. In approximately a third of these cases the course is that of a sub-acute liver failure (SHF). The latter patients are usually older and seldom develop cerebral edema, but have a high incidence of renal failure. Mortality exceeds 85%. Thus the onus is on the attending physician to refer these patients early for possible liver transplantation.

OTHER INFECTIONS

Severe septicemia may result in a clinical syndrome indistinguishable from acute liver failure. Several cases of ALF ascribed to massive replacement of the liver with tuberculous granulomas have been reported.

TOXINS AND DRUGS

Anti-tuberculous therapy is an important cause of acute liver failure in areas with a high prevalence of tuberculosis. Pyrazinamide, rifampin and isoniazid, singly or in combination, account for the majority of cases. While liver disease usually occurs within the first 3 months, ALF has been described up to 12 months after starting therapy. Failure to stop anti-tuberculous drugs sufficiently early results in a high mortality. ALF may also follow the use of aldomet, anti-convulsant agents (in particular sodium valproate which gives a characteristic microvesicular steatosis), non-steroidal anti-inflammatory agents, certain antibiotics or anti-microbial agents and exposure to halothane. Any drug, herbal remedy or homeopathic treatment, however, may induce hepatitis in susceptible individuals and these should be considered as possible causes in patients presenting with acute liver failure.

Paracetamol (acetaminophen) toxicity, a leading cause of acute liver failure in the UK is less frequently seen elsewhere. Usually 16–20 g have to be ingested, but prior use of enzyme-inducing agents or chronic alcohol ingestion may potentiate paracetamol toxicity so that acute liver failure may occur with doses below 6–8 g. Any patient suspected of having taken an overdose of paracetamol should immediately receive intravenous *N*-acetylcysteine. Therapy should not be delayed while awaiting blood levels. In a controlled trial of patients with established paracetamol-induced ALF, continuous infusion of *N*-acetylcysteine significantly improved survival and reduced cerebral edema and hypotension. *N*-Acetylcysteine is given as an initial 15-minute bolus consisting of 150 mg/kg body-weight in 200 ml of 5% or 10% dextrose-water followed by an infusion of 150 mg/kg/24 hours. This is maintained until recovery or death (Chapter 10).

PREGNANCY-RELATED LIVER DISEASE

Acute fatty liver of pregnancy, the HELLP syndrome (hemolysis, elevated liver enzymes and low platelets) as well as hepatic hemorrhage and/or rupture may lead to acute liver failure in pregnancy. Acute fatty liver of pregnancy was once thought to be rare, but more cases are being recognized as awareness of the condition improves. Any patients with epigastric discomfort and raised liver enzymes in the third trimester of pregnancy, should be closely monitored for the development of ALF (Chapter 23).

VASCULAR AND OTHER CAUSES

Systemic hypotension, especially in the presence of a pre-existing hepatic congestion due to right heart failure, the Budd–Chiari syndrome, or veno-occlusive disease may cause acute liver failure (Chapter 15).

Massive infiltration of the liver by lymphoma and other types of malignant cells may also occasionally cause ALF.

While many causes of ALF have been described, it is worth emphasizing that the etiology of the ALF seldom influences its management, once liver failure is established. However, the etiology is often the best indicator of the prognosis in that 'non-A, non-B, non-C' hepatitis and idiosyncratic drug reactions have a significantly lower survival than other causes.

CLINICAL FEATURES AND MANAGEMENT

The cornerstone of management is liver-oriented intensive care, which ideally involves close cooperation between hepatologists, intensive care specialists, microbiologists, nephrologists, hematologists and transplant surgeons.

Management consists of anticipating and treating each complication that arises while awaiting recovery of the liver. Patients with very little chance of recovery should be identified and placed on the urgent liver transplant list. Where liver regeneration ensues, recovery is generally complete and without residual effects. In ALF that has been caused by an acute, short-lived and self-limited insult to the liver, e.g. hepatitis A (or B), paracetamol (acetaminophen) ingestion, acute fatty liver of pregnancy, etc., the prognosis depends on the pattern and severity of complications and the supportive management given. Prognosis in this group has been greatly improved by intensive supportive care. The main complications leading to death are cerebral edema and sepsis. Where the insult to the liver is more prolonged or ongoing, as in SHF, NANB hepatitis or idiosyncratic drug reactions, the outlook is grave and has not been greatly influenced by intensive management. Best results in this group are achieved with liver transplantation.

HEPATIC ENCEPHALOPATHY

Recognition of hepatic encephalopathy, the defining characteristic of ALF, is vital to ensure early transfer of these patients to a specialized center. Both the severity and the rate of onset of hepatic encephalopathy are of prognostic importance. The grade may fluctuate in the early stages, and many cases do not progress beyond stage 1 (confusion) or 2 (drowsiness), where the prognosis is excellent. Progression to stage 3 (coma) and 4 (deep coma with incontinence) is associated with multiple complications and a worsening prognosis (Chapter 13).

The earliest features of encephalopathy include subtle personality changes, delirium, hyperactivity, myoclonus and seizures, and occasionally precede all other manifestations of liver disease, including jaundice. Fetor hepaticus is common but not invariable. Tendon reflexes may be brisk and plantar responses upgoing, but abnormal pupillary, oculocephalic, oculovestibular responses, dysconjugate eye movements, focal neurological signs, focal seizures and decerebrate or decorticate posturing indicate the presence of intracranial structural or metabolic abnormalities, e.g. hypoglycemia or brain swelling.

Treatment consists of removing blood and excess protein from the bowel and giving sufficient lactulose or lactitol to cause two loose stools per day. In patients who are unable to take by mouth, a lactulose enema (300–500 ml in 500 ml water, 30 min retention) may be used. Diarrhea should be avoided as this may cause electrolyte disturbances and nursing problems, and there is little advantage in aggressively treating the encephalopathy once more advanced stages are reached. There is no proof that intravenous or oral branched-chain amino acids, α-keto acids or gamma-aminobutyric acid (GABA) antagonists, e.g. flumazenil, have any role in treating acute hepatic encephalopathy.

CEREBRAL EDEMA

This occurs in up to 80% of ALF patients with grade 3 and 4 encephalopathy and is one of the leading potentially treatable causes of death. It may be caused by vasogenic mechanisms where disruption of the blood–brain barrier results in exudation of fluid from the vascular to the cerebral interstitial compartment or by cytotoxic mechanisms where neuroglial cells lose their ability to maintain an osmotic gradient, resulting in fluid moving intracellularly from the interstitial space.

Clinical features

The risk of a patient developing raised intracranial pressure (ICP) varies with the time of onset of hepatic encephalopathy (70–80% in hyperacute, 50–60% in acute, 10–15% in sub-acute liver failure), the presence of fever, arterial hypertension and psychomotor agitation. Initially raised ICP is episodic, precipitated by suctioning or tactile stimuli. Clinical features which usually occur when intracranial pressure exceeds 30 mmHg (normal <12 mmHg) include arterial hypertension, a relative bradycardia, increased tone, decerebrate posturing, opisthotonos and trismus and ST segment elevation on ECG. Initially the pupils respond sluggishly to light; later they dilate and finally they become

unresponsive. Loss of oculocephalic and oculovestibular responses indicates that brainstem compression has occurred. However, patients with loss of oculocephalic responses (but not oculovestibular responses) can recover. Continuous blood pressure monitoring with an intra-arterial line and careful clinical monitoring of neurological features are essential. When raised ICP is suspected, intracranial pressure should be monitored, using an ICP transducer inserted extradurally over the fronto-parietal region of the non-dominant hemisphere (the right hemisphere if dominance is unknown). The procedure may be performed under local anesthesia in the intensive care unit. Mean arterial pressure, intracranial pressure and the derived cerebral perfusion pressure (mean arterial minus mean intracranial pressure) are monitored continuously. ICP monitoring is more sensitive than clinical signs in detecting early pressure increases. It is a valuable adjunct to guiding management and is vital in patients treated with barbiturates in whom all clinical signs are abolished. It also allows measurement of intracranial perfusion pressure which has to be maintained above 50 mmHg to prevent permanent brain damage, may help in identifying patients with the potential to recover without transplantation and is a critical part of anesthetic management of patients undergoing transplantation. The procedure is relatively safe, provided that extradural probes are used and the operator is experienced.

Management of cerebral edema

Patients should be nursed in a quiet environment with the head elevated no more than 20°. Fluid balance and hemodynamic status must be carefully managed to maintain cerebral perfusion pressure. Hypoxia, hypercapnea, hyponatremia and reduced serum osmolality are potent causes of raised ICP and should be prevented or corrected.

Moderate hyperventilation to maintain a P_{CO_2} of 3.0–3.5 kPa may acutely reduce intracranial pressure by up to 20 mmHg, but prolonged hyperventilation is ineffective in maintaining this lowered ICP.

Mannitol is the first line of treatment for brain swelling. In a prospective, randomized controlled trial comparing mannitol with steroid-treated controls, survival was only 5.9% in controls but 47.1% in patients receiving mannitol. A dose of 0.3–0.4 g/kg is used to avoid nephrotoxicity caused by higher doses. It is given as a rapid bolus infusion over 5–10 minutes and this should be followed by a diuresis of >250 ml. The dose is repeated as frequently as half to one hourly until ICP is reduced to below 25 mmHg and signs of intracranial hypertension disappear. If the patient does not have a diuresis, and measured plasma osmolality is below 310, the dose should be repeated. Concomitant use of a loop diuretic is often effective and has the added benefit of increasing free water clearance. If there is coexisting renal failure, a volume of fluid equal to three to four times the volume of mannitol given, should be removed by hemofiltration or continuous arteriovenous hemofiltration (CAVHF), 15–30 minutes after the mannitol infusion. Rebound increases in ICP caused by mechanical ultrafiltration may be circumvented with the use of CAVHF.

In patients with renal failure and intracranial hypertension unresponsive to mannitol and ultrafiltration, who have a very poor prognosis, barbiturate anaesthesia may improve survival. A bolus infusion of 250 mg of thiopentone is given followed by a continuous infusion of thiopentone at a rate sufficient to cause a reduction in intracranial hypertension. The thiopentone is temporarily stopped if systemic hypotension or hypothermia occur and is restarted at a reduced dose. Confirmation of the benefit of this therapy in a controlled trial is awaited. Corticosteroids are of no benefit and may be detrimental in the treatment of brain swelling due to fulminant hepatic failure. Recovery of cerebral function in survivors, even in those with severe intracranial hypertension, is usually excellent.

HEMORRHAGIC COMPLICATIONS

Coagulopathy is almost universal in patients with fulminant liver failure (Chapter 3). This is due to a combination of reduced synthesis of clotting factors made by the liver and their increased consumption as a result of diffuse intravascular coagulation (DIC). Factor VIII–von Willebrand factor, which has procoagulant activity, is released by endothelial damage. Coagulation inhibitors including protein C and S, anti-thrombin III and α-2 macroglobulin are markedly reduced in fulminant hepatic failure. The platelet count is less than $100 \times 10^9/l$ in 75% of patients. In addition, abnormalities of platelet function and structure have been described.

Treatment

Oral sucralfate or intravenous H_2 blockers should be given to prevent gastric erosions. Prothrombin time, partial thromboplastin time, fibrinogen levels, fibrin(ogen) degradation products (FDP) and platelet count should be monitored regularly. Where necessary vitamin K should be administered but clotting factors and platelets should only be replaced where there is active bleeding or where an invasive procedure is contemplated. There is no evidence that prophylactic replacement of clotting factor deficiency has any clinical benefit and the practice is costly. Fresh-frozen plasma is used to correct the international normalized ratio (INR) while cryoprecipitate is required to replace fibrinogen. Random platelet concentrates are infused if bleeding continues despite the adequate replacement of other clotting factors. Platelet counts in excess of 50 x 10^9/l should be obtained before any invasive procedure is performed. Antithrombin III infusions restore blood levels to normal and improve heparin control with hemodialysis, but do not prevent intravascular coagulation, microvessel plugging or improve prognosis when given to patients with stage 3 or 4 coma. There is no role for the use of ε-amino caproic acid or other anti-fibrinolytic therapies.

INFECTION

The exceedingly high prevalence (up to 90% of all patients) of bacterial and fungal infection in ALF is due to both host and environmental factors. Deficiency of complement, fibronectin, and abnormalities of chemotaxis, neutrophil adherence and locomotion, blockade of leukocyte adhesive interactions by fibronectin or fibrinogen fragments, abnormal mononuclear phagocyte function, impaired mucosal barriers and portal systemic shunting may all contribute to the greatly increased susceptibility to infection. Most infections occur within the first 3 days of the onset of ALF, but fatal infections may also occur late in the course of the disease. Gram-positive cocci account for approximately half to two-thirds of infections, the most important of these being staphylococci. Clinical features of infection such as fever and leukocytosis are frequently absent and the diagnosis depends on early and repeated radiological examination of the chest and on culture of blood, urine and tracheal aspirates. Fungal infections, especially with candida, occur in up to one-third of patients surviving 5 days. These patients typically have concomitant bacterial infection, established renal failure, a markedly elevated white cell count, and a pyrexia unresponsive to antibiotics, and show a deterioration in coma grade after initial improvement.

Management

Treatment of established infection is based on the sensitivities of the cultured organism. If therapy is initiated without a bacteriological diagnosis, it should include anti-staphylococcal and Gram-negative cover. Specific choice of antibiotics depends on antibiotic sensitivities at the center in question. Antifungal therapy with amphotericin B and flucytosine is relatively non-toxic in these patients and should be used where fungal infection is suspected or proved.

Features such as opacification on chest X-ray, temperature exceeding 38°C, white cell count >11 x 10^9/l, evidence of inflammation at wound or catheter sites or laboratory evidence of infection in urine, wound blood or sputum samples, should be treated aggressively with specific antibiotics. Peripheral catheters should be replaced every 1–2 days and indwelling urinary catheters should be removed from anuric patients. Topical oral and vaginal antifungal therapy is inexpensive, safe and may be effective in reducing the incidence of late candida infection.

Selective intestinal decontamination with nystatin and oral non-absorbable antibiotics or oral norfloxacin may be effective in reducing enterobacterial infection. In addition, prophylactic use of selective parenteral and enteral antibiotics significantly reduces the incidence of infection and reduces mortality compared with patients who only received antibiotics for established infection.

METABOLIC ABNORMALITIES

HYPOGLYCEMIA

Hypoglycemia occurs in up to 60% of patients with fulminant hepatic failure and may be difficult to control, even with large doses of intravenous glucose. Pancreatic hypersecretion of insulin and glucagon, peripheral insulin resistance and disordered gluconeogenesis contribute to this disorder.

ELECTROLYTE AND ACID–BASE IMBALANCE

Dilutional hyponatremia is common but sodium depletion may also occur due to inadequate replacement of losses caused by mannitol and other diuretics. Dilutional hyponatremia is treated by fluid restriction and avoiding the use of hypotonic intravenous fluids. Normal saline should be used for replacement in sodium-depleted patients, as hypertonic saline may cause osmotic shifts and aggravate brain swelling. Metabolic acidosis is usually associated with renal failure or paracetamol (acetaminophen) toxicity and is a poor prognostic feature.

HYPERNATREMIA

Hypernatremia usually results from the inappropriate use of isotonic or hypertonic fluid replacement in patients with osmotic diarrhea (e.g. from lactulose) or following diuretic use. It is avoided by careful monitoring of electrolytes. Correction should be slow (1–2 mmol/h) using hypotonic fluid. Rapid correction may aggravate cerebral edema by creating dysequilibrium in osmolality between intra- and extracellular brain tissue.

OTHER ELECTROLYTES

Hypokalemia and hypophosphatemia are particularly prevalent in paracetamol-induced ALF. Hypokalemia may aggravate metabolic alkalosis.

CARDIOVASCULAR COMPLICATIONS

Most patients with ALF have hypotension that responds to fluid replacement. Fluid balance should be monitored by measuring pulmonary wedge pressure. Inotropic agents may be required but tend to diminish tissue oxygen delivery.

RESPIRATORY COMPLICATIONS

Hyperventilation, bacterial and aspiration pneumonia, non-cardiogenic pulmonary edema, atelectasis and ventilation perfusion defects causing hypoxemia are the most frequent respiratory abnormalities found in patients with ALF. Some 50–60% of patients may develop pneumonia. Non-cardiogenic pulmonary edema is commonly seen in patients with paracetamol overdose, particularly in the presence of metabolic acidosis. Peripheral oxygen utilization at tissue level may be impaired leading to a relative tissue hypoxia.

Most patients with grade 3 and 4 encephalopathy require ventilation. Positive end-expiratory pressure (PEEP) should not exceed 5 cm H_2O to avoid impairing venous return and aggravating cerebral edema.

RENAL FAILURE

Renal impairment develops in up to 80% of patients with ALF and is most common in sub-acute (late onset) hepatic failure. Pre-renal uremia, acute tubular necrosis (ATN) and functional renal failure (hepatorenal failure) account for the majority of cases. Renal failure may also result directly from paracetamol (acetaminophen) toxicity, acute fatty liver of pregnancy, and the use of nephrotoxic drugs. Pre-renal uremia may be indistinguishable from the hepatorenal syndrome. Management consists of optimizing fluid and hemodynamic status, ideally with the aid of pulmonary capillary wedge pressure monitoring. Colloid and crystalloids are infused until the plasma space is replete as shown by a sustained rise in the pulmonary capillary wedge pressure after fluid challenge. In the presence of established renal failure, hemodialysis is performed for standard indications. In ALF this is usually done for volume overload and hemofiltration is required in the management of cerebral edema. Chronic arteriovenous hemofiltration

(CAVHF) may be preferable in view of the rebound intracranial hypertension that occurs after mechanical hemofiltration.

LIVER TRANSPLANTATION

Liver transplantation is the only effective therapy currently available for the management of patients with a poor prognosis. Prognostic indicators used by the King's College group are given in Table 12.2. Additional indicators of prognosis include the presence of actin-containing complexes in blood (which indicates severe liver damage), an estimated liver volume of <700 ml on CT scan and histology showing >50% hepatocyte necrosis. The most important feature is the presence of an ongoing insult, e.g. with NANB–ALF and idiosyncratic drug reactions that progress after withdrawal of the drug. Liver transplantation should be considered early, even before hepatic encephalopathy has progressed to the severe grades, to ensure that the patient is in an optimal condition for transplantation and to allow time for finding a donor. Unfortunately, patients frequently develop irreversible complications while awaiting surgery because of problems of donor organ availability. Orthotopic liver transplantation remains the procedure of choice, although heterotopic liver transplantation has been used in a few cases.

While transplantation is technically less difficult in ALF than in patients with chronic liver disease, major intraoperative problems relate to hemodynamic instability and intracranial hypertension. Postoperatively the major problem is the increased incidence of pre-existing infections. Results in fulminant hepatic failure are poorer than in chronic liver disease but survival is still in the order of 60% to 70% at 1 year.

OTHER FORMS OF THERAPY

N-Acetylcysteine

A retrospective study of patients with paracetamol (acetaminophen)-induced fulminant hepatic failure showed that those who received late *N*-acetylcysteine therapy had a better prognosis than those who did not receive it, with a lower incidence of renal failure and less prolongation to deeper levels of coma despite similar prolongation of prothrombin time. A prospective controlled trial has confirmed the beneficial role of *N*-acetylcysteine, even when patients had established liver failure as evidenced by encephalopathy and coagulopathy. The mechanism of action was unclear but patients had a significantly lower incidence of multi-organ failure. Recent work has demonstrated that infusion of *N*-acetylcysteine improves cardiac

Table 12.2 King's College poor prognostic criteria for acute liver failure

---

Paracetamol (acetaminophen)-induced acute liver failure

1. pH <7.30
2. Prothrombin time > 100 s and serum creatinine >300 µmol/l and grade 3 or 4 encephalopathy

Acute liver failure not due to paracetamol (acetaminophen)

1. Prothrombin time >100 s
2. Any three of the following:
    (a) Age <10 or >40 years
    (b) NANB hepatitis or idiosyncratic drug reaction
    (c) Prothrombin time >50 s
    (d) Serum bilirubin >300 µmol/l

---

output, oxygen delivery and tissue oxygen consumption in patients with fulminant hepatic failure both following paracetamol overdose and due to viral hepatitis. *N*-Acetylcysteine infusion also improved cerebral blood flow and cerebral oxygenation. These improvements in tissue oxygenation may improve organ function and hence outcome, as survival is inversely related to the number of failing organs and the duration of dysfunction.

Liver support systems

A great deal of enthusiasm has been expressed for a variety of liver support systems based on columns containing cultured hepatocytes. It is the hope that liver assist devices may be helpful in supporting liver function and promoting regeneration of the native liver. Initial studies have shown much promise although no controlled data are yet available.

RECOMMENDED READING

Bernuau, J. and Benhamou, J.P. (1993) Classifying acute liver failure. *Lancet*, **342**(2), 252–3.

Bernuau, J., Rueff, B. and Benhamou, J.-P. (1986) Fulminant and subfulminant liver failure: definitions and causes. *Semin Liver Dis*, **6**(2), 97–106.

Canalese, J., Gimson, A.E.S., Davis, C. *et al.* (1982) Controlled trial of dexamethasone and mannitol for the cerebral oedema of fulminant hepatic failure. *Gut*, **23**, 625–9.

Ede, R.J. and Williams, R. (1986) Hepatic encephalopathy and cerebral oedema. *Semin Liver Dis*, **6**, 107–18.

Forbes, A., Alexander, G.J.M., O'Grady, J.G. *et al.* (1989) Thiopental infusion in the treatment of intracranial hypertension complicating fulminant hepatic failure. *Hepatology*, **10**, 306–10.

Gimson, A.E.S., O'Grady, J., Ede, R.J. *et al.* (1986) Late onset fulminant hepatic failure: clinical, serological and histological features. *Hepatology*, **6**, 288–94.

Keays, R., Harrison, P.M., Wendo, J.A. *et al.* (1991) Intravenous acetylcysteine in paracetamol induced fulminant hepatic failure: a prospective controlled trial. *Br Med J*, **303**, 1206–9.

Liang, T.J., Hasegawa, K., Rimon, N. *et al.* (1991) Hepatitis B virus mutant associated with an epidemic of fulminant hepatitis. *N Engl J Med*, **324**, 1705–9.

Lidofsky, S.D., Bass, N.M., Prager, M.C. *et al.* (1992) Intracranial pressure monitoring and liver transplantation for fulminant hepatic failure. *Hepatology*, **16**(1), 1–7.

O'Grady, J.G. and Williams, R. (1989) Acute liver failure. *Ballière's Clinical Gastroenterology*, **3**(1), 75–89.

O'Grady, J.G., Schalm, S.W. and Williams, R. (1993) Acute liver failure: redefining the syndromes. *Lancet*, **342**(2), 273–5.

O'Grady, J.G., Gimson, A.E.S., O'Brien, C.J. *et al.* (1988) Controlled trials of charcoal hemoperfusion and prognostic factors in fulminant hepatic failure. *Gastroenterology*, **94**, 1186–92.

O'Grady, J.G., Langley, P.G., Isola, L.M. *et al.* (1986) Coagulopathy of fulminant hepatic failure. *Semin Liver Dis*, **6**, 159–63.

Randomized trial of steroid therapy in acute liver failure. Report from the European Association for the Study of the Liver. *Gut*, **20**, 620–3.

Rolando, N., Gimson, A., Wade, J. *et al.* (1993) Prospective controlled trial of selective parenteral and enteral antimicrobial regimens in fulminant liver failure. *Hepatology*, **17**(2), 196–201.

Rolando, N., Harvey, F., Brahm, J. *et al.* (1990) Prospective study of bacterial infection in acute liver failure: an analysis of 50 patients. *Hepatology*, **11**, 49–53.

Rolando, N., Harvey, F., Brahm, J. *et al.* (1991) Fungal infection: a common, unrecognised complication of acute liver failure. *J Hepatol*, **12**, 1–9.

Wright, T.L., Mamish, D., Combs, C. *et al.* (1992) Hepatitis B virus and apparent fulminant non-A non-B hepatitis. *Lancet*, **339**, 952–5.

13

Hepatic encephalopathy

MICHAEL VOIGT and HAROLD CONN

INTRODUCTION

Hepatic encephalopathy is a reversible state of impaired cognitive function or altered consciousness which occurs in subjects with liver disease or portal systemic shunts. Hepatocellular insufficiency and portal systemic shunting may act separately or in combination to cause encephalopathy. Thus, encephalopathy may be due entirely to shunting (portal vein thrombosis), may result from both shunting and liver cell failure (cirrhosis), or may be due mainly to hepatocellular insufficiency (acute liver failure).

EPIDEMIOLOGY

Almost all cases of clinically apparent hepatic encephalopathy occur in patients with cirrhosis. Fewer than 5% occur in non-cirrhotic forms of portal hypertension. However, a disproportionately large proportion of patients with surgical and radiological portal systemic shunts develop severe, frequently intractable, hepatic encephalopathy.

FACTORS PRECIPITATING ENCEPHALOPATHY

The combination of impaired hepatic and renal function is frequently associated with hepatic encephalopathy (Fig. 13.1). Roughly half of these patients have diuretic-induced renal impairment and half have functional renal failure. This association may be due to nitrogen retention but is equally likely to reflect advanced liver decompensation which is common to both conditions.

Drugs are implicated in approximately 25% of patients with hepatic encephalopathy. Most common are benzodiazepines, barbiturates, analgesics and other sedatives. Unusual drugs that may precipitate hepatic encephalopathy include propranolol, which may act by reducing portal venous blood flow, and sodium valproate, which is thought to produce a drug-induced type of Reye's hyperammonemic encephalopathy.

Another 20% of cases of encephalopathy are precipitated by gastrointestinal tract hemorrhage. This is frequently associated with deep and prolonged coma. The combination of gastrointestinal hemorrhage and hepatic encephalopathy indicates a poor prognosis. Only 15% of such patients survive 1 year compared with 65% of those with hemorrhage alone.

There should be a very low threshold for treating with antibiotics in patients without an obvious precipitant, as infections are common and frequently occur without the

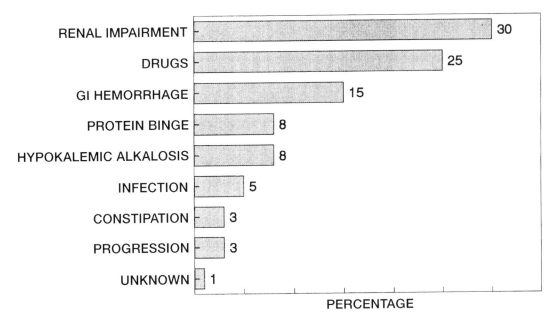

Figure 13.1 Precipitating factors of hepatic encephalopathy.

usual manifestations of fever and leukocytosis.

Finally, a small proportion of cases are precipitated by dietary protein excess, hypokalemic alkalosis, constipation and deterioration of liver function secondary to drugs, toxins, viruses or the presence of hepatocellular carcinoma.

CLINICAL FEATURES

The typical features of hepatic encephalopathy – monotonous speech, flat effect, metabolic tremor, muscular incoordination, impaired handwriting, asterixis, fetor hepaticus, coma, upgoing plantar responses, hypo- or hyperactive reflexes and decerebrate posturing, are listed in Table 13.1.

However, any metabolic or structural insult to the brain may precipitate hepatic encephalopathy in patients with chronic liver disease. Thus the presence of hepatic encephalopathy does not exclude an associated disease which may call for a specific treatment. It is therefore important to recognize features that are not typical of uncomplicated hepatic encephalopathy. These include changes in pupillary responses and oculocephalic reflexes which normally remain intact and may be brisk in the early stages of hepatic encephalopathy.

Patients with liver disease hyperventilate. Respiratory depression should alert one to the possibility of drug-induced coma. Focal neurological signs, seizures, signs of raised intracranial pressure, tonic upward and downward gaze and dysconjugate eye movements are rare in uncomplicated chronic hepatic encephalopathy and all point to an associated complication or alternative diagnosis.

The diagnosis of hepatic coma, especially in alcoholic patients, should only be made once intracranial space-occupying and vascular lesions, trauma, infection, metabolic, endocrine, drug-induced and post-epileptic coma have been excluded.

Table 13.1 Typical features of hepatic encephalopathy; atypical features usually indicate that another neurological process, e.g. drug intoxication or sub-dural hematemia trauma, has caused the coma

Typical	Atypical
Monotonous speech	Focal neurological signs
Flat effect	Seizures
Apraxia	Raised intracranial pressure
Fetor hepaticus	Tonic upward and downward gaze
Flap/myoclonus	Dysconjugate eye movements
Upgoing plantars	Hypoventilation (drug coma)
Abnormal reflexes	
Decerebrate posture	
Intact pupillary and oculocephalic responses	

ASTERIXIS

Asterixis is characterized by the intermittent loss of tone or posture in a muscle group. A slight flicker of the metacarpophalangeal joint is more typical than the gross wrist flap often illustrated in text books. Although it may be asynchronous, the flap is usually bilaterally present. Asterixis present on one side only generally indicates a focal neurological abnormality. Electrophysiologically it is characterized by 50–100 ms electrical silences on the electromyogram (EMG) of active muscle groups and follows on a sub-clinical cortical myoclonus. Asterixis is an insensitive and non-specific sign of hepatic encephalopathy. It may be absent in mild encephalopathy and in deep coma, and is also found in uremia, hyperkalemia, and in respiratory and cardiac failure.

FETOR HEPATICUS

Fetor hepaticus is a sour feculent odor smelt on the breath of patients with hepatic encephalopathy. It is thought to be caused by the volatile mercaptans methan-ethiol, dimethyl sulfide and dimethyl disulfide, which are derived from the action of gut bacteria on precursors such as methionine. Once absorbed they bypass liver extraction. Cirrhotics fed methionine develop typical fetor hepaticus. In chronic liver disease, the absence of fetor does not exclude hepatic encephalopathy, and it is not a useful prognostic sign.

STAGING OF HEPATIC ENCEPHALOPATHY

Formal staging of the grade of encephalopathy is of value in monitoring disease progression or response to treatment but is a simplified descriptive shorthand for a complex and changing situation. Detailed, structured clinical notes are of far greater value in the day-to-day assessment of patients with encephalopathy. Patients with stage 1 encephalopathy have subtle alterations in personality, sleep disturbance and lethargy. In stage 2 somnolence is present, in stage 3 there is stupor which progresses to coma, in stage 4 the patient is incontinent and unrousable. EEG, motor and other changes are variable and are of limited value in grading encephalopathy.

DIAGNOSIS OF HEPATIC ENCEPHALOPATHY

Physicians faced with a patient with liver disease and an altered mental state need to be able to: (1) identify the cause of the delirium/stupor/coma; (2) detect low-grade and sub-clinical hepatic encephalopathy; (3) identify precipitating factors; and (4) monitor the progress of their patient.

Correct use of clinical and laboratory procedures requires an appreciation of both the sensitivity and specificity of the procedure and their diagnostic accuracy in each of these settings.

HISTORY

A history of mental slowing or personality change (aggression or apathy), obtained from close family members of the patient, is the most sensitive test of low-grade and sub-clinical hepatic encephalopathy. This is more sensitive than psychometric, electrophysiological and biochemical studies, although changes are not specific for hepatic encephalopathy.

Another important clue to early hepatic encephalopathy is sleep–wake inversion or insomnia. Injudicious prescription of benzodiazepines may aggravate hepatic encephalopathy if given to patients with this complaint.

LABORATORY TESTS

Measurement of the blood ammonia, preferably arterial, and CSF glutamine are of limited use in the diagnostic work-up of liver patients in coma. Abnormal values are at best supportive of the clinical diagnosis. Although CSF glutamine and α-ketoglutaramate levels correlate statistically with the grade of coma, they are of little use in individual cases. Arterial ammonia levels correlate poorly with the grade of hepatic encephalopathy. All may be abnormal in uremia and in respiratory failure and thus lack both sensitivity and specificity.

PSYCHOMETRIC TESTS

These are tests of memory, visuo-spatial coordination, praxis and other cognitive functions. Simple psychometric tests, such as testing constructional praxis with the five-pointed star, are used in every practice. The number connection test (in which the patients are timed while they connect in ascending order randomly placed numbers on a sheet of paper) has been popularized as a means of monitoring encephalopathy. Indeed, the number connection (Reitan A and B), block design and digit symbol tests have been shown to be of particular value in detecting early hepatic encephalopathy. Unfortunately, the performance and interpretation of these tests is time-consuming and ideally they require administration by a trained psychologist. Since they require patient cooperation they are only of use in the detection of sub-clinical or low-grade encephalopathy. Normal ranges vary and are age- and education-dependent. Serial testing at short intervals results in a significant learning effect. Thus, psychometric tests should be reserved for the diagnosis of subclinical or mild hepatic encephalopathy.

NEUROPHYSIOLOGICAL ASSESSMENT

A variety of neurophysiological tests have been used in hepatic encephalopathy. These include the EEG, visual, auditory and somatosensory evoked potentials and, more recently, the latency of the P300. These tests are all readily performed by a competent neurophysiological laboratory. It is important to note that none of these tests will distinguish hepatic encephalopathy from other causes of encephalopathy. However, the main value of neurophysiological tests in hepatic encephalopathy is not in diagnosis but in monitoring the response to treatment. Here they are objective, quantifiable, and not altered by learning.

PATHOPHYSIOLOGY

The pathogenesis of hepatic encephalopathy is not well understood. A variety of substances have been implicated. Ammonia – which has been claimed to act directly on synaptic transmission, and affects brain energy metabolism, increases brain inhibitory neurotransmitter concentration and damages astrocyte foot processes, thus disrupting the blood–brain barrier – remains a major candidate. Synergism between ammonia, the mercaptans and fatty acids and phenols (with or without hypoxia, hypoglycemia, and abnormal acid–base balance) has also been proposed as the mechanism of encephal-

opathy. These theories have formed the theoretical basis for the use of lactulose, lactitol, neomycin and, more recently, ammonia-sparing agents.

A false neurotransmitter hypothesis has also been proposed. This holds that the effects of liver disease on amino acid balance alters the flux of amino acids across the blood–brain barrier, thus increasing the production of false (non-functional) neurotransmitters. This has led to patients receiving either the branched-chain amino acids or bromocriptine.

More recently attention has focused on the GABA/endogenous benzodiazepine ligand theory which suggests that hepatic encephalopathy results from excess GABA-ergic tone. This has led to the use of benzodiazepine antagonists, e.g. flumazenil.

Studies on the mechanism of hepatic encephalopathy have been hampered by the lack of a suitable animal model, possible differences in the pathogenesis of encephalopathy in acute and chronic liver disease and the inability to study brain biochemistry *in vivo*. To date, there is insufficient evidence to allow one to favour any of the above theories (Table 13.2).

Table 13.2 Hypotheses for the pathogenesis of hepatic encephalopathy

Theory	Mechanism	Application
Ammonia	Synaptic transmission Brain energy metabolism Neurotransmitters Blood–brain transport Astrocyte toxicity	Lactulose Lactitol Antibiotics
Synergism	Merceptans, phenols Fatty acids Hypoglycemia/hypoxia Glutaramate	Benzoate Phenylacetate
False transmitter	Octopamine B/Hydroxyphenylalanine	BCAA Bromocriptine
GABA-BZ	Endogenous BZ-ligand Increased GABA-ergic tone	Flumazenil GABA-antagonists

144

TREATMENT

The treatment of hepatic encephalopathy remains empirical and relies largely on establishing the correct diagnosis, identifying and treating precipitating factors, emptying the bowels of blood, protein and stool, attending to electrolyte and acid–base balance and the selective use of benzodiazepine antagonists.

Non-absorbable disaccharides, such as lactulose or lactitol, remain the mainstay of therapy. Antibiotics and protein restriction (40 g/day) may be advised if there is no response. In intractable cases, closure of surgical shunts and liver transplantation should be considered.

LACTULOSE

This is an artificial, non-absorbable disaccharide, for which the body has no disaccharidase. It passes unchanged to the colon, where bacteria break it down to small organic acids including lactate. The postulated mechanisms of action include: catharsis; acidification of colonic contents with reduced absorption of ammonia (however, it has not been possible to demonstrate increased ammonia excretion in the stool although stool nitrogen excretion is increased); and changing the colonic bacterial flora in favor of forms which utilize ammonia nitrogen. Lactulose more than doubles fecal bacterial output, causing a marked reduction in colonic absorption of soluble nitrogen.

In acute episodes of encephalopathy the dose is titrated to give two to three loose stools per day. If oral therapy is not possible, lactulose enemas (350 g lactulose with 500 ml water) may be used. In chronic therapy, small volumes not sufficient to produce loose stools are effective and better tolerated. The side effects of lactulose include flatulence and discomfort which often influence compliance.

LACTITOL

Beta-galactoside sorbitol is a second-generation disaccharide produced in powder form. It is as effective as lactulose and is said to be more convenient, but no patient preference has been shown when the agents were compared.

Because of the high cost of these agents, a trial of lactose is worthwhile, especially where lactase deficiency is common.

ORAL ANTIBIOTICS

Metronidazole (200 mg three times daily) is probably the most useful antibiotic for treating hepatic encephalopathy. Neomycin (1 g four times daily) and, indeed, most other antibiotics may be effective therapy for hepatic encephalopathy. Side effects, including those due to the slight absorption of neomycin, make this a second-line agent. Despite theoretical reasons against the combination of antibiotics and non-absorbable sugars, controlled trials have shown that they act synergistically and should be combined when the sugar alone is ineffective.

OTHER THERAPIES

There is limited evidence that branched-chain amino acids may influence hepatic encephalopathy. L-Dopa and bromocriptine have been shown to have no beneficial effect. Benzodiazepine antagonists may be of benefit in selected cases and improvement appears to occur independently of the prior use of benzodiazepines.

Several randomized controlled trials have shown sodium benzoate (4–10 g/day) and phenylacetate to be effective in reversing hepatic encephalopathy by stimulating the incorporation of ammonia into non-toxic excretable substances.

CLINICAL VARIANTS

Two important clinical variants of hepatic encephalopathy, namely sub-clinical hepatic encephalopathy and acquired hepatocerebral degeneration, may be under-diagnosed in patients with liver disease.

SUB-CLINICAL HEPATIC ENCEPHALOPATHY

Sub-clinical hepatic encephalopathy is characterized by cognitive impairment including altered visuo-spatial coordination, impaired constructional praxis and impaired motor skills and learning ability, but they do not have features of overt hepatic encephalopathy such as altered level of consciousness or asterixis. Personality changes are frequent. Verbal skills are typically well preserved and electrophysiological abnormalities, if present, are subtle. Sub-clinical hepatic encephalopathy is partially or wholly reversible by treatment with lactulose or following liver transplantation.

This syndrome is common but is frequently missed, most often because the patient's verbal skills are well maintained. However, it has been shown to have a significant impact on the lives of patients with chronic liver disease in whom it results in loss of employment, social and marital problems and higher accident rates. The incidence is difficult to assess, but up to 60% of unselected patients with cirrhosis may have abnormal psychometric tests. Indeed, a study of unselected cirrhotic patients showed that 60% were totally unfit to drive and another 15% were found to be unfit to drive except under ideal circumstances. In a separate study the impact of sub-clinical encephalopathy was assessed in 29 patients undergoing surgical shunting. Nine of the 29 developed overt encephalopathy, while 19 of the 20 remaining patients who had no features of overt hepatic encephalopathy, were mentally slower. Of these, 11 were markedly

aggressive and eight became placid and uncaring about family problems. Eight patients retired prematurely and 20 out of the original 29 experienced marital problems.

Management

Physicians caring for patients with chronic liver disease should be aware of the entity and should ask their patients about their performance at work, should interview their families, and enquire about difficulties with driving or the operation of industrial machinery. When in doubt lactulose should be given. Any history of accidents should be taken seriously. If impairment remains despite therapy, appropriate steps should be taken to prevent further accidents and the patient should be assessed for transplantation.

ACQUIRED HEPATOCEREBRAL DEGENERATION AND SHUNT MYELOPATHY

While minor structural neurological changes are probably present in many if not all patients with chronic liver disease and portal–systemic shunting, a small number develop severe permanent neurological deficits. These are similar clinically, pathologically and radiologically to those found in Wilson's disease. The most severe forms are found almost exclusively in patients with large surgical or spontaneous portal systemic shunts. The condition is found with distal as well as portacaval shunts, and neurological signs may develop at any time from 6 months to 8 years after surgery. Hepatocerebral degeneration is usually preceded by hepatic encephalopathy, but its progress is not influenced by the treatment of the latter.

Patients may have some or all of the following: dementia, cortical blindness, gaze palsies, grasp and pout reflexes, tremor, dysarthria, grimacing, choreoathetosis, cerebellar ataxia and spasticity. The condition is relentlessly progressive, with the longest reported survival being less than 4 years.

Pathologically, the condition is characterized by laminar necrosis at the junction of the cortex and white matter and degeneration of neurones in the basal ganglia and cerebellum. Central pontine myelinolysis may occur. Occasionally the emphasis is on the spinal cord and such patients are labeled as having shunt myelopathy. This starts with difficulty in walking and progresses to spastic paraparesis with loss of sphincter control. Sensation is generally preserved. Although a peripheral neuropathy is not clinically apparent, EMG studies may show its presence. The lateral corticospinal tract degeneration which is the pathological hallmark of this condition results from the primary degeneration of the cortical motor neurones.

Findings on magnetic resonance imaging are identical to Wilson's disease with increased signal intensity in the basal ganglia on T2-weighted images.

Management

The diagnosis should only be made after a thorough search for treatable conditions such as Wernicke's encephalopathy, and vitamin B12 deficiency. Slit lamp examination and biochemical studies should always be done to exclude Wilson's disease. An adequate trial of therapy for hepatic encephalopathy should be given. However, changes are progressive and unresponsive to standard treatment for hepatic encephalopathy. The ability of vitamin E therapy to prevent progression is currently being examined. Embolization of shunts should be considered. Finally, orthotopic liver transplantation has been shown to improve spastic paraparesis, dementia, dysarthria, ataxia, tremor and neuropsychiatric symptoms in a patient with this condition.

CONCLUSION

This review has concentrated on selected aspects of the epidemiology, clinical features and management of hepatic encephalopathy, including new methods of treatment. It has emphasized the variable clinical spectrum of hepatic encephalopathy and has stressed the importance of recognizing the impact of sub-clinical encephalopathy and the impact which this potentially reversible condition has on the lives of patients with chronic liver disease.

RECOMMENDED READING

Basile, A.S., Hugues, R.P., Harrison, P.M. *et al.* (1991) Elevated brain concentrations of 1–4 benzodiazepines in fulminant hepatic failure. *N Engl J. Med*, **325**, 473–8.

Basile, A.S., Jones, E.A. and Skolniek, P. (1991) The pathogenesis and treatment of hepatic encephalopathy: evidence for the involvement of benzodiazepine receptor ligands. *Pharmacol Rev*, **43**, 27–71.

Butterworth, R.F. (1992) Pathogenesis and treatment of portal-systemic encephalopathy: an update. *Dig Dis Sci*, **37**(3), 321–7.

Pomier-Layrargues, G., Giguere, J.F., Perney, P. *et al.* (1994) Flumazenil in cirrhotic patients in hepatic coma: a randomized double-blind placebo controlled cross-over trial. *Hepatology*, **19**, 32–7.

Schomerus, H. and Schreiegg, J. (1993) Prevalence of latent portasystemic encephalopathy in an unselected population of patients with liver cirrhosis in general practice. *Z Gastroenterol*, **31**(4), 231–4.

Tarter, R.E., Switala, J., Plail, J. *et al.* (1992) Severity of hepatic encephalopathy before liver transplantation is associated with quality of life after transplantation. *Arch Int Med*, **152**(10), 2097–101.

14

Pathophysiology and management of portal hypertension

MICHAEL VOIGT, DIDIER LEBREC and JOHN TERBLANCHE

INTRODUCTION

The portal vein carries blood from the small and large bowel, spleen, pancreas and stomach to the liver. Normal portal blood flow is approximately 1500 ml/min. Any obstruction to flow along the course of the valveless portal system, the hepatic veins, inferior vena cava, right atrium and right ventricle, or rarely increased portal flow *per se*, may cause portal hypertension. The causes of portal hypertension are listed in Table 14.1.

Manifestations and complications of portal hypertension differ according to the site of obstruction. Portal hypertension leads to the formation of portal systemic collaterals in transition zones between squamous and glandular epithelium and in retroperitoneal regions. Increased portal pressure and the resultant compensatory portal systemic shunting and disturbed intrahepatic circulation of blood, contribute to many of the important complications of liver disease including variceal bleeding, hepatic encephalopathy (Chapter 13), coagulopathy (Chapter 3), ascites (Chapter 16), the hepatorenal syndrome, immune dysfunction and recurrent infections. Since most of these are discussed

Table 14.1 Etiology of portal hypertension

Pre-hepatic
    Portal and splenic vein thrombosis
    Non-cirrhotic portal hypertension
    Tropical splenomegaly

Intrahepatic
    Cirrhosis
        Alcohol
        Biliary
        Viral
        Alpha-1 antitrypsin deficiency
        Hemochromatosis, Wilson's disease
        Autoimmune
        Cryptogenic

    Non-cirrhotic
        Idiopathic
        Schistosomiasis
        Chronic hepatitis
        Nodular regenerative hyperplasia
        Granulomas and infiltrative diseases
        Vitamin A intoxication

Post-hepatic
    Budd–Chiari syndrome
    Veno-occlusive disease
    Cardiac and pericardial disease

elsewhere this chapter will focus on the pathophysiology, the natural history and the emergency, long-term and prophylactic medical and surgical management of variceal hemorrhage and portal hypertensive intestinal vasculopathy. Variceal hemorrhage occurs most frequently as a result of portal hypertension caused by cirrhosis and as such is a marker for severe liver disease with a high mortality rate. Although bleeding may be controlled by injection sclerotherapy and re-bleed rates reduced by pharmacological means, survival may not be significantly improved. All patients with this complication should thus be assessed for liver transplantation (Chapter 27).

ESOPHAGEAL VARICES AND PORTAL HYPERTENSIVE GASTROPATHY

NATURAL HISTORY

The risk of cirrhotic patients developing varices and portal hypertensive gastropathy, and of the varices enlarging and bleeding, increases with time, the severity of the liver disease and its rate of progression. With sufficiently long follow-up over 90% of Child's C patients will experience variceal hemorrhage. A minority of patients with large spontaneous shunts may be protected from or have regression of their varices, but this is usually at the expense of increased hepatic encephalopathy. Regression also occurs in the rare patient with improvement of the liver disease, e.g. abstinent alcoholics and chronic active hepatitis treated with steroids.

The risk of bleeding if varices are present (i.e. in all Child's A, B and C patients) is 20–40% at 3–10 years' follow-up, with approximately 70% of bleeds occurring within the first 2 years of the varices developing. Mortality during the first bleed varies from 25–50%, although half to two-thirds of these patients die from causes other than hemor-

rhage. Mortality depends on the degree of liver decompensation which may be roughly assessed using the Child–Pugh scoring system and is approximately 5% for Child's A patients, less than 25% for Child's B and more than 50% for Child's C patients. The risk of re-bleeding exceeds 70% over the next 3–10 years in those surviving the initial episode, but mortality from the second bleed is less than 25% as the high risk patients are selected out at the first bleed.

Predicting the likelihood of a first bleed in those with varices is of importance in analyzing the risk-to-benefit ratio of prophylactic therapy in patients with portal hypertension. The severity of the liver disease (including Child–Pugh class, presence of ascites, rate of progression of disease and ongoing alcohol abuse), the appearance of the varices at endoscopy (size of the varices and possibly the presence of red weal and cherry red marks), and intraportal and intravariceal pressure may be predictive of a bleed occurring. Bleeding seldom occurs in patients with a wedged hepatic venous pressure gradient (i.e. the difference between the free hepatic venous pressure and the pressure measured when the catheter is moved into a wedged position in the hepatic vein) of less than 12 mmHg, but above 12 mmHg, the pressure does not correlate well with the likelihood of bleeding.

EMERGENCY MANAGEMENT OF ACUTE VARICEAL BLEEDING

Variceal hemorrhage accounts for approximately 10% of gastrointestinal hemorrhage and should be suspected in anyone presenting with hematemesis who has features of chronic liver disease or portal hypertension. Patients with suspected acute variceal bleeding should be admitted to hospital, preferably to an intensive care unit, and resuscitation for massive hemorrhage instituted. Many have hepatic decompensation, with coagulopathy, ascites, encephalopathy and sepsis. Coagulopathy should be corrected using fresh–frozen plasma, and excess crystalloids should be avoided, as these, combined with vasopressin or its analogs, may lead to marked edema and hyponatremia. Pharmacological control is instituted early in cases suspected of bleeding from varices. Thereafter, when possible, patients should be transferred to a hospital with appropriate facilities and expertise, as subsequent management can be complex. Once circulating blood volume has been restored, emergency endoscopy is mandatory since it is vital to ensure that the patient is actually bleeding from varices. Up to 50% of patients with known varices will have another source of blood loss. Ideally the initial therapeutic procedure, such as sclerotherapy, is performed during this first endoscopy. Alternative therapy, including balloon tube tamponade, transjugular intrahepatic portal systemic stent-shunt (TIPSS) insertion, transhepatic sclerotherapy, esophageal transection with or without devascularization procedures, and selective or non-selective portacaval shunts have more limited application, depending on the local experience, the enthusiasm for these procedures in some centers and on special patient-related circumstances.

PHARMACOLOGICAL CONTROL

Pharmacological therapy, which may help with the immediate control of bleeding, resuscitition and emergency endoscopy, should be started when variceal bleeding is suspected. This therapy is effective as a holding procedure and may temporarily stop bleeding in up to 80% of cases of variceal hemorrhage, but has no role in long-term management as re-bleed rates are very high on withdrawal. Definitive therapy, usually sclerotherapy, should always be used as soon as the patient has been adequately resusci-

tated. Intravenous vasopressin 0.4 U/min (2.75–5.5 mU/kg/min) plus glyceryl trinitrate 0.5–1 mg sub-lingually every 30 minutes for 4–6 hours, is the primary therapy used. Vasopressin constricts the splanchnic vasculature, thus reducing portal pressure and flow. Bolus injections may increase toxicity without significant benefit, while intra-arterial injection is difficult, increases side effects and has little advantage over intravenous therapy. It is essential to combine nitrates with vasopressin, as they have been shown to reduce the cardiac and peripheral side effects of vasopressin, may have an additive effect on lowering portal pressure, and are easy and safe to administer. Pharmacological therapy, which is usually continued for 4–6 hours, may be stopped abruptly without rebound effects.

Glypressin (triglycyl lysine–vasopressin) a synthetic pro-analog of vasopressin, has a longer duration of action, may be less cardiotoxic and is equally effective, but more expensive, than vasopressin. Somatostatin (250–450 μg/h), a potent and safe splanchnic vasoconstrictor when given in supraphysiological doses, is also effective in temporarily stopping bleeding and is probably the most effective agent available today. The long-acting and potent somatostatin analog octreotide is effective at doses of 50 μg/h.

Drugs with other actions, for example metoclopramide (which constricts the lower esophageal sphincter), pentagastrin and cisapride are also being evaluated.

BALLOON TAMPONADE

Because balloon tube tamponade is associated with high re-bleeding rates after removal and may be associated with significant complications, its use is generally reserved for controlling active variceal bleeding where technical expertise for emergency sclerotherapy is not available, where emergency sclerotherapy has failed, or where torrential bleeding prevents definitive emergency endoscopic control. The four-lumen Minnesota modification of the Sengstaken–Blakemore tube is preferred. One lumen each goes to the stomach for aspiration, to the nasopharyngeal region to minimize pulmonary complications from aspiration, and to the stomach and esophageal balloons. After checking the balloons for leaks, the tube is passed through the nose (or mouth) to the stomach. Thereafter the stomach balloon is inflated using 100–200 ml air (or water with added radiocontrast material). Siting may be checked by auscultation over the stomach while injecting air, or radiologically. It is perfectly adequate to check radiologically if air is used in the balloon as it is well visualized. Injections of 50 ml boluses at a time are used, with resistance to injection being a sign of possible incorrect siting in the esophagus. Thereafter the balloon is drawn up tightly to the esophagogastric junction. The esophageal balloon is then inflated to 40 mmHg and the tube fixed at the nose or mouth. In patients with impaired consciousness, an endotracheal tube should first be passed to protect the airway.

Balloon tube tamponade is successful in controlling bleeding in more than 90% of patients. In cases of failure, tube position and diagnosis of the source of bleeding should be re-assessed by an expert. The tube is generally left in place for 4–6 hours (up to 24 hours) to allow for resuscitation and transfer to a center where appropriate expertise is available. Patients should be carefully nursed, with at least hourly aspiration of the stomach and nasopharyngeal tubes and sedation is best avoided. Injection sclerotherapy should be performed at the time of removal of the tube, as tamponade does not prevent re-bleeding. The most important complications of the use of balloon tube tamponade include aspiration pneumonia, esophageal tear or rupture and cardiac arrest.

EMERGENCY SCLEROTHERAPY

Emergency endoscopy should be performed as soon as the patient is adequately resuscitated. If a balloon tube is inserted, sclerotherapy should be performed within 6–12 hours. At the time of endoscopy, approximately one-third of patients will be actively bleeding from their varices, one-third will have stopped and one-third will be bleeding from a source other than varices. In those who have stopped bleeding, a diagnosis of variceal bleed is made if there is adherent clot on a varix, or if varices are present and no other source of bleeding is found on panendoscopy. Sclerotherapy is ideally performed at the time of the first emergency endoscopy in patients who have stopped bleeding and, where feasible, in actively bleeding patients. Blind injection is contraindicated in actively bleeding patients but visibility may be improved by lavage and tilting the patient 30°.

Sclerotherapy is as effective at stopping bleeding as balloon tube tamponade, but in addition provides definitive therapy to prevent further bleeding. A variety of sclerosants may be used including ethanolamine oleate, sodium morrhuate, polidocanol, sodium tetradecyl sulfate, alcohol and more recently Histoacryl ('Superglue' tissue adhesive). Our group prefers a combined intravariceal and paravariceal injection technique using 5% ethanolamine oleate injected freehand via a fiberoptic endoscope. Definitive control of variceal hemorrhage is achieved in up to 95% of patients, although only approximately 70–80% of patients are controlled by a single injection, the remainder requiring a second injection.

If initial sclerotherapy fails, temporary control of bleeding should be obtained using balloon tube tamponade with the patient being subjected to sclerotherapy subsequently. Any patient who re-bleeds after two emergency sclerotherapies during a single hospital admission should be subjected to alternative definitive therapy, such as esophageal transection or emergency portacaval shunt, as he or she has a very poor prognosis. The admission mortality depends on the Child's grade of the patient. Death from uncontrolled continued acute variceal hemorrhage is uncommon.

PORTACAVAL SHUNT SURGERY FOR EMERGENCY MANAGEMENT OF BLEEDING

Shunt surgery is generally reserved for patients who have continued to bleed despite at least two sclerotherapy treatments. It has been used as the primary treatment in bleeding patients. Here, it is effective in stopping variceal bleeding but is more expensive and demanding than sclerotherapy and may be associated with an operative mortality of up to 56%, and a high incidence of postoperative hepatic encephalopathy. When used as a rescue procedure, the side-to-side shunt is preferred, but end-to-side shunt, or a narrow diameter PTFE interposition H-graft and, very rarely, distal splenorenal shunts, may be used. Although operative mortality is very high in emergency shunting, subsequent survival is similar to that after elective shunting.

The use of transvenous intrahepatic portal systemic shunts as a rescue procedure appears to be promising (see below). Preliminary reports suggest that it is highly effective at stopping bleeding, and that the procedure is not accompanied by the high morbidity and mortality associated with surgical procedures. It is currently being evaluated in clinical trials.

ESOPHAGEAL TRANSECTION (AND DEVASCULARIZATION)

The automatic anastomotic staple gun is used to transect and re-anastomose the lower esophagus, thereby transecting and stapling bleeding varices. It is a relatively simple procedure and may be the procedure of choice in patients with failed sclerotherapy. We favor the use of simple transgastric esophageal transection without extensive devascularization procedures. Those patients who present later with recurrent varices after an emergency esophageal transection are subsequently treated with sclerotherapy. The value of staple-gun transection as an alternative to sclerotherapy has been demonstrated by Burroughs *et al.* (1989).

In conclusion, management of acute variceal bleeding includes admission of the patient to hospital with resuscitation, usually making use of vasopressin and nitrates or somatostatin. Emergency endoscopy is mandatory to diagnose the source of bleeding. Sclerotherapy should preferably be performed at the time of the first emergency endoscopy, but if this is not possible it should be performed early after temporary balloon tube tamponade to control initial bleeding and to allow for resuscitation. Between 5% and 10% of patients will fail to respond to sclerotherapy. We recommend that any patient in whom acute variceal bleeding is not controlled by two injection treatments be subjected to a surgical procedure, preferably simple staple-gun esophageal transection, or portacaval shunting, preferably by the transjugular route.

LONG-TERM THERAPEUTIC MANAGEMENT

This is defined as the management of a patient who has had a variceal bleed with the aim of preventing recurrences.

The management options include liver transplantation, repeated sclerotherapy, portacaval shunting, esophageal devascularization and transection operations and long-term beta-blockade or nitrates.

LIVER TRANSPLANTATION

The only definitive treatment for patients

with portal hypertension and end-stage liver disease is liver transplantation (Chapter 27). This not only cures the liver disease but also eradicates the portal hypertension and improves survival dramatically in these patients. All Child's B and C patients should be considered for liver transplantation after their first variceal bleed, although only very few will ultimately be subjected to transplantation because of contraindications and lack of organ availability. Child's A patients generally have a better prognosis and sclerotherapy or other conservative methods are preferred for long-term control of bleeding. Patients who are likely transplant candidates should initially be treated by sclerotherapy or transvenous intrahepatic portal systemic stent-shunt (TIPSS) since major surgery, particularly portacaval shunting involving the hepatic hilum, may make subsequent transplant surgery more difficult.

SCLEROTHERAPY

Various trials have indicated that approximately 25% of patients will never bleed again, but long-term intervention is required to prevent re-bleeding in the remaining 75%. Repeated sclerotherapy is preferred as it is less invasive than surgery, does not induce hepatic encephalopathy, has a relatively low procedure-related mortality, does not adversely affect liver function and is effective in eradicating esophageal varices and preventing re-bleeding in the majority of patients. Following initial control of bleeding, sclerotherapy is performed at weekly intervals until varices are eradicated, unless prevented by complications such as local slough.

The University of Cape Town group has recently published the 10-year results of long-term sclerotherapy in 304 consecutive patients, with 245 patients being available for assessment. Eradication of varices was achieved in 92% of patients who survived for longer than 3 months. Varices remained eradicated in 70% with a mean follow-up of 19 months. Recurrent variceal bleeding after the first admission only occurred in 17% of patients. Survival was dependent on Child's grading and the etiology of the liver disease, with little difference between alcoholic and non-alcoholic patients and between Child's B and C patients. Thus sclerotherapy usually eradicates esophageal varices and bleeding is significantly diminished. However, it is not certain that this improves survival, particularly if the best available treatment is used to manage subsequent acute variceal bleeding.

Because sclerotherapy does not correct the portal hypertension, varices tend to recur following initial eradication, necessitating life-long surveillance, and possibly pharmacological therapy, to prevent recurrent bleeds. Following initial eradication, a further endoscopy should be performed at 3 months to check that the diagnosis of eradication was correct. Thereafter, 6-monthly or yearly endoscopy should be performed and recurrent varices treated with the identical sclerotherapy regimen until eradication is achieved again.

ENDOSCOPIC VARICEAL LIGATION

Esophageal variceal ligation or banding was devized by Stiegmann of Denver. A modified endoscope pre-loaded with an elastic rubber band is passed through an over tube onto the varix to be banded and after suctioning the varix into the tip of the endoscope, the rubber band is slipped over the tissue bolus causing subsequent necrosis and a superficial ulceration of the varix. The endoscope is removed and reloaded for each varix requiring banding.

Banding has been shown, in four controlled trials, to be effective in controlling variceal bleeding and to have fewer treatment-related complications than sclerotherapy. It may become the treatment of choice for endoscopic management of varices. The combination of variceal ligation with simultaneous low volume sclerotherapy may result in more rapid eradication of varices than either technique alone. The major disadvantages include the need to repeatedly withdraw and re-insert the endoscope for each ligation, trauma to the esophagus due to pinching of the esophageal wall in the gap between the over tube and the endoscope, and engorgement of the distal esophageal varices due to the insertion of the over tube. Complications related directly to elastic banding are remarkably few although bleeding from the ulcer site has been recorded. Ulcers after banding are generally shallower than those after sclerotherapy and are re-epithelialized more quickly.

In summary, endoscopic variceal ligation may be superior to injection sclerotherapy in the management of both acute variceal bleeding as well as the long-term eradication of varices, either alone or in combination with low-volume sclerotherapy, but the technique is still under evaluation and requires confirmation of the promising early controlled data.

PORTACAVAL SHUNTS

Transvenous intrahepatic portal systemic stent-shunt (TIPSS)

The recently described radiological placement of an intrahepatic shunt may have significant advantages over invasive surgical techniques in managing patients with recurrent variceal bleeds. Transjugular intrahepatic portal systemic shunting is performed by cannulating a hepatic vein via the jugular route and creating a tract through the liver parenchyma, from hepatic to portal vein, using a needle under ultrasound and fluoroscopic guidance. The tract is then catheterized, dilated and an expandable metal stent placed, preventing its collapse and maintaining shunt patency over a

prolonged period. Obstructed shunts may be re-expanded and thus long-term patency may remain high. Technical success rate for the procedure is excellent and hemodynamic effects are similar to those seen in surgical shunt procedures, without the attendant morbidity and mortality associated with surgery. It may be the preferred procedure for patients who could undergo subsequent liver transplantation, as it does not disturb the surgical field, although migration to the inferior vena cava (IVC) may occasionally cause a fibrotic reaction making removal of the recipient organ difficult. Preliminary reports indicate that TIPSS is highly effective at stopping acute variceal hemorrhage (>95%) as a salvage procedure if sclerotherapy and beta-blockers have failed to control recurrent variceal bleeds, and to control bleeding from gastric varices and congestive gastropathy after failure of standard medical therapy. However, because encephalopathy occurs in up to 25% of cases, and up to 50% of shunts may occlude by 1 year, its primary role may be as a bridge to liver transplantation. Long-term trial results are awaited to determine its efficacy, safety and effect on mortality. The main complications are listed in Table 14.2.

Surgical portal systemic shunts

Of the various surgical portacaval shunts, the distal splenorenal shunt described by Warren is the most widely used. In their controlled trial which compared the Warren shunt with sclerotherapy, the originators of the technique found that early sclerotherapy was preferable to shunting. However, in the sclerotherapy group, the 30% of failures needed to be salvaged with a Warren shunt.

Failure of sclerotherapy is defined as either repeated severe variceal bleeds or varices that are difficult to eradicate. Such patients should be subjected to either a portal systemic shunt or a devascularization and transection proce-

Table 14.2 Complications of transvenous intrahepatic portal systemic stent-shunt (TIPPS)

Early complications
Intra-abdominal hemorrhage (perforation of hepatic capsule)
Hepatic encephalopathy
Hemobilia
Sepsis
Shunt infection
Shunt occlusion
Portal vein thrombosis
Cardiac failure
Electrolyte disturbance
Stent migration
Hemolysis

Long-term complications
Hepatic encephalopathy
Sepsis
Shunt occlusion
Vena-caval fibrosis
Stenosis of hepatic vein proximal to shunt

dure. Where a shunt is performed, the TIPSS has become popular but proof of its superiority over other techniques is awaited. Where the technique is not available, most groups prefer the distal splenorenal shunt, although in alcoholic patients a standard portacaval shunt appears to produce good results.

PROPHYLACTIC MANAGEMENT

Prevention of the first bleed

Options for prophylactic management include pharmacological prevention (using beta-blockers, nitrates, and possibly diuretics), sclerotherapy, shunts or devascularization and transection operations. The natural history in patients with varices that have not bled indicates that 20–40% of those with varices will bleed at up to 5 years' follow-up. Bleeding varices are a marker for severe liver disease and hemorrhage is often not the primary cause of death in these patients, i.e. there are competing causes for death which

are not altered by preventing variceal hemorrhage. There are no good markers for those at particular risk of bleeding (Table 14.3), so high-risk patients are difficult to identify to allow their specific targeting for prophylactic therapy.

However, evidence from numerous trials has indicated that beta-adrenergic antagonists are of proven efficacy in preventing first and recurrent variceal bleeds in patients with portal hypertension and varices. We believe that major surgery is unjustified in prophylaxis. In the multiple trials comparing prophylactic sclerotherapy with conservative management there have been conflicting results and conclusions. However, there are problems in that sclerotherapy may precipitate bleeding in a patient who has never bled before and this may be associated with mortality.

Pharmacological prevention of first variceal bleed

A review of nine placebo-controlled trials for the prevention of the first bleed in patients with cirrhosis and esophageal varices indicates

Table 14.3 Factors associated with increased risk for first variceal hemorrhage

Clinical factors
Child's B/C patients
Interval after diagnosis of varices (those who will bleed do so in first 12 months)
Ascites
Rate of progression of disease

Endoscopic factors
Large varices
Cherry red or hematocystic spots
Red weal markings
Associated concomitant fundic varices

Hemodynamic factors
Hepatic venous pressure gradient >12 mmHg
High portal and intravariceal pressure

that beta-adrenergic antagonists reduced the incidence of initial bleeding in compliant patients. Between 0–46% of the patients in these trials were in Child's C category, more than 70% had alcoholic liver disease; in four studies the varices were large, while in five studies both small and large varices were studied. The non-selective beta-adrenergic antagonists propranolol (40–300 mg/day) (seven studies) or nadolol (two studies) were used in doses sufficient to reduce heart rate by 25%. Bleeding occurred in only 0–18% and 6–26% of the beta-blocked group at 1 and 2 years respectively, but in 12–30% and 5–61% in the placebo group at 1 and 2 years. One study showed significantly increased survival at 2 years. Three meta-analyses showed that beta-adrenergic antagonists significantly reduced the risk of initial gastrointestinal bleeding and of fatal hemorrhage in patients with cirrhosis and esophageal varices, while mortality was found to be decreased in one meta-analysis based on individual data. Side effects, mainly dizziness (3%), Raynaud's phenomenon (2%), hepatic encephalopathy (<2%) requiring withdrawal of therapy, occurred in approximately 5% of patients. Resuscitation after bleeding was not compromised in any of these studies.

In conclusion, non-selective beta-adrenergic antagonists are of proven efficacy in preventing the initial variceal hemorrhage in selected patients with cirrhosis and varices, and may reduce fatal bleeds and improve survival in compliant patients. Although a variety of other pharmacological agents have been studied, beta-blockers are currently the only agents of proven value in the prevention of first variceal hemorrhage.

Pharmacological prevention of recurrent variceal hemorrhage

Twelve trials have studied the use of beta-blockers in the prevention of recurrent variceal hemorrhage or bleeding from portal hypertensive gastropathy, with 2 years' follow-up in patients with cirrhosis. A further two studies have included patients with cirrhosis, idiopathic portal hypertension and schistosomiasis. The risk of re-bleeding varied between 33% and 76% at 1 year, and between 50% and 87% at 2 years in the placebo groups. In contrast, patients receiving beta-blockers had a risk of re-bleeding at 1 year of 10–71% and at 2 years of 21–72%. Moreover, a significant reduction was found in the risk of recurrent hemorrhage from portal hypertensive gastropathy. Two meta-analyses confirmed that the use of beta-blockers reduced the risk of re-bleeding at 2 years by 20% compared to placebo, and a significant difference in mortality was found in one of these studies. Beta-blockers were ineffective in reducing re-bleed rates in patients who developed hepatocellular carcinoma, were not compliant, had no reduction in heart rate and did not abstain from alcohol. It has been shown that the combination of endoscopic sclerotherapy with beta-blockade is more effective in preventing recurrent gastrointestinal hemorrhage than either form of therapy alone. Beta-blockers were well tolerated in studies of prevention of recurrent hemorrhage.

CONCLUSIONS

Sclerotherapy remains the procedure of choice in the acute management of bleeding varices and should be performed at the earliest opportunity, preferably at the initial emergency endoscopy. Subsequently, long-term sclerotherapy combined with the use of beta-blockers, in doses sufficient to reduce heart rate by approximately 25%, and endoscopic surveillance are required to maintain eradication of varices. Variceal banding procedures may supplant sclerotherapy as this procedure is more effective in variceal eradication and may cause fewer mucosal and esophageal motility problems. Failure of sclerotherapy with beta-blockade is best managed by insertion of a shunt or an esophageal transection and devascularization procedure. Liver transplantation should be considered in all Child's B or C patients presenting with variceal hemorrhage as this is the only management that significantly improves prognosis. Prophylactic therapy with beta-blockers is indicated in patients with cirrhosis and portal hypertension with varices.

RECOMMENDED READING

Bornman, P.C., Terblanche, J., Kahn, D. *et al.* (1986) Limitations of multiple injection sclerotherapy sessions for acute variceal bleeding. *S Afr Med J*, **70**, 34–6.

Burroughs, A.K., Hamilton, G., Phillips, A. *et al.* (1989) A comparison of sclerotherapy with staple transection of the esophagus for the emergency control of bleeding from esophageal varices. *N Engl J Med*, **321**, 857–62.

Conn, H.O. (1993) Transjugular intra-hepatic portal systemic shunts: state of the art. *Hepatology*, **17**, 148–58.

Hayes, P.C., Davis, J.M., Lewis, J.A. and Bouchier, I.A.D. (1990) Meta-analysis of value of propranolol in prevention of variceal haemorrhage. *Lancet*, **336**, 153–6.

Kahn, D., Bornman, P.C. and Terblanche, J. (1989) A 10-year prospective evaluation of balloon tube tamponade and emergency injection sclerotherapy for actively bleeding esophageal varices. *HPB Surg*, **1**, 207–19.

Lebrec D. (1993) Pharmacologic prevention of variceal bleeding and rebleeding. J *Hepatology*, **17** (suppl 2), S29-S33.

McCormick, P.A., Dick, R., Chin, J. *et al.* (1993) Transjugular intrahepatic portal systemic stent-shunt. *Br J Hosp Med*, **49**(11), 791–8.

Pagliaro, L., D'Amico, M.D., Thorkild, I. *et al.* (1992) Prevention of first bleeding in cirrhosis. A meta-analysis of randomized trials of nonsurgical treatment. *Ann Int Med*, **117**, 59–70.

Shields, R. (ed.) (1992) Portal Hypertension. *Ballière's Clinical Gastroenterology*, **6**(3), 425–634.

Terblanche, J. (1989) The surgeon's role in the management of portal hypertension. *Ann Surg*, **209**, 381–95.

Terblanche, J., Burroughs, A.K. and Hobbs, K.E.F. (1989) Controversies in the management of bleeding esophageal varices. *N Engl J Med*, **320**, 1393–8, 1469–75.

Terblanche, J., Kahn, D. and Bornman, P.C. (1989) Long-term injection sclerotherapy treatment for esophageal varices. A 10-year prospective evaluation. *Ann Surg*, **210**, 725–31.

Terblanche, J., Krige, J.E.J. and Bornman, P.C. (1990) Endoscopic sclerotherapy. *Surg Clin North Am*, **70**, 341–59.

The North Italian Endoscopic Club for the Study and Treatment of Esophageal Varices (1988) Prediction of the first variceal hemorrhage in patients with cirrhosis of the liver and esophageal varices: a prospective multicenter study. *N Engl J Med*, **319**, 983–9.

van Stiegmann, G. (1993) Endoscopic ligation: now and the future (editorial). *Gastrointest Endosc*, **39**(2), 203–5.

van Stiegmann, G.V. and Goff, J.S. (1988) Endoscopic oesophageal varic ligation (EVL): preliminary clinical experience. *Gastrointest Endosc*, **34**, 105–8.

15

Vascular disorders of the liver

SIMON ROBSON, RICHARD HIFT and IAN BOUCHIER

ANATOMY OF THE HEPATIC BLOOD SUPPLY

The liver has a dual circulation. It receives low-pressure venous blood via the portal vein and high-pressure arterial input from the hepatic artery. The terminal portal vein branches open into the hepatic sinusoids where flow is unidirectional from the periportal to centrilobular hepatocytes (Fig. 15.1).

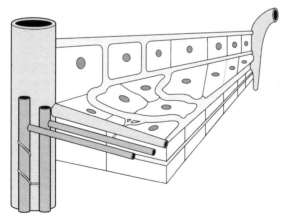

Figure 15.1 Diagramatic representation of microcirculation of liver and sinusoidal blood flow. Note arterial twigs to bile ductule.

The microcirculation of the liver is specialized for the uptake and modification of nutrients and to allow hepatocytes free access to plasma. Sinusoids possess a fenestrated endothelial barrier with no distinct basement membrane: this facilitates the exchange of nutrients and metabolites between the incoming blood and hepatocytes via the space of Disse. From the central veins of the liver, blood flows into the three main hepatic veins. These lie within the incissurae which divide the liver into four functional segments, and each receives a portal pedicle (Fig. 15.2).

The common hepatic artery usually arises from the celiac axis together with the left gastric and splenic arteries. Variant arrangements are common. In most cases the hepatic artery enters the porta hepatis with the portal vein and common bile duct and divides into right and left branches. The hepatic arteries give rise to the portal tract capillaries to form an arteriolar plexus around the bile ducts (Fig. 15.1).

The hepatic artery supplies up to 35% of the hepatic blood flow. Hepatic artery blood flow will increase should portal venous inflow decrease for any reason. The reverse does not hold true as portal flow cannot

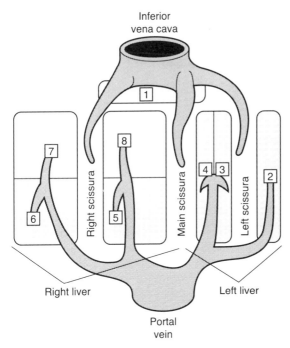

Inferior
vena cava

Right scissura

Main scissura

Left scissura

Right liver

Left liver

Portal
vein

Figure 15.2 Diagramatic representation of hepatic and portal veins. Three hepatic veins which lie within the incissivae divide the liver into four functional segments, each of which receives a portal pedicle. Venous outflow from the caudate loop (segment 1) drains directly into the inferior vena cava.

increase where hepatic arterial input is reduced. Similarly, the portal circulation does not adapt to increases in hepatic venous pressure. The latter has important consequences in the setting of heart failure and hepatic venous outflow obstruction which result in rapidly developing portal hypertension. Humans lack resistance sphincters in the three hepatic veins draining into the inferior vena, which might otherwise regulate efferent blood flow under pathological conditions. Indeed, the hepatic microcirculation appears extremely sensitive to small increases in pressure in the hepatic venous outflow, which result in increased intrasinusoidal pressures and enhanced fluid filtration

through the fenestrated endothelial barrier, rapidly leading to increased interstitial tissue pressures and increased rates of liver lymph flow. Where transcapsular filtration of fluid exceeds clearance by diaphragmatic and other mesenteric lymphatics, ascites will develop (Chapter 16).

HEPATIC EFFECTS OF SYSTEMIC CIRCULATORY DISTURBANCES

CIRCULATORY FAILURE

Systemic hypotension and shock may give rise to acute liver injury, sometimes known as ischemic hepatitis. Mild cases present with cholestatic jaundice and a minor rise in transaminases, while more severe cases may manifest deep jaundice, very high transaminase levels – measuring in the thousands – and may progress to fulminant hepatic failure with encephalopathy. In contrast to the kidney, where renal failure is commonly encountered following episodes of shock or hypotension, clinically apparent hepatic ischemic injury is relatively rare. The risk is however increased in the presence of elevated right atrial pressure from pre-existing cardiac disease, where the decreased hepatic inflow is compounded by reduced drainage because of high inferior vena caval and hepatic venous pressures. Such circumstances are commonly encountered in patients with valvular lesions who develop a tachyarrhythmia, patients with pericardial tamponade, or those undergoing cardiac surgery. Shock and ischemic necrosis should always be considered in the differential diagnosis of unexplained hepatitis or hepatic failure in such patients. The liver lesion is potentially reversible and must not be seen as a contraindication to treatment of the cardiac lesion even when this involves surgery in a patient with fulminant hepatic failure with all the associated complications.

159

PASSIVE VENOUS CONGESTION

Venous congestion with impaired drainage via the hepatic veins is encountered in severe congestive heart failure and constrictive pericarditis. The Budd–Chiari syndrome, where drainage is impaired as a result of obstruction of the hepatic veins themselves is discussed later in this chapter. The liver is commonly enlarged in uncontrolled heart failure, and acute distension may lead to a tender hepatomegaly. Biochemical abnormalities are not uncommon and usually include features of cholestasis and a slight rise in transaminases. Severe, chronic hepatic congestion can lead to the development of fibrosis and ultimately cardiac cirrhosis, an outcome that is now rare in developed countries as a result of improved treatment of heart failure.

ABNORMALITIES OF THE HEPATIC ARTERIES

HEPATIC ARTERIAL OCCLUSION

Occlusion of the arterial circulation will result in hepatic infarction when the onset is sufficiently rapid to preclude the development of adequate collaterals, or where the artery is obstructed proximally, before the origins of the right gastric and gastroduodenal vessels. Pre-existing disturbances of the portal circulation or a low cardiac output will potentiate liver ischemia and increase the risk of death even with incomplete occlusions.

Liver infarction usually follows surgical ligation or radiological intervention with embolization. Hepatic artery occlusion currently arises most frequently in liver transplant recipients. Other causes of spontaneous occlusion of the hepatic artery include widespread atherosclerosis, polyarteritis nodosa, embolization as in infective endocarditis and encasement of vessels by tumors at the hepatic hilum. Myeloproliferative disorders, the prolonged use of oral contraceptives, the anti-

phospholipid syndrome with or without other features of systemic lupus erythematosus and other thrombophilic conditions may also result in spontaneous hepatic infarction.

Patients may present with right upper quadrant pain. Complete occlusions are usually followed by shock and fulminant liver failure. The diagnosis may be suggested by computed tomography (CT), ultrasonography with Doppler or isotope scanning of the liver (Chapter 4). Angiography or surgical exploration will confirm the diagnosis and delineate the extent of obstruction.

Though fulminant hepatic failure is the usual outcome of complete arterial obstruction, incomplete occlusion is often tolerated, particularly in young children. Incomplete obstruction or obstruction with compensating collaterals may present as biliary strictures, giving rise to the radiographic appearance of sclerosing cholangitis, with anastomotic aneurysms or, in liver transplant recipients, as a delayed bile leak with the development of fistulae, recurrent bacteremia or fungemia.

HEPATIC ARTERY ANEURYSMS

Such aneurysms are rare. They may complicate trauma, neoplasia or vascular disease. The condition is usually silent until complicated by rupture. Extrahepatic aneurysms will present with intraperitoneal hemorrhage, while a ruptured intrahepatic aneurysm may present with hemobilia, jaundice and abdominal pain. Treatment of extrahepatic aneurysms is by ligation or resection and reconstruction. Intrahepatic aneurysms may be effectively managed in some cases by selective transcatheter embolization.

ARTERIOPORTAL FISTULAE

These may arise where an aneurysm ruptures into the portal venous system, or following blunt trauma or iatrogenic misadventure, including liver biopsy. They may also arise in neoplastic disease, particularly hepatocellular carcinoma. Patients with this condition may be asymptomatic or present with a rapid onset of features of portal hypertension. An arterial bruit is often audible and the diagnosis can be confirmed by angiography.

ABNORMALITIES OF THE EXTRAHEPATIC PORTAL VEIN AND ITS TRIBUTARIES

EXTRAHEPATIC PORTAL VENOUS THROMBOSIS (PVT)

This is the most common cause of portal hypertension in many parts of the developing world. With schistosomiasis, it accounts for most cases of pre-sinusoidal portal hypertension. It most commonly occurs in children and adolescents but may present for the first time in later life. Occasionally a history of omphalitis or umbilical vein catheterization in infancy will suggest a cause for the thrombosis. However, most cases in children are idiopathic. The association with umbilical sepsis has been questioned and a developmental origin for portal vein obstruction has been postulated. It is also possible that episodes of severe diarrhea, dehydration, and portal pyemia in early infancy or childhood predispose to the condition. In contrast, in adult-onset PVT in the Western world, a cause may be established in up to 50% of cases. The more common etiological factors include intra-abdominal sepsis, trauma, pancreatitis, malignancy, pregnancy or oral contraceptive use, as well as the numerous medical conditions favoring thrombophilia such as the anti-phospholipid syndrome, anti-thrombin III or protein C deficiency and the myeloproliferative disorders. It has been suggested that latent myeloproliferative disorders are a significant factor underlying idiopathic PVT. This is unproven and in any

event appears to have little clinical or prognostic significance.

PVT occasionally occurs as a complication of end-stage cirrhosis, where it may be an agonal event precipitating further increases in portal hypertension with variceal bleeding. It may also complicate hepatocellular carcinoma or operations on the portal venous system, such as splenectomy, particularly in the setting of liver disease and portal hypertension.

PVT rarely presents acutely; when it does, the diagnosis may be suggested by unexplained abdominal distension, ileus and even intestinal infarction. Following orthotopic liver transplantation, early portal venous obstruction may be suggested by the development of coagulopathy in an otherwise stable patient. However, most cases present with established portal hypertension, ascites, splenomegaly and variceal bleeding. Variceal hemorrhage in these patients is usually well tolerated as hepatic synthetic function is normal and the patients are usually young individuals who are otherwise fit. Typically biochemical indices of liver function, such as the plasma albumin and prothrombin time, are normal. Interestingly, many of these patients demonstrate systemic hemodynamic, hemostatic and immunological abnormalities comparable to those seen in cirrhosis, suggesting that some of the abnormalities seen in cirrhosis are features of portosystemic shunting *per se* rather than of hepatocellular dysfunction.

The diagnosis may be suggested by ultrasound, with failure to visualize the portal vein or when collateral vascular channels, so-called cavernous transformation, are demonstrated. Doppler ultrasound is diagnostic and will reveal an absence of flow in the region of the portal vein. Angiography may be used to confirm the diagnosis in selected cases. Splenoportography, though diagnostic, is seldom used because of the risk of hemorrhage (Chapter 4).

Treatment is largely directed at control of variceal bleeding and ascites. Variceal bleeding is treated similarly to that associated with cirrhosis. The prognosis of these patients is favorable but is balanced by the fact that this condition is more frequently seen in geographical areas where sophisticated follow-up and procedures are limited. Therapeutic options for the long-term control of bleeding are controversial. They include endoscopic sclerotherapy or ligation and splenorenal shunts. The latter can only be performed where the splenic vein is patent, and patents may be predisposed to thrombosis of the surgical shunt because of underlying thrombophilia or abnormal flow conditions.

Pharmacological therapy with beta-blockers has not been adequately explored in this condition but evidence from animal models of prehepatic portal hypertension suggest that this option may have clinical benefit.

We have noted an increased incidence of significant bacterial infections and tuberculosis in the patients with PVT, perhaps as a result of immunological abnormalities and poor nutritional status secondary to spontaneous portosystemic shunting. In contrast with cirrhotic patients, however, the long-term prognosis of patients with PVT is more favorable since hepatocellular function is essentially normal. Variceal bleeding may even remit spontaneously as a result of the development of spontaneous portosystemic collaterals.

SPLENIC VEIN THROMBOSIS

Splenic vein thrombosis may occur independently or in association with portal vein occlusion. Where the portal vein is patent, it is important to recognize the condition, as splenectomy may cure the portal hypertension. Gastrointestinal bleeding is commonly from gastric varices since the left coronary vein

may drain the esophageal plexus adequately, preventing the development of esophageal varices. The main causes of isolated splenic vein thrombosis include chronic pancreatitis, pancreatic carcinoma, renal cell carcinoma and retroperitoneal fibrosis.

CONGENITAL ABNORMALITIES OF THE PORTAL VEIN

Before birth, umbilical venous blood from the placenta largely bypasses the hepatic sinusoids via the ductus venosus which leads directly to the inferior vena cava. Following birth, the fibrosis which leads to the obliteration of the umbilical vein may extend and result in portal vein stenosis. This condition may present as prehepatic portal hypertension. Associated congenital cardiac defects or other circulatory anomalies may be present.

COMPRESSION OF THE PORTAL VEIN

Partial nodular transformation of the liver, hepatic adenomas or retroperitoneal fibrosis may result in extrinsic compression of the portal vein with portal hypertension. These are uncommon disorders.

HEPATIC VENOUS OUTFLOW OBSTRUCTION

Post-sinusoidal portal hypertension may occur when the venous drainage of a region of the hepatic parenchyma corresponding to two or three hepatic veins is obstructed. This portal hypertension is associated with a decrease in sinusoidal blood flow and the development of centrilobular congestion with liver injury and ischemia. As the caudate lobe drains directly to the inferior vena cava (Fig. 15.2), it tends to undergo compensatory hypertrophy where the hepatic veins are obstructed.

The etiological factors may be conveniently

classified by the site and mechanism of obstruction according to Valla and Benhamou (1991) and include: thrombogenic conditions of the main hepatic veins, malignant invasion of the hepatic veins and vena cava, compression of hepatic veins, lesions of the vena cava and the intrahepatic lesions of the veno-occlusive disorders.

EXTRAHEPATIC VENOUS OBSTRUCTION

The most common cause of hepatic venous outflow obstruction, the Budd–Chiari syndrome, follows obstruction of the hepatic veins. The etiological factors are similar to those resulting in portal vein thrombosis. Although myeloproliferative disorders are commoner in older males, they appear to be complicated by hepatic vein thrombosis more frequently in women under the age of 40. Paroxysmal nocturnal hemoglobinuria (PNH), congenital or acquired abnormalities of the coagulation and fibrinolytic systems, oral contraceptives and pregnancy have all been linked to the Budd–Chiari syndrome. In some parts of the world, up to 50% of cases are considered idiopathic.

Primary lesions of the inferior vena cava include the entity termed membranous obstruction of the inferior vena cava which is more frequent in southern Africa than in other parts of the world. Hepatocellular carcinoma has been associated with this condition, but a causal relationship has not been proven.

Veno-occlusive disorders of the liver are characterized by initial injury to intrahepatic veins with subsequent thrombosis. Eventually the main hepatic veins may be involved as the thrombotic process extends distally. This disease is classically seen following bone marrow transplantation, cytotoxic drug administration and hepatic irradiation. Predisposing factors include repeated bone marrow grafts and the presence of viral hepatitis with liver injury prior to conditioning for bone marrow grafting.

Anti-neoplastic or immunosuppressive drugs have been implicated in the development of veno-occlusive disease. Azathioprine may cause centrilobular liver injury in cardiac, renal or liver transplant recipients, usually after months of continuous administration. Alcoholic liver disease may be associated with hepatic venous injury and perivenular thrombosis with centrilobular sclerosis. Pyrrolizidine alkaloids from heliotropes or senecio plant species used as herbal remedies may result in acute or chronic forms of veno-occlusive disease depending upon the levels and tempo of administration. The diagnosis should be suspected in the correct clinical context as described above.

Acute Budd–Chiari syndrome presents with intense right upper quadrant pain, tender hepatomegaly, elevated transaminases and ascites. In contrast to most other forms of portal hypertension, the ascitic fluid usually resembles an exudate, with a high protein content. The picture may progress to one of fulminant or sub-fulminant liver failure with circulatory shock, the rapid accumulation of ascites, variceal bleeding and encephalopathy. With the development of collateral vessels, ischemia is usually averted and the picture is that of severe portal hypertension. A mortality of 50% is quoted, death commonly being secondary to fulminant liver failure. Complete recovery can occur but progression to hepatic fibrosis and even cirrhosis has been noted.

CT and magnetic resonance imaging (MRI) scanning are often suggestive though not always diagnostic for the Budd–Chiari syndrome. Filling defects may be shown in the inferior vena cava (IVC) or hepatic veins. Patchy changes in the hepatic parenchyma and an enlarged caudate lobe may be seen. Failure to demonstrate a flow signal in the hepatic veins on Doppler ultrasound is diagnostic. Venous angiography, showing obstruction of the IVC or a failure to demonstrate or cannulate the hepatic veins is highly suggestive (Chapter 4). Liver biopsy shows a characteristic picture of centrilobular congestion. Veno-occlusive disorders are diagnosed by demonstrating the typical histological venous lesions in the presence of patent main hepatic veins.

Treatment is largely supportive. Any underlying procoagulant disorder, such as thrombophilia, the anti-phospholipid syndrome or myeloproliferative state, should be treated and corrected as far as possible. Fibrinolytic therapy is controversial but may be considered for the acute clinical presentation. Anticoagulation with heparin and warfarin is usually introduced and should be continued long term. Because of the liver injury, patients may be unduly sensitive to warfarin therapy and may develop coagulopathy. Ascites is managed in the usual fashion (Chapter 16). Ascites is refractory in up to one-half of cases; hence shunting procedures or transplantation are often considered. With the establishment of a surgical portosystemic shunt, the portal vein is transformed into an outflow tract. With caudate lobe hypertrophy and consequent compression of the inferior vena cava or pre-existing caval thrombosis, a mesoatrial interposition graft, which effectively bypasses the vena cava, is the recommended option. Liver transplantation should be considered for patients where shunting has failed, and is often the only option in patients with the chronic forms of hepatic venous outflow tract obstruction and established cirrhosis. A further reason for considering transplantation is the long-term risk of hepatocellular carcinoma in the Budd–Chiari syndrome. Shunt surgery, by prolonging survival, may allow this to develop.

RECOMMENDED READING

Cardin, F., Graffeo, M., McCormick, P.A. *et al.* (1992) Adult 'idiopathic' extrahepatic venous thrombosis. Importance of putative 'latent' myeloproliferative disorders and comparison with cases of known aetiology. *Dig Dis Sci*, **37**(3), 335–9.

Cohen, J., Edelman, R.R. and Chopra, S. (1992) Portal vein thrombosis: a review. *Am J Med*, **92**(2), 173–82.

Jaskiewicz, K. and Robson, S.C. (1991) Noncirrhotic portal hypertension. *S Afr Med J*, **79**, 268–70.

Kahn, D., Krige, J., Robson, S.C. *et al.* (1994) A 15 year experience with injection sclerotherapy in patients with extrahepatic portal vein thrombosis. *Ann Surg*, **219**, 34–9.

Robson, S.C., Kahn, D., Kruskal, J. *et al.* (1993) Disordered hemostasis in extrahepatic portal hypertension. *Hepatology*, **18**, 853–7.

Scrobohaci, M.L., Drovet, L., Monem-Margi, A. *et al.* (1991) Liver veno-occlusive disease after bone marrow transplantation: changes in coagulation parameters and endothelial markers. *Thromb Res*, **63**(5), 509–19.

Valla, D. and Benhamou, J.P. (1991) Disorders of the Hepatic Veins, in *Oxford Textbook of Clinical Hepatology* (eds N. McIntyre, J.P. Berhanou, J. Bircher, M. Rizzetto and J. Rodes), vol. 2, Oxford University Press, Oxford, pp. 995–1012.

Vidal-Vanaclocha, F., Rocha, M.A., Asumendi, A. and Barbera-Guillem, E. (1993) Role of periportal and perivenous sinusoidal endothelial cells in hepatic homing of blood and metastatic cancer cells. *Semin Liver Dis*, **13**, 60-71.

16

Ascites

MICHAEL VOIGT and LAWRENCE BLENDIS

INTRODUCTION

Cirrhotic ascites results from excess renal sodium and water retention associated with sinusoidal portal hypertension and disordered systemic and splanchnic hemodynamics. The development of ascites is a sign of moderate to severe liver disease and may be the forerunner of renal failure; it indicates a limited prognosis. However, because aggressive therapy may be dangerous, with up to 10% of cirrhotic patients dying from iatrogenic complications, treatment should always be approached cautiously. Appropriate management requires an accurate etiological diagnosis, exclusion of complications such as tuberculous or spontaneous bacterial peritonitis and the rational use of salt restriction and diuretics. This chapter will deal with the etiology of ascites, its pathogenesis, clinical and radiological features, the investigation of patients with ascites and finally its stepwise management at home and in hospital.

ETIOLOGY AND EPIDEMIOLOGY

Cirrhosis, malignant disease, tuberculous peritonitis (in Africa and the Indian sub-continent) and cardiac failure are the commonest causes of ascites. The etiology varies geographically. Chronic hepatitis B, tuberculous peritonitis and hypoproteinemic states are more common in underdeveloped countries, while alcoholic and hepatitis C-related cirrhosis and malignancy predominate in developed communities.

PATHOGENESIS

The formation of ascites in liver disease is usually associated with both sinusoidal portal hypertension and systemic splanchnic and renal hemodynamic changes.

The peripheral vasodilation model of ascites formation is most consistent with the abnormalities observed in the early and intermediate stages of ascites formation. The 'underfill' theory of ascites formation, which states that sodium retention is initiated by loss of fluid from the vascular space into the peritoneal cavity due to portal hypertension, is inconsistent with the observations that plasma volume is increased in cirrhosis and that sodium retention precedes ascites formation. The 'overflow' theory, which states that vascular overfill initiates ascites formation, is also not consistent with the findings that the renin–angiotensin, sympathetic nervous system and other markers of volume depletion are hyperstimulated and are not suppressed, as should be the case if the overfill theory were correct.

Current evidence suggests that the initiating event in ascites formation is peripheral vasodilation which occurs early in the course of liver disease causing relative underfilling of the circulatory system (Chapter 14). This leads to baroreceptor-mediated stimulation of the renin–angiotensin and sympathetic nervous system and altered renal pressure natriuresis which cause sodium retention and volume expansion. The intravascular volume is re-established but the combination of peripheral vasodilation and volume expansion with increased venous return causes increased cardiac output, which may aggravate portal hypertension (forward flow theory). Facts supporting this model are that sodium retention has consistently been shown to occur before the onset of ascites in animal models of liver disease. In addition, recent studies have shown that this sodium retention follows vasodilation, which occurs within hours of the onset of portal hypertension or surgically created portal systemic shunting. The cause of the peripheral vasodilation remains speculative. Sodium retention ceases and renin–angiotensin–aldosterone and sympathetic nervous system activity return to normal in the compensated phase of cirrhosis. It is unclear why some patients subsequently decompensate with further sodium retention and ascites formation, but there have been suggestions from a variety of animal models that liver function has to deteriorate below a certain threshold (as measured for instance by aminopyrine clearance) for this to occur.

ANTI-NATRIURETIC MECHANISMS

Sodium retention, the primary abnormality in ascites formation, is not due to reduced glomerular filtration rate (GFR), which is normal in most patients with ascites. It thus follows that sodium retention must result from increased tubular re-absorption, which is influenced by tubular hydrostatic and oncotic pressure and several local and humoral factors including the renin–angiotensin–aldosterone system (RAAS), sympathetic nervous system (SNS), atrial natriuretic factor, brain natriuretic peptide and natriuretic hormone, which modulate transepithelial transport of sodium. While the RAAS is normal in compensated cirrhosis, levels are usually markedly raised in patients with ascites. Sodium retention, as shown by urinary sodium excretion, correlates closely with the degree of hyperaldosteronism and is relieved by aldosterone antagonists; there is a close chronological correlation of RAAS activation with sodium retention in experimental models of cirrhosis. The sympathetic nervous system activity is also markedly increased in ascitic patients, and may contribute to sodium retention by altering renal hemodynamics and its effects on renin production.

THE HEPATORENAL SYNDROME

The hepatorenal syndrome (HRS) may be defined as acute oliguric renal failure resulting from intense intrarenal vasoconstriction in otherwise normal kidneys. It occurs in patients with advanced liver disease, usually with cirrhosis and ascites or acute liver failure; a clinical cause is often not found, treatment is usually ineffective and prognosis is poor (Table 16.1).

PATHOGENESIS

The pathogenesis is complex and poorly understood, but a variety of factors have been implicated. Systemic abnormalities implicated include central nervous system effects on the kidneys that are induced by hepatic encephalopathy or related metabolic disturbances, peripheral vascular dilation and volume

166

Table 16.1 Characteristic findings associated with hepatorenal syndrome

---

1. Patients usually have advanced cirrhosis or acute liver failure, are in hospital at the onset of hepatorenal syndrome, and a precipitating cause is seldom identified

2. Ascites (but not necessarily jaundice) is usually present

3. Hyponatremia is usual

4. Hepatic encephalophathy is commonly present

5. Blood pressure is reduced compared with previous pressures recorded in the patient

6. There is marked oliguria

7. Renal sodium concentration is very low (<10 mmol/l)

8. Urinary protein and casts are minimal or absent

---

depletion, diminished venous return due to raised intra-abdominal pressure and high levels of circulating endotoxin.

Neurohumoral abnormalities implicated include increased circulating catecholamines, increased renal sympathetic activity and high circulating levels of renin and angiotensin. Derangements of intrarenal vasoconstrictor and vasodilator balance include reduced production of renal vasodilators, such as kallikrein and prostaglandin E2 production, and increased production of renal vasoconstrictors especially renal Endothelin-1 and Endothelin-3. The role of many of these pathogenetic factors is controversial.

TREATMENT

The majority of patients with liver disease who develop azotemia will have pre-renal failure or acute tubular necrosis (ATN). The diagnosis of HRS is one of exclusion, and should never be made until all potentially reversible causes of renal failure have been excluded. The more common potentially reversible causes are listed in Table 16.2.

All patients suspected of having HRS should have intravenous colloid infusions in an attempt to exclude intravascular hypovolemia as a cause of pre-renal azotemia. Prostaglandin E1 (misoprostal) 400 mg four times daily coupled with albumin infusions may be effective in some patients. Perioneovenous shunting has been successful in rare patients in improving renal function. Liver transplantation, if otherwise appropriate and feasible, is the only truly effective therapy in these patients who have a very poor prognosis

MECHANICS OF CIRRHOTIC ASCITES FORMATION

In cirrhosis, ascitic fluid arises predominantly from the liver where increased hepatic sinusoidal pressure plus a low plasma oncotic pressure (due to decreased albumin concentration) result in fluid shifts to the extravascular space. The rate of extravasation exceeds the capacity of lymphatic drainage and fluid exudes through the liver capsule into the peritoneal cavity.

The hepatic sinusoids are unique in that there are large fenestrations in the endothelial lining which normally allow protein-rich fluid

Table 16.2 Common causes and precipitants of pre-renal azotemia and acute tubular necrosis in patients with liver disease

---

1. Sepsis: this common cause of impaired renal function may not manifest with fever or abnormally raised white cell count

2. Over diuresis or lactulose-induced diarrhea

3. Volume depletion due to vomiting, diarrhea or gastrointestinal blood loss

4. Use of non-steroidal anti-inflammatory drugs (NSAIDS) which may block vasodilatory renal prostaglandins

5. Electrolyte disturbance

6. Nephrotoxic drugs, especially aminoglycosides

7. Large-volume paracentesis without adequate intravenous colloid replacement

---

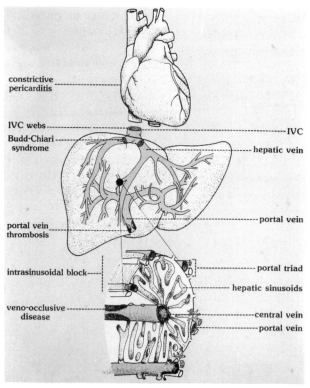

Figure 16.1 Schematic presentation of the sites of hepatic sinusoidal outflow obstruction which may lead to ascites formation.

into the space of Disse where it comes into contact with the sinusoidal surface of the hepatocytes (Fig. 16.1).

Pressure in the hepatic sinusoids is normally very low and extravascular fluid is efficiently removed by lymphatics. When sinusoidal outflow is obstructed, lymph flow increases linearly with intrasinusoidal hydrostatic pressure. In early cirrhosis, osmotic pressure has little effect on ascites formation because of the free flow of albumin through the large fenestrations. Thus the rate of fluid exudation is primarily dependent on sinusoidal pressure. It has been estimated that a 4 mmHg increase in sinusoidal pressure will cause a 14-fold increase in hepatic lymph flow. The fenestrations disappear as liver disease progresses (capillarization of the sinusoids), but low serum albumin and

increasing portal pressure maintain the imbalance in the Starling forces across the hepatic sinusoids, and hemodynamic changes in the splanchnic microcirculation impair the autoregulation of flow in this region.

Impaired sinusoidal outflow may be due to a variety of lesions involving the heart (congestive cardiac failure, pericardial tamponade or constriction), inferior vena cava (thrombosis, webs), hepatic veins (Budd–Chiari syndrome, veno-occlusive disease) and the hepatic parenchyma (cirrhosis) (Fig. 16. 1).

In contrast to the hepatic sinusoids, omental and intestinal capillaries are relatively impermeable to protein, and compensatory mechanisms such as increased oncotic pressure, pre-capillary vasoconstriction and post-capillary vasodilatation effectively protect against extravasation of fluid until the Starling forces are grossly disturbed by the combination of hypoalbuminemia, markedly raised portal pressure and impaired autoregulation found in cirrhosis. Thus pre-sinusoidal portal hypertension (schistosomiasis, portal vein thrombosis) is an uncommon cause of ascites.

NON-CIRRHOTIC ASCITES

The mechanism of ascites formation in diseases other than cirrhosis is less well studied. Understanding the pathogenesis of these forms of ascites is helpful in the interpretation of diagnostic tests and in guiding management. All forms of post-sinusoidal portal hypertension, including veno-occlusive disease, Budd–Chiari syndrome, inferior vena cava (IVC) thrombosis and webs, constrictive pericarditis and right heart failure have in common a marked increase in sinusoidal hydrostatic pressure which, together with the initially high permeability of the hepatic sinusoids, leads to extravasation of fluid from the liver. This fluid may be protein-rich and create diagnostic difficulty. A variety of different mechanisms may contribute to malignant ascites formation including lymphatic obstruction, cytokine-mediated permeability changes in peritoneal and splanchnic capillaries, raised portal pressure due to hepatic infiltration, and, in adenocarcinomas, secretion of mucinous fluid by the tumor. Lymphatic disruption, particularly due to lymphoma, irradiation, trauma or surgical mishap, gives rise to chylous ascites, with leakage of triglyceride-rich chyle into the peritoneum. Pancreatic ascites usually occurs when a pancreatic duct is disrupted and pancreatic fluid leaks into the peritoneal cavity.

CLINICAL FEATURES

Cirrhotic ascites develops in patients with advanced liver disease. Thus the overwhelming majority of these patients have stigmata of chronic liver disease including jaundice, spider angiomata, ecchymoses, white nails, clubbing, palmar erythema, Dupuytren's contractures, parotomegaly, muscle wasting, gynecomastia and testicular atrophy (Chapter 1). Edema is often present. The liver, if palpable, is often firm to hard and splenomegaly, which is suggestive of portal hypertension, is present in many patients. Tense ascites may preclude assessment of liver and spleen size and consistency. The presence of ascites, suggested by abdominal distension, flank fullness and dullness, is best confirmed by demonstrating shifting dullness and by ultrasonic examination which is extremely useful in cases where there is doubt about the presence of fluid. Patients with ascites often complain of flatulent discomfort and may experience mild dyspnea. Pleural effusions and basal atalectasis are not uncommonly seen on chest radiographs, and lung functions tests may reveal restricted lung volumes which improve following large-volume paracentesis. Abdominal distension is due to dilated bowel as well as accumulation of fluid. Examination of the abdomen frequently reveals dilated superficial veins draining outwards from the umbilicus, but caput medusae and umbilical venous hum (Cruvelier–Baumgarten syndrome) are rare. Although tense ascites may be associated with an elevated jugular venous pressure (JVP), cardiac causes of ascites must be excluded in these cases.

APPROACH TO MANAGEMENT OF THE PATIENT WITH ASCITES

DIAGNOSIS

The two objectives of the diagnostic work-up are firstly to diagnose the primary cause of the ascites and secondly to establish whether any complications are present.

Diagnosis is based on a thorough clinical evaluation and a diagnostic paracentesis. All patients with newly diagnosed ascites, and all patients with pre-existing ascites who have any clinical deterioration, should have a diagnostic paracentesis. Infective complications may give few classical signs in the chronically ill and are easily missed.

CLINICAL EVALUATION

In the absence of typical features of hepatic disease other causes of the ascites should be sought. Cardiac failure causing ascites will usually manifest with tricuspid incompetence causing large 'cv' waves in the neck veins, an enlarged heart, abnormal apex beat, murmurs and added sounds, while constrictive pericarditis and restrictive cardiomyopathy may cause markedly raised jugular venous pressures with rapid 'y' descents. IVC obstruction usually manifests with dilated collaterals over the back and lateral chest wall with large azygous veins on chest X-ray. Tuberculous ascites should be suspected in patients with AIDS and in areas of high TB prevalence, where it is responsible for up to 20% of cases of ascites. In adults it occurs more frequently in alcoholics and manifests as a chronic wasting illness, with fever, night sweats, weight loss, abdominal pain and a doughy abdomen. While these features may suggest the diagnosis, they are frequently absent, especially where cirrhotic ascites was present prior to the onset of tuberculosis infection. Malignant ascites has protean clinical manifestations which depend on the primary site, but weight loss and constitutional symptoms with an enlarged hard nodular liver or other abdominal masses may be present.

DIAGNOSTIC PARACENTESIS

TECHNIQUE

Prior to paracentesis the International Normalized Ratio (INR) should be measured and, if necessary, corrected using vitamin K or, where appropriate, fresh-frozen plasma. Platelet numbers and function should also be assessed. Ascitic tap should be done under ultrasound guidance if there is less than 4 cm shifting dullness or if the ascites is difficult to assess because of obesity. Paracentesis is performed using full sterile technique, preferably after correction of significant coagulation disturbance. The bladder is emptied and patients are placed in a semi-recumbent position. After the skin has been cleaned and anesthetized, a standard 3.8 cm, 22-gauge metal needle (for obese patients longer 22-gauge needles may be used) is inserted into the abdominal wall over an area of maximal dullness. Usually this is below the umbilicus in the left iliac fossa, but the right side or the midline may be used. Care must be taken to avoid surgical scars (as bowel may be adherent) and dilated veins. The skin is pulled downwards during needle insertion so that the tract through the abdominal wall is acutely angled and seals spontaneously, preventing subsequent leakage (the so-called Z-technique). Approximately 100 ml of fluid should be withdrawn for diagnostic purposes. The procedure is safe and ascitic fluid leaks and infection are rare complications.

FLUID ANALYSIS

The following ascitic fluid studies are essential and should be performed expeditiously.

White cell count

A white cell total and differential count must be performed on every patient. Ideally this should be done in a laboratory by appropriately experienced staff, but if this is not immediately available, the clinician should perform a cell count using a white cell counting chamber. It has been clearly shown that the neutrophil count is the most sensitive method for detecting bacterial peritonitis (which is frequently clinically occult). Ascites is derived from hepatic and peritoneal lymph and should not contain neutrophils. A neutrophil count of 0.025×10^9 cells/l (250 cells/ml) is highly suggestive of peritonitis, while neutrophil cell counts of $0.05 \times 10^9/l$ (500 cells/ml) are 90–95% specific for spontaneous bacterial peritonitis (SBP). The white cell count is the most sensitive method of detecting spontaneous peritonitis and a count of greater than $0.025 \times 10^9/l$ (250 cells/ml) associated with a negative culture (called culture-negative neutrocytic ascites) is indistinguishable from culture-positive SBP with regard to patient profile, symptoms, response to antibiotics, mortality and prognostic importance.

Failure to perform the white count in sufficient time may result in the diagnosis of SBP being missed or delayed as the clinical features of peritoneal infection, e.g. peritonitonism, fever, rebound tenderness and guarding are frequently absent. Delay in instituting antibiotic therapy may result in death. A marked lymphocytosis is highly specific for tuberculosis, although it is fairly insensitive.

Fluid culture

A 5 ml sample of ascitic fluid should immediately be inoculated into each of the aerobic and anaerobic blood culture bottles. This system improves the pick-up rate of ascitic fluid bacterial infections from less than 50% (not using blood culture bottles) to approximately 95% (Runyon, Canawati and Akriviadis, 1988). Direct, bedside inoculation of fluid into double-strength Kirschner (DSK) culture medium improves the bacteriological culture yield for *M. tuberculosis* by at least 30%, and is cheaper than the BACTEC radiometric mycobacterial culture system. Two aliquots each of 5 ml should be placed in DSK bottles. Conventional Ziehl–Neelsen stains

should also be requested. A separate 10 ml sterile bottle should be used for this.

Biochemistry

The biochemical investigation of ascitic fluid should always include the following.

Serum ascites albumin gradient (SAAG)

A SAAG of greater than 11 g/l is the best test for distinguishing hypertensive (transudative) from exudative processes. A serum–ascites albumin difference of less than 11 g/l usually indicates an exudative process while that of more than 11 g/l suggests a transudative process. An ascites : serum albumin ratio of 0.8 is both less sensitive and less specific than the serum–ascites albumin difference. The ascites : serum total protein ratio of 0.5 has poor diagnostic accuracy. Prolonged treatment with diuretics results in a greater loss of fluid than protein from the abdominal cavity and may increase the ascites albumin concentration. The use of ascitic fluid total protein has poor discriminatory value in distinguishing a transudative ascites from an exudative process, although ascites total protein concentration below 15 g/l indicates that those patients have an increased risk of developing SBP. Ascites lactate dehydrogenase (LDH) levels have little diagnostic value and should not be measured.

Adenosine deaminase (ADA)

This is a highly sensitive and specific and inexpensive test for the presence of tuberculosis. ADA activity should be measured on every patient since alcoholics have an increased incidence of tuberculous peritonitis and there is an increasing incidence of extrapulmonary TB related to AIDS. Patients who develop tuberculous peritonitis frequently have underlying liver disease and the presence of pre-existing cirrhotic ascites does not exclude this complication.

Amylase

Amylase should be measured when pancreatic ascites is suspected. The amylase activity is usually more than 10 times normal and the ascites : serum amylase ratio is greater than 1 in pancreatic ascites.

Ascites triglyceride levels should be measured if ascitic fluid is turbid or milky to distinguish chylous from pseudochylous ascites, where turbidity is due to malignant or inflammatory cells. Chylous ascites has triglyceride levels >2.5 mmol/l (200 mg/dl) but usually levels are >11 mmol/l (1000 mg/dl). Fat globules may be demonstrated on microscopy using Sudan stains.

Other tests such as ascites electrolytes, total protein, pH and LDH have very little discriminatory diagnostic value, are not cost-effective and should thus not be performed. Similarly, while raised ascites fibronectin and cholesterol levels may help distinguish carcinomatosis from chronic liver disease, this distinction rarely poses a clinical problem as the clinical presentation and progression of the diseases differ, and these tests are too non-specific to assist clinical management or to assess prognosis.

Cytology

A 5 ml sample of ascitic fluid should be mixed with 5 ml of 50% alcohol for cytology. Cytological yield may be as high as 73–95% for peritoneal carcinomatosis.

TUBERCULOUS ASCITES

The most useful test for tuberculous ascites is the adenosine deaminase (ADA) activity of the ascitic fluid. ADA is an enzyme released by peritoneal mononuclear cells which are recruited in response to TB infection. Activity of greater than 33 IU/ml is approximately 98% sensitive and specific for TB peritonitis. The ascites lymphocyte count is only raised in approximately 70% of cases, and raised ascites and serum : ascites ratios of protein, LDH and reduced glucose concentrations are insensitive and non-specific tests. If the ascites ADA activity is raised in a patient with typical clinical features and a raised lymphocyte count and albumin concentration, treatment for tuberculosis may be started. However, if atypical features are present, a mini-laparotomy or laparoscopy should be done. An unexpectedly raised ADA should always prompt a diligent search for tuberculosis. Laparotomy or laparoscopy is performed where there is doubt and should always include biopsy and culture as visual diagnosis is less than 70% specific.

SPONTANEOUS BACTERIAL PERITONITIS (SBP)

SBP and its variants, culture-negative neutrocytic ascites (negative ascitic cultures but raised neutrophil count) and bacterial ascites (positive ascitic culture but neutrophil count below 250 cells/ml) occur in approximately 10–25% of patients admitted with ascites. This condition is easily missed if appropriate tests are not done. Although patients with cirrhotic ascites are most frequently affected, SBP occurs also in ascites due to the nephrotic syndrome, malignancy, the Budd–Chiari syndrome, etc. This is usually a monomicrobial, blood-borne, spontaneous infection of the peritoneum and must be distinguished from the secondary peritonitis that arises from an intra-abdominal source. The latter is usually a polymicrobial infection and generally requires surgical treatment. Secondary peritonitis is associated with more florid signs and high (usually polymicrobial) bacterial loads. The ascites protein is often more than

10 g/l (unlike SBP where it is usually less than 10 g/l), ascitic : serum glucose concentration is less than 50%, LDH concentration is often higher than normal, the Gram stain is frequently positive (which is unusual in SBP), the neutrophil count often does not decrease with treatment and cultures frequently remain positive despite antibiotic therapy.

Prevalence

Between 10% and 25% of patients admitted to hospital with ascites are found to have SBP on admission and an additional 10–15% may develop it in the course of their hospital stay. Thus SBP should be actively sought with every new episode of clinical deterioration in patients with cirrhotic ascites, even while in hospital.

Clinical features

The typical patient has advanced liver disease. Indeed, only one-quarter to one-third of patients with SBP survive 1 year after the event. Patients usually have voluminous ascites, but SBP may occur in small volumes of ascites. The serum albumin is usually less than 30 g/l and there may be evidence of renal impairment and of severe portal hypertension.

Typical clinical features of SBP are given in Table 16.3. These features may be misleading as fever, pain, rebound and guarding are frequently absent and, when present, may be mild. Clinical deterioration, especially hepatic encephalopathy, diarrhea, gastrointestinal hemorrhage or constipation may be the only indication of SBP and should prompt an evaluation for peritoneal infection.

The organisms responsible are most commonly *E. coli* or streptococci. Anaerobic infections are uncommon while polymicrobial infections occur in 10% of cases (Table 16.4).

Table 16.3 Characteristics of subjects susceptible to spontaneous bacterial peritonitis

Severe liver disease
Large volume of ascites
Serum albumin <30 g/l
Ascites albumin <10 g/l
Creatinine >130 µmol/l
Varices and severe portal hypertension

Table 16.4 Microbiology of spontaneous bacterial peritonitis

Organism	Proportion of cases (%)
E. coli	43
Streptococcus pneumoniae	8
Streptococcus A, B, D	18
Klebsiella	8
Enterobacteriaceae	2
Staphylococcus	2
Polymicrobial*	10
Other	9

* Consider secondary peritonitis

Diagnosis

An ascitic fluid polymorphonuclear count greater than 0.05×10^9/l (500 cells/ml) has 90% sensitivity and 98% specificity in diagnosing SBP. Over 90% of these patients have counts in excess of 1000 cells/ml. A presumptive diagnosis of SBP should be made and treatment initiated with broad-spectrum intravenous antibiotics in all patients with:

1. An ascitic fluid polymorphonuclear count $>0.05 \times 10^9$/l (500 cells/ml);
2. A polymorphonuclear count $>0.025 \times 10^9$/l (250 cells/ml) plus a compatible clinical picture (i.e. exclusion of other causes of neutrophilic ascites, e.g. carcinomatosis, pancreatitis, penetrating peptic ulcer, etc.

Ascitic fluid levels and ascitic fluid-to-blood gradients of pH lactate, glucose, albumin and cholesterol are non-specific findings and have insufficient diagnostic accuracy in SBP but, if grossly abnormal, may indicate secondary peritonitis or severe infection.

A repeat tap at 24 hours will show a diminishing neutrophil count if the appropriate antibiotic is being used. The majority of cases will yield a positive culture, provided appropriate culture techniques are used.

Culture technique

The bacterial count in ascites is often very low (1 per 1 ml of fluid) and conventional culture techniques are negative in half to two-thirds of cases. A 10 ml sample of fluid inoculated into aerobic and anaerobic blood culture bottles yields a positive culture in 93% of patients with SBP. Standard culture techniques, direct inoculation into broth and centrifugation of large volumes all have very poor sensitivities (approximately 50%). Blood cultures should be performed simultaneously as greater than 50% of patients will have a positive culture.

Treatment is best guided by the knowledge of the organism. Aminoglycosides should be avoided because of their markedly increased renal toxicity in these patients. Amoxil/clavulanic acid has been shown to be an effective and relatively inexpensive treatment.

Prevention of SBP

Patients with SBP are at markedly increased risk of repeated infections. Low-dose oral therapy with quinolone antibiotics (ofloxacin) reduce bacterial translocation from the gut and hence reduce the risk of recurrent peritonitis. Most authorities recommend their use as prophylaxis against SBP (ofloxacin 200–250 mg/day), but this practice has not been shown

to improve mortality when compared with treatment of infections as these occur. The risk of SBP and the cost of hospitalization must be weighed against the cost of long-term antibiotics and the potential for inducing antibiotic resistance.

TREATMENT OF UNCOMPLICATED CIRRHOTIC ASCITES

A sequentially increasing intensity of treatment is given, aimed at creating a negative balance between sodium intake and excretion. Only 500–1000 ml of ascitic fluid can be reabsorbed into the vascular compartment in 24 hours. Thus any extra loss in non-edematous patients will result in depletion of intravascular volume and may result in hypotension, encephalopathy and further renal impairment. Most patients with mild to moderate ascites can be managed as outpatients. However, those with tense ascites, respiratory impairment, infection, renal impairment or hepatic encephalopathy, or refractory ascites should be admitted. Patient education and participation in therapeutic decision-making is important. We have found that most patients will purchase reasonably accurate bathroom scales and can be trained to adjust their medication according to their daily weights. Target losses, e.g. 0.5 kg/day, and a target weight, where ascites is asymptomatic, can be identified and achieved.

OUTPATIENT MANAGEMENT

Patients with mild to moderate ascites, normal renal function, serum electrolytes, and serum albumin, with no complications such as hepatic encephalopathy or gastrointestinal hemorrhage and a urine sodium excretion greater than 30 mmol/day respond well to therapy and do not require admission. A careful history may reveal a precipitating event, e.g. alcoholic binge, excess salt intake (such as salted meat, etc.), or a recent bleed or infection. Non-steroidal anti-inflammatory agents, alcohol-containing tonics or cough mixtures, and antibiotics or antacids containing salt may all be involved and should be stopped.

Sodium restriction

Many patients with ascites excrete less than 10 mmol of sodium per 24 hours. To achieve a negative sodium balance in these patients sodium intake would need to be severely restricted. In practice this is difficult and severe sodium restriction makes food unpalatable and may aggravate malnutrition. A knowledge of sodium balance is helpful in planning treatment of ascites. A urinary sodium excretion of less than 10 mmol/24 hours usually indicates that potent diuretic therapy will be required while excretion of more than 30 mmol/24 hours suggests that the patient may respond to sodium restriction alone. A relatively low salt diet (50–60 mmol/day) is practical to institute. Potassium salt ('No-salt') should generally be avoided especially if potassium-sparing diuretics are used, or renal impairment is present. Food should be prepared without adding salt. This includes meat tenderizers and onion, garlic and celery salts. Vegetable and meat extracts, all varieties of spreads (cheese, peanut butter, fish and meat spreads), cheeses, sauces (tomato, mayonnaise, Worcestershire), canned and pickled meats, instant soups and 'fast' foods contain excess salt and should be avoided. It is usually not necessary to use salt-poor bread, salt-free butter and margarine, or to avoid foods containing baking powder or baking soda.

Restricted fluids

Fluid intake should only be restricted if there is evidence of an inability to excrete a water load that manifests as dilutional hypona-

tremia. Mild restriction to approximately 500 ml more than insensible loss, i.e. approximately 1 litre in cold weather and 1.5 litres in hot weather, is usually adequate. Beverages containing caffeine, including coffee, tea and cola, should be avoided as patients with cirrhosis retain caffeine which activates the sympathetic nervous system and raises renin and aldosterone levels, thus stimulating sodium and fluid retention.

Diuretics

Approximately 10% of patients with ascites will respond to the above measures alone. Non-responders, and those who find sodium restriction difficult, require diuretic therapy. Aldosterone antagonists (spironolactone and potassium canrenoate) alone have been shown to be more effective than loop diuretics in non-azotemic subjects with ascites. Spironolactone is recommended as a first-line agent starting at doses of 100 mg/day and increasing (every 4–5 days to allow effects to manifest) to 400 mg daily. It is successful in up to 65% of patients, but high doses may cause gynecomastia, impotence and decreased libido, and spironolactone is also expensive. Amiloride may be substituted for spironolactone if necessary. Addition of a loop diuretic, e.g. furosemide (and more recently torasemide, which is more potent), achieves a response in approximately 85% of patients, and the 'spironolactone-sparing effect' of loop diuretics reduces the cost of medication. Not only is the combination of spironolactone with a loop diuretic more effective than the administration of either alone, but electrolyte disturbance and complications are diminished.

RESISTANT ASCITES

Resistant ascites may be defined as ascites that persists in the face of salt restriction plus maximum diuretic therapy, or where side effects (usually renal impairment, hepatic encephalopathy or hyperkalemia) preclude the use of adequate doses of diuretics. The 10–15% who fall into this group should be carefully re-examined for any complication such as SBP, hepatoma, renal failure, tuberculosis, etc. Compliance should be assessed and an initial period in hospital on the same treatment as prescribed outside is necessary. Bed rest may be beneficial. When patients with ascites assume the upright position there is marked activation of the renin–angiotensin and of the sympathetic nervous systems. Portal venous blood flow and renal perfusion are reduced and glomerular filtration diminished. These result in sodium retention and a diminished response to diuretics.

Salt-poor human albumin infusions, although still advocated by some, have not been subjected to clinical trials of efficacy in diuretic-resistant patients. It is our impression that it is expensive and any benefit is usually short-lived.

Therapeutic paracentesis

The primary indications for therapeutic paracentesis are failed diuretic therapy and the relief of tense or markedly symptomatic ascites. Use of large-volume paracentesis has also been shown to be a cost saving and safe method for treating hospitalized patients with severe ascites. Large-volume paracentesis should always be combined with the best medical therapy possible, because the procedure only provides temporary removal of fluid which rapidly recurs unless effective medical therapy is instituted.

Large-volume paracentesis has been evaluated in six randomized controlled trials to date. The following facts have emerged:

1. Repeated large-volume paracentesis (4–6 l/day) combined with intravenous albumin infusion (40 g after each tap) was more effective than diuretic therapy alone, significantly shortened hospital stay, and reduced complications. There were no differences in patient survival or the likelihood of re-admission in the paracentesis and diuretic groups. Single large volume paracenteses are safe, provided 6–8 g albumin are given for each litre of fluid removed.

2. Changes in plasma volume, cardiac output, renal function, serum sodium level and activation of sodium-retaining neurohumoral mechanisms occur following large-volume paracentesis if intravenous plasma volume expansion is not given. The abnormalities occur 12–24 hours after completion of the paracentesis and, contrary to previous wisdom, the presence of peripheral edema actually aggravates renal function and hyponatremia, rather than protecting against these complications. These complications of paracentesis are prevented by infusion of intravenous albumin.

3. As a cheaper alternative to albumin infusion, both Dextran 70 and Hemaccel prevented clinically significant hemodynamic deterioration (although significant neurohumoral activation occurred in subjects receiving Dextran 70). Dextran 40 was not effective as a plasma volume expander because the plasma contraction only occurs approximately 12 hours after paracentesis and the plasma expander must still be present in the circulation at this stage to prevent these volume changes. Dextran 40 is filtered and metabolized by then. A disadvantage of Hemaccel and Dextran 70 is that they do not replace protein in these malnourished patients, who lose considerable amounts of albumin with each tap. This is mainly a problem in patients requiring repeated taps.

4. When compared to peritoneovenous shunt in the management of refractory ascites,

patients receiving repeated paracentesis had a reduced duration of hospital stay, but re-admission occurred earlier and was more frequent. No differences in survival between the two groups were noted.

Technique

Full sterile technique is essential. A blunt needle with side holes, introduced with the aid of a trocar, is generally used to perform the paracentesis. Alter-natively, peritoneal dialysis catheter systems may be used as they have been shown to be safe (Wilcox, Woods and Mixon, 1992), and are widely available. Bowel perforation has not been reported and infective complications are extremely rare.

Peritoneovenous shunt

Peritoneovenous shunts (PVS) conduct ascitic fluid from the peritoneal cavity to the superior vena cava. PVS undoubtedly relieves ascites but there is a high rate of complications, including blockage, bacterial infections, especially staphylococcus, intravascular coagulopathy, pulmonary edema and gastrointestinal hemorrhage. Clinical trials have not shown any benefit in terms of survival using this form of treatment. Thus, use of PVS should be limited to a highly selected group of patients in whom the benefits might outweigh the risks.

RECOMMENDED READING

Garcia-Tsao, G., Conn, H.O., Lerner, E. *et al.* (1985) The diagnosis of bacterial peritonitis. Comparison of pH, lactate concentration and leukocyte count. *Hepatology,* **5**, 91–6.

Hoefs, J.C. (1990) Spontaneous bacterial peritonitis: prevention and therapy (editorial). *Hepatology,* **12**, 776–81

Hoefs, J.C. and Runyon, B.A. (1985) Spontaneous bacterial peritonitis. *Dis Month,* **31**, 1–48.

Levy, M. (1993) Hepatorenal syndrome. *Kidney Intl,* **43**, 737–53.

Moore, K., Wendon, J., Frazer, M. *et al.* (1992) Plasma endothelin immunoreactivity in liver disease and the hepatorenal syndrome. *N Engl J Med,* **327**(25), 774–8.

Naccarato, R., Messa, P., D'Angelo, A. *et al.* (1981) Renal handling of sodium and water in early chronic liver disease. *Gastroenterology,* **81**, 205–10.

Runyon, B.A., Canawati, H.N. and Akriviadis, E.A. (1988) Optimization of ascitic fluid culture technique. *Gastroenterology,* **95**, 1351–5.

Strang, G., Latouf, S., Commerford, P. *et al.* (1991) Bedside culture to confirm tuberculous pericarditis. *Lancet,* **338**, 1600–1.

Voigt, M.D., Kalvaria, I., Trey, C. *et al.* (1989) Diagnostic value of ascitic fluid adenosine deaminase in tuberculous peritonitis. *Lancet,* **i** (8641), 751–3.

Wilcox, C.M., Woods, B.L. and Mixon, H.T. (1992) Prospective evaluation of a peritoneal dialysis catheter system for large volume paracentesis. *Am J Gastroenterol,* **87**(10), 1443–46.

17

Gallstone disease

JAKE KRIGE

INTRODUCTION

The vast majority of diseases of the extrahepatic biliary system are associated with gallstones. Gallstone disease occurs in approximately 10% of the adult population in Western countries. The incidence of cholelithiasis increases progressively with age so that approximately one-third of people in their eighth decade of life have calculi. Gallstones associated with hemolytic anemia may occur in children. Biliary calculi develop about four times more frequently in women than in men, although with age the incidence in males approaches that of females.

A combination of environmental and genetic factors explains the varying prevalence of gallstones among different ethnic groups. A high prevalence of gallstones is seen in American Pima Indian women who secrete excessive amounts of cholesterol in their bile. Obesity, rapid weight reduction, prolonged bowel rest, hypertriglyceridemia, total parenteral nutrition and loss of terminal ileal function through disease or substantial resection are all associated with an increased incidence of gallstones. There is probably no increased risk of gallstones in hypercholes-

terolemia, diabetes or in women receiving oral contraceptives. Pigment gallstones occur more commonly in patients who have disorders of the hepatobiliary system, including chronic hepatocellular disease or infection and/or obstruction of large bile ducts. Pigment stones may also occur in patients with chronic hemolytic anemia.

PATHOGENESIS

In general, gallstones are classified as either cholesterol stones (composed primarily of cholesterol) or pigment stones (containing less than 25% cholesterol). Cholesterol stones are present in more than 75% of patients with cholelithiasis in Western countries. However, in some parts of the world such as Japan, two-thirds of gallstones are of the pigment type.

CHOLESTEROL GALLSTONES

The pathogenesis of cholesterol gallstones is related to an acquired or hereditary defect in the hepatic metabolism of lipids and bile acids. Increased activity of the hepatic microsomal enzyme 3-hydroxy-3-methylglutaryl-coenzyme-A (HMGCoA) reductase, rate-limiting for cholesterol synthesis and diminished activity of the hepatic microsomal enzyme cholesterol 7-alpha-hydroxylase, rate-limiting for bile acid synthesis, can lead to increased secretion of cholesterol and decreased secretion of bile acids respectively.

Under normal conditions and at normal rates of bile acid secretion, cholesterol is solubilized in mixed micelles which consist of lecithin and bile acids. At lower rates of bile acid secretion, as occur during fasting, cholesterol is transported primarily in lecithin vesicles. This constitutes an essential stage in the development of gallstones. The precipitation of cholesterol crystals is preceded by the conglomeration of cholesterol-rich vesicles. In the majority of patients, cholesterol supersaturated bile is the result of enhanced cholesterol secretion, while in some patients the major defect is a decrease in bile acid secretion.

Although cholesterol supersaturation is necessary for the development of cholesterol gallstones it can be present without gallstones being formed. Recent studies have identified nucleating and anti-nucleating proteins in human bile. These promote and antagonize cholesterol crystallization. Rapid crystal formation is due to the presence of nucleating proteins in the gallbladder. In addition, cholesterol gallstone production is related to the secretion of mucus in the gallbladder as well as to decreased gallbladder contractility. Mucus provides a matrix on which cholesterol crystals aggregate to form stones. Decreased contractility results in gallbladder stasis providing nucleation of cholesterol crystals.

PIGMENT STONES

Pigment stones represent less than a quarter of gallstones in most populations. As with cholesterol stones, the incidence of pigment stones increases with age. Intrahepatic gall-

stones and stones caused by stasis or cirrhosis are usually pigment stones. An increased incidence of pigment stones also occurs in hereditary spherocytosis and sickle cell anemia.

Dietary factors have been implicated in the pathogenesis of pigment stones. The incidence of pigment stones decreases among Japanese women taking a Western diet. Other factors, including parasites, especially *Ascaris lumbricoides*, have been detected in the pigment stones of Japanese patients.

In contrast to cholesterol stones, the mechanisms for the formation of pigment stones remain largely unproven. When compared to the bile from patients with cholesterol stones, the bile of patients with pigment stones generally contains less cholesterol but similar amounts of bile acid, phospholipid and total bilirubin. In the Far East, gallbladder bile is often infected (usually with *E. coli*) which liberates the enzyme beta-glucuronidase that deconjugates bilirubin mono- and diglucuronide to form unconjugated bilirubin. The latter combines with calcium to produce insoluble calcium bilirubinate stones. In contrast to patients in the Far East, the majority of patients in Western countries with chronic cholecystitis and cholelithiasis have sterile bile within the gallbladder. Here stasis appears to be a major factor in the formation of pigment stones, which suggests that incomplete emptying may lead to increased concentrations of bilirubin and calcium within the gallbladder, favoring the precipitation of sparingly soluble compounds.

NATURAL HISTORY

The widespread use of diagnostic ultrasonography has led to the discovery of an increasing number of silent gallstones during life. It is unknown why some gallstones become symptomatic and others do not. This may relate to a chance mechanical event depending upon the movement of stones and their impaction in Hartmann's pouch or the cystic duct or their passage into the common bile duct. The relative size of the stones and the caliber of the various components of the biliary tree may be important. The concept of stasis is considered relevant in the etiology of postoperative cholecystitis.

ASYMPTOMATIC GALLSTONES

The decision whether to perform a cholecystectomy for silent stones depends on a knowledge of the natural history of such stones and weighing the risks of expectant management against the hazards of surgery. Early studies all concluded in favor of cholecystectomy. However, in these studies, gallstones were initially detected at laparotomy for other conditions. Other studies which recommended prophylactic cholecystectomy in good risk surgical patients did not strictly consider asymptomatic patients at the outset.

Two subsequent major studies have strongly recommended the expectant management of silent gallstones. Gracie and Ransohoff (1982) in a study of 123 patients with asymptomatic stones found that only 18% became symptomatic during a follow-up period of 15 years. Their subjects were identified by cholecystographic screening of a healthy population. However, their study group, faculty members of the University of Michigan, comprised 110 men and 13 women, a male : female ratio substantially different to that of the usual gallstone population. The authors concluded that routine prophylactic surgery for silent gallstones in white American men was neither necessary nor advisable. More recently McSherry *et al.* (1985) followed 135 patients for a mean of 5 years and found that only 10% developed symptoms. They recommended expectant management for silent stones. Current evidence suggests that since the majority of patients remain asymptomatic, and given the low present-day mortality rate following prompt treatment of those who develop symptoms, elective cholecystectomy is not indicated in patients with asymptomatic gallbladder stones.

ACUTE CHOLECYSTITIS

In the vast majority of patients, acute cholecystitis is associated with gallstones and results from obstruction of the neck of the gallbladder or cystic duct due to gallstones impacted in Hartmann's pouch. Direct pressure of the calculus on the gallbladder mucosa results in ischemia, necrosis and ulceration with consequent edema and impairment of venous return. These processes in turn increase and aggravate the associated inflammation. If the stone becomes dislodged, the inflammatory process subsides rapidly. However, if the calculus remains impacted, the inflammation may progress to pressure necrosis of the gallbladder mucosa and wall with perforation and pericholecystic abscess formation, free perforation with generalized peritonitis or a combination of these events.

About 5% of patients with acute cholecystitis have no gallstones in their gallbladder. Acute acalculous cholecystitis tends to occur in critically ill and severely traumatized patients. Intravenous hyperalimentation, sepsis, hypotension, multiple blood transfusions, prolonged fasting and ventilatory support have been implicated as possible causative factors in the pathogenesis of acute acalculous cholecystitis. Impaired emptying secondary to hyperalimentation or protracted starvation with alterations in the enterohepatic circulation of bile salts may affect biliary lipid synthesis and contribute to the secretion of lithogenic bile supersaturated with cholesterol. Prolonged exposure of gallbladder mucosa to high concentrations of cholesterol or bile salts or both may result in mucosal inflammatory changes that progress to acute cholecystitis. Rarely acalculous cholecystitis may result from cystic artery occlusion or primary bacterial infection.

Several etiological factors are involved in the pathogenesis of acute calculous and acalculous cholecystitis. The combination of chemical irritants and cystic duct obstruction are responsible for the development of acute inflammation of the gallbladder in most cases. At the onset of acute cholecystitis in the majority of cases, the initial inflammation is chemical and no microorganisms are obtained on culture. However, with unresolved obstruction and progression of cholecystitis, most patients have a positive culture with a greater risk of perforation and spread of infection.

CLINICAL MANIFESTATIONS

The patient with acute cholecystitis usually presents with moderate to severe pain in the right upper quadrant or epigastrium which may radiate to the right infrascapular area. The patient is often febrile and vomiting may be pronounced. Tenderness, usually below the right costal margin, is often associated with rebound tenderness and guarding. A mass may be palpable in one-third of cases. Mild jaundice may be present and is related to calculi within Hartmann's pouch and edema encroaching upon the common duct.

Patients who develop suppurative complications, including empyema or localized pericholecystic abscess are toxic with fever, rigors and a marked leukocytosis. Rarely, patients with acute cholecystitis may present with septic shock and minimal abdominal tenderness. Progression of disease with transmural gangrenous changes and perforation of the gallbladder wall may result in either a localized pericholecystic collection or free perforation with generalized peritonitis.

DIFFERENTIAL DIAGNOSIS

In view of the common nature of gallstones in the Western world, radiological demonstration of gallstones, especially in suspected acute cholecystitis, does not necessarily imply that the acute pain is due to the gallstones. The clinical findings must substantiate the radiographical and biochemical changes before a confident clinical diagnosis can be made.

Other abdominal emergencies to be considered, especially when the pain remains diffuse, include perforated high retrocecal appendicitis and pancreatitis. Viral hepatitis, Fitz-Hugh–Curtis syndrome, and alcoholic-related liver disease should also be excluded. A pyogenic or amebic liver abscess or neoplasm may present with acute right upper quadrant pain indistinguishable from acute cholecystitis.

Calculi, infection or neoplasms in the urinary tract may be difficult to exclude without careful radiological investigation (Chapter 4).

Both pulmonary and cardiac disease may need to be excluded in some situations by X-ray and electrocardiogram. The right hemidiaphragm may not move freely on screening, and there may be fluid above the inflamed gallbladder mass on either side of the diaphragm.

LABORATORY TESTS

There is generally a neutrophil leukocytosis accompanied by minor elevations in liver function tests. Even in the absence of clinically apparent jaundice, the serum bilirubin, together with the transaminases, may be elevated. The presence of bile in the urine on testing is a useful pointer to disease of the biliary tract. A substantial increase in bilirubin and alkaline phosphatase levels indicates obstruction of the common duct. Mild elevation in serum amylase is consistent with uncomplicated cholecystitis, but higher values suggest acute pancreatitis. Biliary sepsis is a common cause of Gram-negative septicemia, especially in the elderly. Blood cultures should be obtained if pyrexia and toxicity are marked. Blood urea may be raised in such patients, who are at risk of developing renal failure.

RADIOLOGICAL DIAGNOSIS

Plain abdominal radiographs reveal calcified gallstones in 10% of patients (Chapter 4). Oral cholecystography and intravenous cholangiography have been supplanted by ultrasonography as the mainstay of diagnosis. Ultrasound is the method of choice for acute imaging of the gallbladder and biliary tree because it is readily available, non-invasive and may be easily repeated, but it is operator dependent. Accuracy is compromised in obese patients and in marked upper abdominal distension. Ultrasonic features suggestive of acute cholecystitis include the presence of stones, thick gallbladder wall with edema and pericholecystic fluid, and the ability to elicit an ultrasonically positive Murphy's sign. Non-visualization of the gallbladder due to overlying gas, especially in patients with acute disease, can be improved with careful real-time ultrasound.

Scintiscanning, using 99m technetium-labeled derivatives of iminodiacetic acid (HIDA, PIPIDA) and pyridoxylidine glutamate, is a simple technique with a specificity approaching 100%. These good results for scintigraphy rely on the fact that the cystic duct is blocked in acute cholecystitis.

SURGERY

Conflicting opinions persist concerning the management of acute cholecystitis with particular reference to optimal timing of surgical intervention. The initial management of acute cholecystitis has usually been conservative with intravenous fluids, antibiotics and analgesia. Emergency surgery is only indicated if perforation of a gallbladder appears imminent or is judged to have occurred. Following resolution of the acute episode and confirmation of the diagnosis on ultrasound, elective cholecystectomy is advised 6–12 weeks later. In the past decade, however, there has been a move towards early surgery for acute cholecystitis. This involves removal of the gallbladder on the next available operating list. Those in favor argue that the surgery may be performed with safety and relative ease. They maintain that with early surgery the duration of illness and the total period of hospitalization is reduced with a reduction in the cost of management. The advocates of the conservative delayed surgery approach argue that the diagnosis of acute cholecystitis is not infrequently in error and that early surgery may result in greater morbidity and possible mortality.

A number of clinical trials comparing early and delayed surgery have been reported and all have shown that, providing the surgeon is experienced, early operation may be performed with safety. Early surgery reduces the period of disability, duration of hospitalization and overall costs when compared with the more conservative approach.

If the diagnosis of acute cholecystitis has been demonstrated unequivocally on ultrasound and the patient presents within 3–5 days of the onset of symptoms, early operation is performed. Emergency cholecystectomy is seldom necessary except in the situation where clinical evidence of localized peritonitis and perforation are apparent or gallbladder perforation has been demonstrated on ultrasound. If the patient who initially is managed conservatively deteriorates with increasing local signs, surgical treatment is usually performed within 48 hours of admission. If a cholecystectomy has been planned but the inflammatory process is so marked that it compromises the dissection and display of the extrahepatic biliary system, a sub-total cholecystectomy is performed. Rarely, a cholecystostomy is necessary.

If the patient presents more than a week after the onset of symptoms and improves during the early stages of hospitalization, surgical intervention is usually deferred and an elective operation is planned 6–12 weeks later.

COMMON BILE DUCT STONES

The majority of common bile duct stones have their origin in the gallbladder and pass through the cystic duct into the common bile duct. Although more frequently encountered in the Far East, primary common bile duct stones are unusual in Western populations and are recognized by their light brown color and soft, friable consistency. The natural history of common duct stones is unpredictable. Stones in the common bile duct may remain asymptomatic for long periods of time but acute pancreatitis, cholangitis, obstructive jaundice, biliary strictures and choledochoduodenal fistulae may develop. Small stones may pass spontaneously to the duodenum without causing symptoms or may briefly obstruct the pancreatic duct, induce an episode of pancreatitis and then pass into the duodenum with relief of symptoms. If stones obstruct the common duct and the bile becomes infected, acute cholangitis ensues. The classic triad of fever, chills and jaundice leads to the suspicion of common duct stones. Hypotension and mental confusion in addition to the triad, confirms the presence of acute obstructive suppurative cholangitis. This is a medical emergency. Appropriate broad-spectrum antibiotic therapy (aminoglycoside, ampicillin and metronidazole) is given and followed by emergency biliary decompression. Ultrasonography (US) has evolved as the primary screening examination because of its reliability in demonstrating gallbladder stones and

detecting dilated bile ducts. Evidence of duct dilatation is almost always indicative of obstruction, but failure to detect dilated ducts on US does not exclude common duct stones.

Endoscopic retrograde cholangiopancreatography (ERCP) and endoscopic sphincterotomy (ES) have transformed the diagnostic and therapeutic approach to biliary disease in general and the treatment of bile duct stones in particular. Endoscopic sphincterotomy and extraction of stones achieves duct clearance in over 90% of patients (Fig. 17.1). Immediate post-sphincterotomy problems are bleeding (1%), pancreatitis (3%), cholangitis (5%) and retroperitoneal perforation (<1%). Extended ES done for large stones has an increased risk of perforation or bleeding. Local anatomical factors affecting endoscopic access may dictate therapy. Patients with esophageal strictures, pyloric stenosis, previous Polya gastrectomy or bile duct strictures are best treated surgically.

About 10% of patients undergoing routine cholecystectomy harbor common duct stones. If undetected or untreated, complications such as jaundice, cholangitis and pancreatitis may result. Operative cholangiography is therefore used to detect common duct stones during cholecystectomy. Optimal management of patients with common bile duct stones depends on the clinical presentation. In patients with symptomatic gallbladder stones and no clinical or laboratory evidence of common duct stones, laparoscopic cholecystectomy is recommended, accompanied by an operative cholangiogram. If stones are found in the common duct during a laparoscopic cholecystectomy, common duct exploration may be performed laparoscopically or ES and common duct clearance performed several days later. If the cholecystectomy is performed via laparotomy and stones are found on cholangiography, the common duct is explored, the stones removed and a T-tube is left in the duct. Post-operative

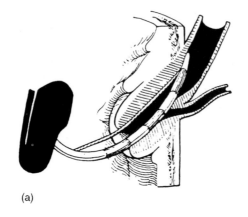

(a)

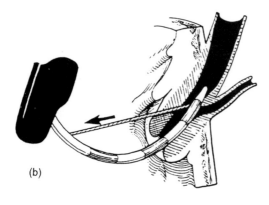

(b)

Figure 17.1 (a) Sphincterotome in position in the lower common bile duct. (b) Sphincterotomy performed by cutting the lower sphincter.

cholangiography is performed a week later to confirm complete duct clearance before removal of the T-tube.

In patients with symptomatic gallbladder stones suspected of having common duct stones because of jaundice, cholangitis or abnormal liver function tests, an ERCP is carried out to confirm or refute the presence of common bile duct (CBD) stones. If present, stones are extracted after ES. Cholecystectomy can then be performed without the need for CBD exploration.

Patients who have had a previous cholecystectomy and present with CBD stones are best managed by ES. When the risk of surgery is high, ES without cholecystectomy is acceptable treatment for common duct stones even when the gallbladder is still present. This procedure eliminates the common duct stones and controls symptoms in 90% of cases. Late gallbladder problems (principally colic) are uncommon (10%) and can be managed electively.

Large common bile duct stones (>2 cm) may be difficult to extract endoscopically, although improved methods of mechanical lithotripsy through the endoscope are now available. Dissolution of common duct stones has only a minor role, since extracorporeal shock-wave lithotripsy can fragment about 80% of stones that cannot be extracted by endoscopy.

GALLSTONE PANCREATITIS

Patients with gallstone pancreatitis characteristically have small cholesterol gallstones and a large patent cystic duct. Most such cases are relatively mild and subside without complications. Affected patients are allowed to recover and are then scheduled for laparoscopic cholecystectomy during the same hospital admission. If cholecystectomy is delayed for 1 or 2 months after resolution of biliary pancreatitis, there is a 60% chance of another attack, which may be severe.

ES is recommended early for severe biliary pancreatitis to allow impacted common duct stones to pass. There is good evidence that the outcome is improved with this procedure, but timing is the key to success. ES is indicated principally in patients whose clinical findings deteriorate 24 to 48 hours after admission or who have evidence of cholangitis or biliary obstruction. ES may also prevent recurrent attacks, and elderly or frail patients may be followed expectantly after ES without removing the gallbladder.

RECOMMENDED READING

Bateson, M.C. (1984) Progress in gallstone disease. *Br Med J*, **289**, 1163–4.

Bruckstein, A.H. (1990) Non-surgical management of cholelithiasis. *Arch Intern Med*, **150**, 960–4.

Finlayson, N. (1989) Cholecystectomy for gallstones. *Br Med J*, **298**, 133–4.

Gibney, E.J. (1990). Asymptomatic gallstones. *Br J Surg*, **77**, 368–72.

Gracie, W.A. and Ransohoff, D.F. (1982) The natural history of gallstones. The innocent gallstone is not a myth. *N Engl J Med*, **307**, 798–800.

McSherry, C.K., Ferstenberg, H., Calhoun, W.F. *et al.* (1985) The natural history of diagnosed gallstone disease in symptomatic and asymptomatic patients. *Ann Surg*, **202**, 59–63.

Salen, G. and Tint, G.S. (1989) Non-surgical treatment of gallstones. *N Engl J Med*, **320**, 665–6.

18

Amebic liver abscess

JAKE KRIGE, SUSAN ADAMS and AHMED SIMJEE

INTRODUCTION

Some 10% of the world's population are chronically infected with *Entamoeba histolytica*. Although *E. histolytica* often exists as a gut commensal it is responsible for approximately 50 million cases of invasive amebiasis with 100 000 deaths annually. Indeed, amebiasis constitutes the third leading parasitic cause of death, surpassed only by malaria and schisto-somiasis on a worldwide basis.

E. histolytica is ubiquitous with a worldwide distribution. The prevalence of infection varies widely, and is most frequently encountered in tropical and sub-tropical climates. Overcrowding and poor sanitation are the major environmental predisposing factors and the brunt of disease is borne by the poor and lower socioeconomic groups within developing nations. Host factors that increase susceptibility to the disease include malnutrition. Particularly severe infections may occur late in pregnancy and during the puerperium. Colonic invasion is more common in the presence of coexistent infection with *Trichuris trichiura*, intestinal schistosomiasis and *Shigella*. Before puberty there is an equal incidence of hepatic amebiasis in both sexes but after puberty the condition is three to 10 times more common in males.

PATHOGENESIS

Parasite transmission is via the fecal–oral route with the ingestion of protozoal cysts. Only the cystic form can resist destruction by gastric hydrochloric acid. The incubation period ranges from 2 days to 4 months, with a mean of 7 days. Excystation occurs in the alkaline medium of the small intestine where the cyst wall disintegrates. Motile trophozoites are released which migrate to the large bowel where pathogenic strains may cause invasive disease. Tissue invasion by *E. histolytica* is accomplished only by the *trophozoite*, the frequency of tissue invasion depending on the strain and virulence of the organism and the host resistance. Two enzymes in particular, hexokinase and phosphoglucomutase, appear to be markers for pathogenicity. Pathogenic strains are also able to evade complement-mediated lysis, which is a major host defense mechanism.

Invasion commences with trophozoite adherence to the colonic mucous blanket. This results in depletion and penetration of the mucus layer. Host-cell lysis follows allowing access to host tissues in the region of the interglandular epithelium. Adherence is mediated by a 170-kDa heavy sub-unit of a galactose and N-acetyl-D-galactosamine inhibitable lectin which has immunological similarity to human adherence receptors. Secretion of proteases by *E. histolytica* facilitates amebic penetration; however, killing of target cells only occurs upon direct contact. Invasion results in colonic ulceration accompanied by blood vessel engorgement, capillary proliferation and thrombosis. Following penetration, which in the early stage occurs without a substantial inflammatory response, the lesions produced by *E. histolytica* spread laterally and initially are confined to the colonic mucosa. With progressive enlargement, the muscularis mucosae is breached and further radial spread through non-resistant sub-mucosal tissue occurs. A typical early colonic mucosal lesion of amebiasis develops with the formation of flask-shaped ulcers. When the muscularis mucosae is penetrated and the sub-mucosa and muscularis are entered by invading trophozoites, the walls of mesenteric venules are penetrated and the amebae gain access to the portal venous system. Lymphatic spread does not appear to play a role in the pathogenesis of the disease.

Intestinal amebiasis is always a precursor of amebic liver abscess. However, liver involvement during an acute episode of intestinal amebiasis varies from 1–25%. Only a minority of patients with liver abscess have active intestinal disease. Some patients may have had recently proven amebiasis or may give a history of resolved diarrhea or dysentry. However, in the majority there is no clue about when the initial phase in the bowel occurred.

The right lobe of the liver is involved in 50–80% of cases, with most lesions developing near the dome. Multiple abscesses are present in 20–40% of cases. The lesions vary from pinpoint size to large masses replacing 80–90% of normal liver tissue. Men are affected more commonly than women. In children the majority of abscesses occur under the age of 3 years and liver involvement is more commonly associated with concurrent intestinal disease.

The cellular basis of amebic liver abscess has been studied experimentally in the hamster with inoculation of trophozoites directly into the portal venous system. Here, liver abscesses are produced by the accumulation and lysis of leukocytes and macrophages around the amebas.

IMMUNITY IN AMEBIASIS

No prospective trials have adequately determined whether patients cured of amebic liver abscess and colitis are resistant to subsequent tissue invasion. However, animals cured of invasive disease or immunized with whole parasite protein show resistance to further tissue invasion on re-challenge.

Within 1–2 weeks of onset of symptoms patients with amebiasis develop rising titers of antibody to the amebas. The specific antigens recognized by immune sera include the 170-kDa heavy sub-unit of the adherence lectin already mentioned and other parasitic glycoproteins. Patients cured of the disease almost all have antibody to the adherence lectin. Antibody to the lectin is able to inhibit adherance to colonic mucins and epithelial cells and inhibit parasite destruction of cell monolayers. Studies on serum from cured patients have demonstrated the presence, *in vitro*, of immunostimulatory factors. In contrast, serum from people with active disease may suppress certain immune response parameters. Finally, experimental evidence from our own studies suggests that there may be immunological similarity between certain amebic adhesive proteins and human integrins or cell adhesion

187

molecules. Its importance lies in the fact that 'autoantibodies' may be produced in invasive disease, binding to both amebic proteins and host immunocompetent cells. Since the long-term goal of much amebiasis research is to produce an effective vaccine, knowledge of the immunostimulatory and suppressive properties of candidate antigens as well as any similarities to human proteins is of considerable importance.

CLINICAL PRESENTATION

The duration of symptoms ranges from a few days to several weeks before presentation (Table 18.1). Pain is an almost invariable and prominent feature and its location is dependent on the position of the abscess in the liver. Thus 73% of patients have right upper quadrant pain, 28% right-sided chest pain, 9% radiation to the right shoulder (diaphragmatic lesion) and 21% epigastric pain. The latter should suggest the possibility of a left lobe abscess.

Fever is characteristically intermittent and associated with night sweats. In patients with gradual onset of symptoms, there may be marked weight loss, nausea and vomiting. Cough and dyspnea may be present and suggest diaphragmatic or lung involvement such as atelectasis, empyema or hepatobronchial fistula.

The physical findings in amebic liver abscess reflect the pathological process. The patient appears toxic, febrile and chronically ill. The liver is enlarged with varying degrees of tenderness. A point of maximum tenderness can often be detected, either in a lower right intercostal space or over the enlarged liver. Occasionally pressure from a right lobe abscess produces bulging of an intercostal space with exquisite localized tenderness to palpation. If the dome of the right lobe is involved, there is a corresponding elevation of the right diaphragm. Dullness to percus-

Table 18.1 Main clinical features in 400 consecutive admissions with amebic liver abscess (Adams and MacLeod, 1977)

Clinical feature	Proportion of cases (%)
Length of history	
0–2 weeks	59
2–4 weeks	20
4–12 weeks	16
>12 weeks	5
Symptoms	
Pain	99
Right hypochondrium	73
Right chest	28
Epigastrium	21
Right shoulder	9
Previous dysentery	19
Present diarrhea or dysentery	14
Cough	11
Dyspnea	4
Signs	
Tenderness right hypochondrium	85
Liver palpable and tender	80
Fever	75
Signs at right lung base	47
Localized intercostal tenderness	38
Epigastric tenderness	22
Localized swelling over liver	10

sion with diminished air entry at the right lung base is present due to the raised diaphragm or accumulation of pleural fluid.

DIAGNOSIS

In endemic areas, typical forms of the disease may be diagnosed clinically, but confirmation is important to exclude tumors, pyogenic abscess or secondarily infected hydatid cysts of the liver.

Common laboratory features include a significant leukocytosis with 70–80% polymorphs (eosinophilia is not a feature), a raised erythrocyte sedimentation rate and moderate anemia. In severe disease with multiple abscesses, elevated alkaline phosphatase and bilirubin levels may occasionally be found. However, even with a large amount of liver parenchymal destruction hepatic dysfunction is seldom a feature. Jaundice is an uncommon clinical finding.

Stool examination may reveal cysts or, in the case of dysentery, hematophagous trophozoites. The examination should be performed on warm, fresh stool as the trophozoites only remain active at room temperature for approximately 30 minutes. The yield in patients with amebic liver abscess is low since only a minority of patients will have concurrent intestinal disease.

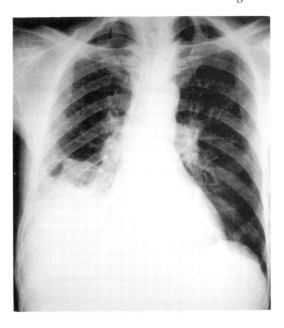

Figure 18.1 Right lower lobe pulmonary collapse consolidation due to underlying amebic liver abscess.

RADIOLOGY

Radiological imaging forms an essential part of the diagnosis (Chapter 4). A raised, poorly moving, right diaphragm is present in half to three-quarters of patients (Fig. 18.1). Atelectasis or pleural effusion at the right base are common. After rupture through the diaphragm, a pleural effusion, lung abscess, consolidation or, rarely, features of a bronchopleural or hepatopleural fistula, may be present; in such cases a fluid level may be seen in the hepatic abscess (Fig. 18.2). Radiological features of pericardial effusion are present if rupture complicates left lobe abscess. There may be features of a pleural effusion which in most cases represents a sterile sympathetic exudate.

The development of improved ultrasonography has facilitated the diagnosis and is the imaging modality of choice. Given the characteristic clinical picture ultrasound is usually the only imaging necessary. It is not, however, possible to distinguish confidently

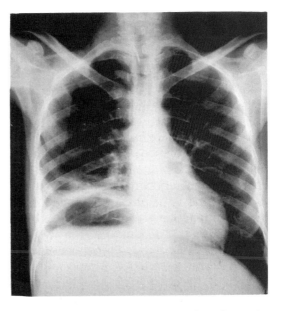

Figure 18.2 Air fluid level under the right diaphragm with adjacent lung changes.

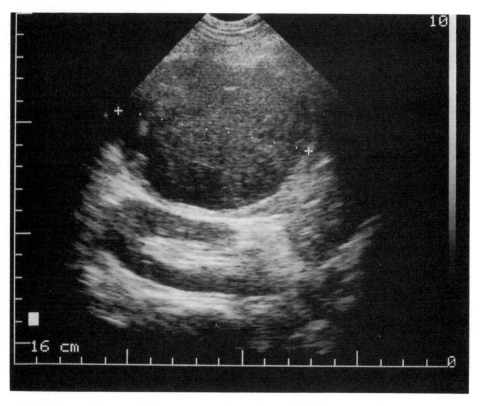

Figure 18.3 Oblique ultrasound view demonstrating a large right lobe amebic liver abscess with echogenic content. The crosses mark the diameter of the abscess.

amebic from pyogenic abscesses on ultrasound or computed tomography (CT) scans. Although abscesses can be distinguished from solid tumors it may not be possible to distinguish them accurately from other liver cysts. This distinction is important because hydatid cysts may also be common in areas where amebiasis is endemic, and uncontrolled aspiration of hydatid cysts may facilitate spread.

Ultrasound is helpful when aspiration is necessary for establishing the diagnosis or for treatment (Fig. 18.3). Ultrasound is also used to assess the response to therapy but may be misleading if used to monitor response to therapy in the short term. Amebic abscesses often remain static or appear initially to enlarge and take many months to resolve completely. Ultrasound has a diagnostic accu-

racy of 95% and is useful in showing the size and position of an abscess. CT also defines the position and extent, but the diagnostic yield is no better than ultrasound which is less expensive (Fig. 18.4).

SEROLOGICAL TESTS

Serological tests for amebiasis are of considerable value in diagnosis and are positive in over 90% of cases. Techniques include gel diffusion, latex agglutination, indirect hemagglutination, enzyme immunoassay, immunofluorescence and cellulose acetate precipitation. The indirect hemagglutination test is widely used for diagnosis. The purified antigen utilized makes it highly specific. The gel diffusion precipitation test is sensitive in invasive disease and

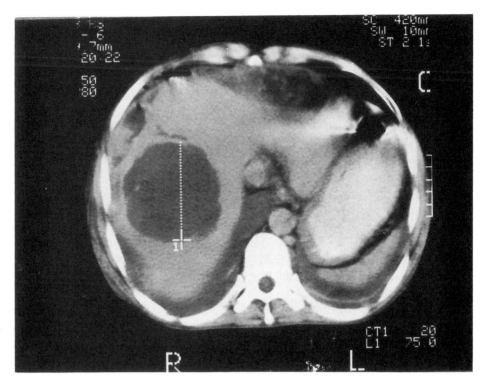

Figure 18.4 Computed tomagraphy scan showing large low-density right lobe amebic liver abscess with ascites. The dotted line indicates the diameter of the abscess.

will be positive in 96% of cases of liver abscess. However, 15–20% of the population in endemic areas have a positive test without any clinical evidence of active disease. It therefore has limited value in distinguishing current infection. The indirect fluorescent antibody test is both specific and sensitive and titers drop rapidly with successful treatment.

The most recently developed ELISA techniques detect specific IgM antibody directed to epitopes on the surface membrane of the ameba in current invasive disease. In comparative serological studies this ELISA was found to be positive on hospital admission in cases of amebic liver abscess when other precipitin tests were negative. Asymptomatic carriers of pathogenic zymodemes all produce IgG antibody to the surface membrane of *E. histolytica*. Absence of IgM response in these patients

would indicate chronicity of infection and probable absence of deep tissue invasion.

DIFFERENTIAL DIAGNOSIS

The diagnosis is based on clinical, serological and radiological features. The patient will usually be resident in an endemic area or have visited such an area recently. A raised right diaphragm, intercostal point tenderness or tenderness over the liver can all occur with pyogenic and amebic liver abscesses as well as with infected hydatid cysts. The patient is usually febrile with evidence of abscess formation on ultrasound. Serological tests may provide a rapid means of confirming the diagnosis. If there is doubt about the diagnosis it is reasonable to aspirate the abscess for culture and microscopy, but this is not

191

usually necessary. It is important to recognize that amebic pus may not have the characteristic 'anchovy sauce' appearance consisting of necrotic liver cells mixed with blood. The appearance may be variable and may be modified by secondary infection.

It can be difficult to distinguish between amebic and pyogenic abscess. The white blood count and the ESR may be elevated in both. In amebic liver abscess the indirect hemagglutination test is positive in almost all cases. Blood cultures may be positive in 50% of pyogenic abscesses.

The distinction between amebic liver abscess and hydatid cysts of the liver is important in areas where both conditions are endemic. Hydatid cysts show a characteristic echo pattern on ultrasonography. In endemic areas, primary hepatocellular carcinoma is also often common and distinction may be difficult clinically.

In areas where amebiasis is uncommon, delay in diagnosis may occur because the disorder has not been considered. Pain or tenderness in the right upper quadrant may lead to a suspicion of other liver, gallbladder, duodenal or pancreatic disease. A history of travel abroad to an endemic area and a raised right diaphragm on X-ray should lead to the diagnosis.

Aspiration of the lesion is used in diagnosis when serological tests are negative and other conditions such as pyogenic abscess or carcinoma need to be excluded. Hydatid cysts should be excluded before aspiration is attempted. The aspirate in amebiasis is usually sterile unless secondarily infected. The parasites occur on the periphery of the abscess, therefore the terminal portion of the aspirate is most successful in yielding positive results for culture or staining.

COMPLICATIONS

The major complications of amebic liver abscess occur either as a result of rupture into adjacent structures or from secondary infection. Extension may occur into the peritoneal cavity, other intra-abdominal organs, chest, pericardium or skin. In general, two-thirds of ruptures occur intraperitoneally and one-third intrathoracically.

PERITONEAL AND VISCERAL INVOLVEMENT

Intraperitoneal rupture can take the form of a localized perihepatic abscess or a free perforation, and is more frequently associated with left lobe abscesses. Intra-abdominal rupture may present with increased toxemia and worsening of previous symptoms, with associated peritonitis.

The pathological process usually involves adjacent structures in continuity and contiguity and the abscess becomes adherent to diaphragm, omentum, small and large bowel and frequently the abdominal or chest wall. If rupture occurs this adherence between liver and other structures tends to confine the area of contamination. Free rupture into the peritoneal cavity is uncommon and usually occurs in an untreated patient. The abscess may also rupture directly into the organ to which it has become adherent, such as the stomach, and lead to spontaneous drainage.

THORACIC AND PLEUROPULMONARY INVOLVEMENT

An abscess involving the upper surface of the liver frequently becomes adherent to the diaphragm. A sympathetic straw-colored effusion may develop in the pleural space with a right lobe abscess, or either a pleural or pericardial effusion if the abscess is in the left lobe of the liver. Because of the greater bulk of the right lobe, abscesses in this lobe cause the majority of clinical problems.

With further spread through the diaphragm

the abscess may rupture into the pleural space with the production of an amebic empyema. Occasionally the lung becomes adherent to the diaphragm and rupture of the abscess occurs into lung parenchyma producing pneumonic consolidation. Further progression may produce rupture into a bronchus leading to a hepatobronchial fistula and decompression of the abscess.

PERICARDIAL INVOLVEMENT

Amebic pericarditis occurs in fewer than 2% of cases of amebic liver abscess but carries a high mortality unless the diagnosis is made and the proper therapy instituted.

Extension from an abscess in the left lobe of the liver is the usual cause. Much less frequently spread is from the right lobe.

Two types of involvement are seen: first, a pre-suppurative or 'sympathetic' phase consisting of a serous effusion resulting from irritation by a neighboring abscess without rupture of its contents into the pericardium, and second, perforation of the liver abscess into the pericardium resulting in a true amebic pericarditis.

The onset can be acute with shock and death within a short time, or the presentation may be gradual with signs of tamponade.

Patients with amebic pericarditis may present in three ways. In the first, the hepatic presentation, symptoms and signs due to abscess in the left lobe of the liver dominate. In the second, cardiac presentation, clinical features of pericarditis and congestive cardiac failure dominate while evidence of liver involvement is inconspicuous. The electrocardiogram may show typical features of pericarditis. In the third mode of presentation, shock, there is sudden collapse due to acute pericardial tamponade. The diagnosis is easily missed and depends on a high index of suspicion. Some patients are first seen because of symptoms of heart failure without

clear evidence of prior involvement of the liver; and in such patients hepatic tenderness is wrongly attributed to venous congestion alone. The diagnosis should be suspect if, in a patient with pericarditis and signs of cardiac failure, tenderness of the liver is much more marked over the left lobe than in the rest of the liver. However, signs of a left lobe abscess can disappear after rupture of the abscess into the pericardium.

When there is a reasonable suspicion of amebic pericarditis, aspiration should not be delayed. Aspiration is conveniently done via the epigastrium. Since the procedure may damage the myocardium and may cause rapid cardiac tamponade, electrocardiographic or ultrasonic control is essential. The finding of serous fluid is consistent with the pre-suppurative stage of the disease but is not diagnostic. The diagnosis can be made with confidence when the aspiration yields typical 'anchovy' fluid. Drainage of the pericardium to relieve cardiac tamponade is essential. When possible this should be done by repeated aspiration rather than by an indwelling tube. If the liver abscess is of appreciable size, it should also be aspirated. If drainage by aspiration proves inadequate for the control of tamponade, surgical intervention becomes necessary. Subsequent development of constriction constitutes an absolute indication for pericardectomy.

TREATMENT

Supportive measures such as adequate nutrition and pain relief are important. The mainstay of drug therapy is metronidazole given in a dose of 800 mg three times daily for 5–7 days. This has a cure rate for amebic liver abscess of 95%. Lower doses are frequently effective in invasive disease but may fail to eliminate the intraluminal infection and so clinical relapse can occur. Other 5-nitroimidazole derivatives, tinidazole and ornidazole, can be used. Clinical symptoms usually improve after 24 hours, if there is no improvement after 48–72 hours alternative measures need to be considered.

Alternative drugs are available but their use is limited by potential toxicity. Emetine hydrochloride is the most potent tissue amebicide and is given by daily intramuscular or deep subcutaneous injections at a dose of 1 mg/kg/day (maximum daily dose 60 mg) for a maximum of 10 days. The course should not be repeated within 28 days. The most serious side effect is cardiovascular toxicity. Dehydroemetine is a less toxic derivative of emetine which is given in a dose of 1.25 mg/kg/day (maximum daily dose 90 mg). Chloroquine is useful in hepatic amebiasis, binding strongly to host proteins within the liver, and can be used in conjunction with metronidazole. The standard course of treatment is a loading dose of 150 mg 6-hourly for 2 days followed by 150 mg twice a day for 19 days (pediatric dose 10 mg/kg/day). Side effects are minimal at this dose and treatment duration.

Following therapy for amebic liver abscess other drugs are occasionally used to eliminate the intraluminal amebas in the intestine. Diloxanide furonate 500 mg, 8-hourly for 7–10 days is recommended. Tetracycline and erythromycin are alternative possibilities.

NEEDLE ASPIRATION

Most uncomplicated abscesses resolve with metronidazole treatment alone, so the only indication for aspiration in these cases is to confirm the diagnosis if this is in doubt. Aspiration should be performed if the abscess is large, if there is point tenderness, or if there is no satisfactory response to treatment.

Decompression of the abscess may relieve symptoms and should be undertaken if there is evidence to suggest that rupture into adjacent structures is likely. Ultrasound-guided percutaneous needle or catheter aspiration is the safest and most reliable technique.

Repeated aspiration may be necessary after an interval of a few days. Specific indications for aspiration of amebic liver abscesses are listed in Table 18.2. Recent work suggests that percutaneous catheter drainage for resistant amebic liver abscess may be more appropriate than repeated therapeutic needle aspiration in terms of hospital stay, morbidity and rapidity of resolution.

Table 18.2 Indications for aspiration of amebic liver abscess (De la Rey Nel, Simjee and Patel, 1989)

- No improvement clinically within 48–72 hours of starting adequate medical therapy
- Abscesses causing marked tenderness or severe pain
- All large abscesses (10 cm diameter) or abscesses increasing in size on therapy
- Marked elevation of the diaphragm
- Negative serological tests

SURGICAL DRAINAGE

Surgical drainage is required only in unusual circumstances. The conservative regimen described above has been adopted in most endemic areas. Open surgical drainage becomes necessary if there is no response to medical treatment in spite of needle aspiration or catheter drainage in left lobe abscesses with signs of impending rupture into the pericardium, or in abscesses with secondary infection not controlled by antibiotics and aspiration.

Despite the availability of very effective treatment for invasive amebiasis, it remains a major cause of morbidity and mortality in the developing world. As with many infectious diseases, the cure is not so much medical as sociopolitical. It is only with an improvement in basic living conditions and education that a significant contribution to the eradication of this disease can be made.

RECOMMENDED READING

Adams, E.B. and MacLeod, I.N. (1977) Invasive amoebiasis. *Medicine, Baltimore,* **56**, 325–34.

De la Rey Nel, J., Simjee, A.E. and Patel, A. (1989) Indications for aspiration of amoebic liver abscess. *S Afr Med J,* **75**, 373–6.

Ravdin, J.I. (1989) Entamoeba histolytica: from adherence to enteropathy. *J Infec Dis,* **159**, 420–9.

Sathar, M.A., Bredenkamp, B.L.F., Gathiram, V. *et al.* (1990) Detection of *Entamoeba histolytica* immuno-globulins G and M to plasma membrane antigen by enzyme-linked immunosorbent assay. *J Clin Microbiol,* **28**, 332–5.

19

Pyogenic liver abscess

JAKE KRIGE

INTRODUCTION

Pyogenic abscess is the commonest cause of hepatic abscess in developed countries, accounting for about three-quarters of all cases. Elsewhere, amebic abscess is more frequent and, worldwide, is the commonest cause of liver abscess. The advent of accurate diagnostic techniques and newer strategies for treatment, including the availability of improved antibiotics and ultrasound-guided aspiration, have influenced the management of pyogenic liver abscess (PLA). Earlier diagnosis and appropriate treatment have substantially reduced the mortality in recent years.

ETIOLOGY

PLA is almost always the result of bacterial infection, although on rare occasions, in immunologically compromised individuals, fungal infection may occur. Immunosuppression due to AIDS, intensive chemotherapy and transplantation has resulted in an increase in the incidence of PLA, especially with involvement by opportunistic organisms.

SOURCE OF INFECTION

The majority of pyogenic liver abscesses are caused by infection originating in the biliary or intestinal tracts. The etiology of liver abscesses can be conveniently divided into categories based on the route of extension of the primary infection. These etiological categories include the following sources of infection.

1. Biliary from ascending cholangitis.
2. Portal vein due to pylephlebitis resulting from appendicitis, diverticulitis, or pelvic sepsis.
3. Hepatic artery from septicemia.
4. Direct extension from a contiguous area of infection.
5. Traumatic from blunt or penetrating injuries.
6. Cryptogenic when no primary source of infection is found.

With the advent of effective anti-microbial therapy, the source of PLA has undergone an important change. During the pre-antibiotic era the portal source was the commonest due to complicated acute appendicitis and diverticulitis. With better control of portal pyemia and a decrease in the incidence of pyelothrombosis and septic pylephlebitis as complications of intra-abdominal sepsis, the biliary tract is now the commonest source of infection (Table 19.1).

Table 19.1 Etiology of pyogenic liver abscess

Biliary
    Stones
    Carcinoma
    Strictures
    Sclerosing cholangitis
    Caroli's disease

Portal pyemia
    Appendicitis
    Diverticulitis
    Regional enteritis
    Pelvic sepsis

Hematogenous
    Renal infection
    Pneumonia
    Bacterial endocarditis
    Intravenous drug abuse

Contiguous
    Gallbladder empyema
    Perforated peptic ulcers
    Sub-phrenic abscess
    Perinephric abscess

Iatrogenic
    Liver biopsy
    Percutaneous biliary stent drainage

Trauma

Septic cholangitis may complicate any biliary obstruction, especially if the obstruction is partial. The abscesses are commonly multiple in these cases. Approximately 40% of PLAs of biliary origin occur in patients with an underlying malignancy. Other routes of spread are by direct extension from an adjacent inflammatory process such as an empyema of the gallbladder or a perinephric abscess, via the hepatic artery as a result of bacteremia or as a result of trauma. Even with the considerable improvement in diagnostic tests, cryptogenic abscesses still constitute a quarter of all cases.

BILIARY TRACT DISEASE

Pyogenic liver abscess may complicate cholelithiasis, strictures or stones in the biliary system, and malignant disease of the pancreas, gallbladder or bile ducts. Cholangitis results in infection ascending into the intrahepatic biliary tree which may spread through the vascular and lymphatic channels to involve the portal vein. These abscesses are usually multiple but may be confined to one lobe of the liver.

PORTAL PYLEPHLEBITIS

Liver abscess may result from infection in any site drained by the portal vein. Intra-abdominal sepsis, particularly appendicitis, diverticulitis and pelvic infection, was previously the most common cause of pyogenic liver abscess. Initially, there is thrombophlebitis of the intramural vessels followed by progressive involvement of the venous drainage. Small septic emboli become detached from the thrombus and reach the liver via the portal vein. Abscesses are usually multiple and are most commonly found in the right lobe of the liver.

CONTIGUOUS INFECTION

Abscesses may result from direct extension of infection from contiguous or adjacent sites including empyema of the gallbladder, sub-phrenic abscess, pleural infection or perinephric abscess.

TRAUMA

Liver abscess may result from either blunt or penetrating injuries of the liver with tissue necrosis and extravasation of bile which predispose to secondary infection. Trauma accounts for up to 10% of pyogenic liver abscesses in some series. If adequate debridement of devitalized tissue is performed during the initial laparotomy and the injured area is effectively drained to avoid accumulation of blood or bile, abscesses are uncommon.

SEPTICEMIA

Generalized septicemia may result in liver abscess formation. Bacterial seeding occurs via the hepatic artery and may complicate bacterial endocarditis or other systemic infection. Up to a quarter of pyogenic liver abscesses may result from septicemia. The abscesses are usually small and multiple and found in both lobes of the liver.

CRYPTOGENIC ABSCESS

No associated disease or cause is found in 15% of liver abscesses. This type of abscess is usually solitary and is commonly found in the right lobe of the liver. In some patients, the etiology of liver abscess remains obscure even after an extensive clinical and pathological investigation. Compromised host defenses have been implicated in the development of cryptogenic abscess and may indeed play a role in the etiology of most hepatic abscesses. Although human portal vein blood is usually sterile, transient portal bacteremia does occur in diminished host resistance from debilitating disease. Liver abscesses occur in children with leukemia and other immune disorders. Diabetes mellitus has been noted in 15% of adult patients with pyogenic liver abscess.

MISCELLANEOUS CAUSES

Abscess may complicate both primary and secondary hepatic malignancy. Such abscesses result from necrosis and secondary infection and are usually solitary. Hydatid cysts of the liver can also become secondarily infected if there is communication with the biliary tract.

BACTERIOLOGY

Data from numerous studies indicate that in most pyogenic liver abscesses multiple microbes are found, endogenous organisms predominate, and anaerobes play a significant role. Gram-negative aerobes are found in over two-thirds of cases. *Escherichia coli* is the most frequently isolated aerobe. *Klebsiella*, *Proteus vulgaris* and *Pseudomonas* are also cultured.

Streptococcal species are found in approximately 35% of cases, 20% are aerobic with half of these enterococci and 15% are anesthetic or microaerophilic. *Streptococcus faecalis* is especially common in association with biliary tract sepsis.

Staphylococcus aureus and *Streptococcus pyogenes* should be considered after trauma and in the immunosuppressed host.

There is a changing pattern in the bacteriology of liver abscess with an increasing incidence of anaerobic infection in recent reports. The most frequently isolated anaerobes include microaerophilic streptococci, *Bacteroides fragilis*, and *Fusobacterium nucleatum*. Because of improved culture techniques many abscesses previously reported as sterile now grow anaerobic organisms. Anaerobes are found in up to a third of cases. Recovery of anaerobic organisms is common in cryptogenic abscesses. The primary site of infection is usually the gastrointestinal tract in these cases. Features suggesting anaerobic infection include foul-smelling pus, gas in the abscess cavity and lack of aerobic growth on culture. Occasionally, there may be superimposed infection on other intrahepatic conditions, such as a tuberculous abscess or ascaris infection.

Streptococcus milleri (Lancefield group F), which is neither a true anaerobe nor a microaerobe, is a common causative organism. *S. milleri* is part of the normal flora found in the pharynx, vagina and gastrointestinal tract. *S. milleri* (also called *Streptococcus intermedius*) is easily mistaken for an anaerobe but in fact grows well only in a CO_2-enriched environment, and is insensitive to metronidazole.

CLINICAL FEATURES

The classic presentation is with abdominal pain, swinging pyrexia and nocturnal sweating, vomiting, anorexia, malaise and weight loss. The pain is mainly in the right lower chest or right upper quadrant of the abdomen and may be pleuritic in nature with referral to the shoulder-tip. There may be an irritating cough if there is involvement of the diaphragm or pleuropulmonary spread. Any pattern of pyrexia may occur and can be intermittent or continuous, depending on the type of abscess and the pathogenic organism involved. Jaundice, ascites and diarrhea may occur. Jaundice is present in 15% to 20% of cases, particularly when the abscess is a complication of biliary tract disease, and usually indicates suppurative cholangitis or multiple abscess formation.

There may be a prodrome of several weeks, but in most patients symptoms have been present for about 2 weeks at the time of presentation. With the advent of antibiotic usage, the clinical presentation is less acute and it is unusual for patients to present with prostration and shock. The onset is particularly insidious or even occult in the elderly. Single abscesses tend to be more insidious in onset and are often cryptogenic. Multiple abscesses are associated with more acute systemic features and the cause is more often identified.

Usually the onset of symptoms is sub-acute with malaise, low-grade fever and dull abdominal pain increased by movement. Fever is present in over 80% of patients. Chills, nausea and vomiting occur in half of patients. Almost 30% of patients have non-specific symptoms. Fewer than one-third of cases have the complete symptom triad of right upper quadrant pain, fever or chills and malaise.

Clinically the liver is enlarged and tender in half of the patients. Percussion over the lower ribs aggravates the pain. The spleen may be palpable in chronic cases. Ascites is uncommon. Clinical jaundice occurs only in the late stage unless there is suppurative cholangitis. It is important to note that some patients do not have right upper quadrant pain or a hepatomegaly and an initial diagnosis is a fever of unknown origin.

LABORATORY INVESTIGATIONS

In two-thirds of cases there is a marked leukocytosis, but the white count may be entirely normal or decreased. The ESR is usually markedly raised, especially in long-standing cases, and there is often the low-grade anemia of chronic infection. The alkaline phosphatase is generally raised and there may be hypoalbuminemia. The serum aminotransferases are marginally elevated.

RADIOLOGY

There is generally elevation or alteration of the contour of the right dome of the diaphragm and this may be associated with a pleural reaction or pneumonic consolidation (Chapter 4). There may also be a right-sided pleural effusion, empyema, lung abscesses or bronchopleural fistula. In early cases, screening may show only reduced diaphragmatic movement. On plain abdominal film, hepatomegaly may be seen, and there may be an air fluid level in the abscess cavity.

Ultrasound and computed tomography

199

(CT) scanning have increased the ability to establish the diagnosis. Ultrasound is the preferred initial diagnostic approach, as it is non-invasive, cost-effective and accurate (80–90% sensitivity). CT scan has a sensitivity of almost 100% and is able to detect PLAs as small as 0.5 cm with a diagnostic accuracy of 90–95%. A negative CT scan virtually excludes PLA and is of added value in identifying underlying intra-abdominal abnormalities or other intra-abdominal abscesses.

Cholangitic abscesses may be diagnosed by percutaneous transhepatic cholangiogram. ERCP is useful in localizing an abscess and defining the site and cause of biliary obstruction.

ASPIRATION

The identification of the organism involved is an essential diagnostic step. A diagnostic aspiration is indicated in all cases with a presumptive diagnosis of pyogenic liver abscess or with uncertainty as to the diagnosis of pyogenic or amoebic abscess.

Bacteria are sought by cultures obtained from the blood or aspirated material. Culture must be done aerobically, anaerobically and in carbon dioxide-enriched media for *S. milleri*.

Culture of aspirated material is positive in 85 to 90% of cases. Adequate culture techniques will reveal anaerobes in over 50% of cases. Blood culture grows the organism less commonly because a substantial number of patients with PLA do not have bacteremia. Blood cultures yield two organisms in up to 15% of cases.

TREATMENT

ANTIBIOTICS

The appropriate antibiotic regimen should be based on the knowledge of the spectrum of organisms likely to be isolated in pyogenic hepatic abscesses. Since pyogenic abscesses may harbor multiple organisms, broad-spectrum antibiotic coverage is indicated until specific bacteria have been isolated and sensitivities are known. With the introduction of newer antibiotics, several combinations provide effective cover against organisms likely to be isolated. Each combination provides a broad spectrum against Gram-negative aerobes, *Streptococcal* species including enterococci, and anaerobes including *Bacteroides fragilis*. In patients allergic to penicillin, the combination of vancomycin, an aminoglycoside, and metronidazole will provide appropriate and effective cover. Metronidazole has the additional advantage of providing treatment for *Entamoeba histolytica* and should be included in the initial antibiotic regimen whenever there is suspicion of an amebic abscess.

The length of antibiotic therapy should be individualized based on the number of abscesses, the clinical response, and the potential toxicity of the chosen regimen. Patients with multiple biliary abscesses should receive 4–6 weeks of antibiotic therapy. A shorter antibiotic course may suffice for a small, solitary abscess that has been adequately drained. Initially, antibiotic therapy should be administered parenterally. In patients requiring a prolonged course of antibiotics, appropriate oral agents may be used after 2 weeks of systemic therapy.

No single therapeutic option is applicable for all pyogenic liver abscesses. The therapy of PLA should take into account whether the abscess is single or multiple, if additional problems requiring surgical therapy are present and the presence of any underlying disease.

Current therapeutic options for PLA include antibiotics in conjunction with aspiration, catheter or surgical drainage. Antibiotic therapy alone is effective only in a small number of cases. There are no controlled studies defining the proper duration of antibiotic administration. Parenteral antibiotic therapy should be continued until the patient is afebrile and asymptomatic. As the mean time for defervescence is about 7 days, initial parenteral antibiotic therapy is recommended for at least 10 days.

DRAINAGE

Most pyogenic liver abscesses require some form of drainage. Pus that initially appears viscous, becomes thinner and drains more easily after careful irrigation of the catheter. Many abscesses that appear loculated on imaging have free communication between the other components of the abscess, and drainage of one area may drain the entire communicating collection.

Ultrasound- or CT scan-guided percutaneous aspiration or catheter drainage have become the most widely used methods of abscess drainage. There is no difference in the time to defervescence or duration of hospitalization in patients treated with either of these percutaneous methods. Percutaneous drainage has several advantages including avoiding general anesthesia and an operative procedure, shorter hospitalization, easier nursing and better patient acceptance. Early effective percutaneous drainage has reduced the mortality and morbidity in PLA and is successful in 75–90% of cases.

Open surgical drainage has a role in patients in whom antibiotic therapy and percutaneous aspiration or catheter drainage have failed or where there is underlying intra-abdominal disease such as biliary tract stones or obstruction or intra-abdominal sepsis that requires surgery. Operation may be necessary for deep radiologically inaccessible abscesses, abscesses that are multiloculated, very large or those not amenable to catheter drainage. Open surgical drainage is now necessary in less than 20% of cases.

Different surgical techniques have been used for drainage of liver abscesses. The specific approach depends on the size, multiplicity and position of the abscesses, the degree of debility of the patient and the presence or absence of incompletely treated antecedent intra-abdominal infection. Extraperitoneal drainage was the procedure of choice before the antibiotic era as it avoided contamination of the peritoneal cavity. Adhesions between liver and parietal peritoneum permitted either an anterior sub-costal approach or a posterior approach through the bed of the 12th rib without anxiety of spreading pus. With more effective antibiotics, spread of infection is of less concern. An inability to explore with the limited exposure for associated intra-abdominal infection precludes the general use of extraperitoneal approaches.

A transperitoneal exploration providing wide access and allowing large bore tube drainage of pyogenic hepatic abscesses with antibiotic therapy is the operative approach used most frequently. Concomitant intra-abdominal disease, multiple hepatic abscesses or sub-phrenic or sub-hepatic collections can be effectively treated using this approach. After a thorough abdominal exploration and treatment of the intra-abdominal disease, the involved area of the liver is isolated from the rest of the peritoneal cavity with laparotomy packs. The abscess cavity is usually fluctuant and apparent on the surface of the liver, but on occasion, needle aspiration under ultrasound guidance is required to locate the abscess. Trocar suction is helpful to empty the cavity and avoid peritoneal contamination. Once the abscess is completely evacuated, this cavity is irrigated thoroughly to allow complete drainage of all loculated collections. Soft penrose or sump catheters are placed within the abscess cavity and brought out through a separate stab wound to the skin via the shortest intraperitoneal route. Such catheters allow post-operative irrigation of the cavity and a sinogram to determine the extent of cavity regression. Drains can usually be removed gradually in 2 to 3 weeks when the cavity has shown suitable progress.

PROGNOSIS

Early diagnosis, treatment with appropriate antibiotics and selective drainage have substantially reduced mortality. In uncomplicated cases, promptly diagnosed and treated with the correct antibiotics and effectively drained, the mortality should not exceed 10%. However, the overall mortality may be as high as 30–40%. This high figure is related to the presence of underlying diseases such as neglected intra-abdominal sepsis, immunodeficiency states and malignancy rather than the abscess itself. Adverse prognostic factors include the presence of shock, adult respiratory distress syndrome, disseminated intravascular coagulation, severe hypoalbuminemia, diabetes, ineffective percutaneous or surgical drainage and associated malignancy.

CONCLUSION

The good results and minimal morbidity after aspiration or catheter drainage compared with open surgical drainage has resulted in an increasingly conservative approach in patients with PLA but without coexistent intra-abdominal disease. Initial empiric parenteral broad-spectrum antibiotic therapy should include penicillin, an aminoglycoside and metronidazole. In the elderly and those with impaired renal function a third-generation cephalosporin should be used instead of an aminoglycoside. Metronidazole is effective against both anaerobes and amebiasis. Penicillin is the drug of choice for *S. milleri* infections which are resistant to metronidazole. An urgent ultrasound or CT scan is the initial investigation of choice to confirm the diagnosis of a liver abscess. Concurrent aspiration of the abscess under ultrasound guidance to provide material for bacteriological culture and sensitivity to guide subsequent antibiotic therapy is an important component of treatment. If sepsis persists, repeat ultrasound and catheter drainage is necessary. Surgical drainage is reserved for failures of aspiration or catheter drainage and is required in patients with coexistent intra-abdominal sepsis. In all cases an underlying cause should be sought and treated. Biliary obstruction must be relieved and can usually be done via endoscopic papillotomy and, if necessary, insertion of a biliary stent.

RECOMMENDED READING

Farges, O., Leese, T. and Bismuth, H. (1988) Pyogenic liver abscess. *Br J Surg*, **75**, 862–5.

Gerzof, S.G., Johnson, W.C., Robbins, A.H. *et al.* (1985) Intrahepatic pyogenic abscess: treatment by percutaneous drainage. *Am J Surg*, **149**, 487–94.

Lee, K., Sheen, P., Chen, J. *et al.* (1991) Pyogenic liver abscess: multivariate analysis of risk factors. *World J Surg*, **15**, 372–7.

McDonald, A.P. and Howard, R.J. (1980) Pyogenic liver abscess. *World J Surg*, **4**, 369–80.

Miedema, B.W. and Dineen, P. (1984) The diagnosis and treatment of pyogenic liver abscess. *Ann Surg*, **200**, 328–35.

Robert, J.H., Mirescu, D., Ambrosetti, P. *et al.* (1992) Critical review of the treatment of pyogenic hepatic abscess. *Surg Gynecol Obstet*, **174**, 97–102.

20

Hepatocellular carcinoma

MICHAEL KEW, ANTON VAN WYK and SIMON ROBSON

INTRODUCTION

Hepatocellular carcinoma (HCC) accounts for more than 90% of all primary hepatic tumors and is one of the most common human cancers. There is a striking geographical variation in its prevalence. In most developed countries HCC is rare or uncommon and usually develops as a late complication of clinically obvious (usually alcoholic) cirrhosis. In contrast, HCC is extremely common in sub-Saharan Africa and in many parts of the Far East where its presence correlates strongly with chronic hepatitis B virus (HBV) infection and clinically unrecognized macronodular cirrhosis. In Japan, a high incidence region of HCC, and Spain and Italy, which have intermediate incidences, the presence of the tumor is closely associated with cirrhosis induced by persistent hepatitis C virus (HCV) infection.

SEX AND AGE DISTRIBUTION

Men are more susceptible to HCC than are women. Male predominance is more evident in high risk populations (male : female ratios range from 2.1 : 1 to 5.7 : 1, mean 3.7 : 1) than

in low or intermediate risk (1.0 : 1.0 to 5.0 : 1, mean 2.4 : 1). The higher incidence in men probably reflects a combination of higher HBV carrier rates, greater exposure to chemical carcinogens in the working environment, and sex differences in the rate of metabolism of chemical carcinogens, such as aflatoxin. The rare fibrolamellar variant of HCC occurs equally in the two sexes.

The incidence of HCC generally increases progressively with age although there is a tendency to level off in the oldest age groups. However, in some sub-Saharan populations HCC occurs at an earlier age. This is most striking in Mozambican Shangaans where HCC occurs at a mean age of 33.4 years and 50% of patients are aged under 30. Fibrolamellar HCC characteristically occurs in young adults.

ETIOLOGY

The etiology and pathogenesis of HCC is multifactorial. The geographical variation in prevalence may reflect differences in frequency of chronic HBV or HCV infection and possibly of exposure to environmental carcinogens such as aflatoxin. Epidemiological evidence of a close association between HBV infection and HCC has been strengthened by studies that have suggested ways in which hepadnaviral integration may induce malignant transformation of hepatocytes. Several lines of study have supported a multistep process in the pathogenesis of HCC which includes several molecular genetic events and stages of initiation, promotion and progression. The recognition that chronic or recurrent necroinflammatory hepatic disease secondary to persistent HCV infection is complicated by the development of HCC emphasizes the importance of hepatocyte regeneration in the multistep process of hepatocarcinogenesis.

HEPATITIS VIRUSES

The evidence for a causal role for HBV in HCC is compelling. More than 80% of all cases of HCC show markers of current or past HBV infection and there is a close geographical correlation between HBV carrier rates and incidence of HCC. HBV infection is the major risk factor for HCC in regions where this virus is endemic. Acquisition of the carrier state in early childhood constitutes the greatest risk for the subsequent development of HCC, irrespective of whether the infection is acquired perinatally, as is true in the Far East, or horizontally, as occurs in sub-Saharan Africa. HBV DNA has been shown to be integrated into cellular DNA in the great majority of HBV-related HCCs. Integration occurs at random sites in the host chromosomes although specific sites in the viral DNA are involved. Integration, mediated in part by topoisomerases, may result in deletions or translocation in the flanking cellular DNA sequences and can induce instability of host DNA distant from the site of insertion. In 50% of woodchucks with HCC, woodchuck hepatitis virus DNA has been shown to be integrated in or adjacent to c-myc or N-myc, but integration of HBV DNA into a known

oncogene has been reported in only three human HCCs. Both the HBV X gene and the truncated preS/S genes are known to have trans-activating properties, and the former has been shown to be capable of inducing HCC in a transgenic mouse model. In another transgenic model, overproduction of the large surface protein results in its accumulation in the smooth endoplasmic reticulum of hepatocytes, where it produces severe and prolonged hepatocellular injury. This initiates a response characterized by inflammation, regenerative hyperplasia, transcriptional deregulation, and ultimate progression to neoplasia. These findings suggest that severe and prolonged injury to hepatocytes *per se* can initiate a chain of events which eventually result in tumor formation.

It has become apparent that a close association exists between chronic HCV infection and the occurrence of HCC. In Japan, Spain and Italy HCV infection is the major risk factor for the tumor, antibody to HCV (anti-HCV) being detected in as many as 80% of patients. A far smaller percentage of black African and Chinese patients are anti-HCV-positive. This is also true in most other countries where HCC is uncommon (HCV and HBV each account for only a minority of the patients). There is no evidence that HCV is directly carcinogenic, and it seems likely that the tumor is the end result of the virally-induced cirrhosis or, less often, chronic hepatitis.

AFLATOXIN

Aflatoxins are mycotoxins produced by *Aspergillus flavus*. Aflatoxin B1 is the most toxic: it is converted to a reactive B1 epoxide by the mixed function oxygenase system. Aflatoxin B1 is a very potent experimental hepatocarcinogen and, in addition, there is convincing epidemiological evidence of a direct correlation between aflatoxin ingestion and the incidence of HCC in some countries in Africa and the Far East. Until recently there have been no measurable criteria to indicate the extent of past exposure to aflatoxin, and this has prevented an evaluation of its precise role in the etiology and pathogenesis of human HCC. Recently, however, it has become possible to measure serum albumin adducts of aflatoxin and these should prove to be a measure of dietary exposure to aflatoxin over a reasonable period of time.

A specific point mutation (guanine to thymine) in the third base of codon 249 of the tumor suppressor gene, p53, has recently been detected in 50% of HCCs from Mozambican Shangaans and Chinese patients from Qudong County in the People's Republic of China. Aflatoxin has previously been shown in mutagenic experiments to bind particularly to guanine residues in GC-rich regions of the gene and, further, that codon 249 is a preferred target: it causes guanine to thymine mutations almost exclusively. These observations suggest a possible mechanism whereby aflatoxin might contribute to hepatocarcinogenesis, i.e. inactivation of a tumor suppressor gene by mutation induction. In a subsequent study HCCs from many parts of the world, some with high aflatoxin exposures and others with no or little exposure, were analyzed for p53 mutations and a good correlation between heavy exposure to aflatoxin and specific codon 249 mutations was confirmed.

ALCOHOL

Alcohol has not been shown experimentally to be a direct carcinogen. The epidemiological correlation between excessive alcohol ingestion and the development of HCC is probably explained by the fact that alcohol abuse causes cirrhosis and the latter is a major risk factor for HCC. In addition, alcohol increases biotransformation of chemical carcinogens by inducing microsomal mixed function oxygenase systems.

CIRRHOSIS

About 80% of all HCCs arise in cirrhotic livers. It has been postulated that either cirrhosis *per se* is a premalignant condition or that the increased cell turnover rate in chronic necroinflammatory hepatic disease renders hepatocytes susceptible to ubiquitous environmental carcinogens. In developing countries with a high incidence of HCC, the associated cirrhosis is of an inactive macronodular or mixed macronodular/micronodular variety and evidence of alcohol-induced hepatic disease is rarely found. In contrast, in developed countries with a low incidence of HCC, evidence for alcoholic hepatic disease is common and the cirrhosis may be micronodular or macronodular.

MISCELLANEOUS

The reported incidence of HCC in subjects with genetic hemochromatosis ranges from 4.5–18.9% and the calculated relative risk exceeds 200. If venesection is commenced before cirrhosis has developed, the risk of HCC is considerably reduced, although rare cases of HCC in the absence of cirrhosis have been reported.

The role of growth factors and cytokines in HCC is currently the subject of many studies. It is thought that they may mediate their effect on cellular growth and differentiation, in part, by altering matrix protein deposition and the expression of cellular adhesion protein receptors. Preliminary research suggests that the expression of certain important integrin heterodimers and matrix proteins in HCC differs significantly from adjacent nonneoplastic liver tissue.

Other minor risk factors for HCC are membranous obstruction of the inferior vena cava, alpha-1 antitrypsin deficiency, porphyria cutanea tarda (although this has recently been shown to be associated with chronic HCV infection), smoking, contraceptive steroids, anabolic androgenic steroids, tyrosinemia and glycogenosis.

CLINICAL PRESENTATION

The clinical features and course of HCC differ in high and low incidence areas. In developed countries HCC usually occurs in elderly patients with long-standing symptomatic cirrhosis. While the symptoms and signs of the tumor may be difficult to distinguish from those of the underlying liver disease, the HCC may declare itself by the appearance of new symptoms or signs, such as pain, fever, or a hepatic arterial bruit, or by a sudden unexplained deterioration in the patient's condition. The course from the time of diagnosis is usually one of moderately rapid deterioration, although survival may be prolonged. The presentation and prognosis are considerably worse in black African and Chinese patients. The former are often young, and the patients often present only when the tumor has reached an advanced stage. The disease always progresses rapidly with increasing pain, hepatomegaly and weight loss. Ascites may worsen and jaundice deepens. Rural southern African blacks survive for a mean of only 11.2 weeks from the onset of symptoms and of 6 weeks from the time of diagnosis.

SYMPTOMS

HCC runs a silent course during the early stages of the disease. Often the earliest symptom is abdominal pain or discomfort, which is usually a dull ache felt in the right upper quadrant or epigastrium but occasionally radiates into the back or right shoulder. The pain is continuous but may be aggravated in certain positions or by jolting. A sudden onset of severe right hypochondrial pain may signify a bleed into the tumor. Severe acute abdominal pain accompanied by pallor and shock suggests that the tumor has ruptured causing a hemoperitoneum. In populations with a high incidence of HCC, tumor rupture is the most common cause of non-traumatic acute hemoperitoneum. Weakness and weight loss, which are often of surprisingly short duration when the extent of the tumor burden is considered, are also prominent symptoms. Other symptoms include postprandial epigastric fullness, anorexia, intermittent nausea, vomiting and constipation. The patient may become aware of an upper abdominal mass, or complain of generalized swelling of the abdomen when ascites is present. Jaundice is an infrequent presenting symptom. Patients with established cirrhosis may present with hepatic decompensation with encephalopathy or with variceal bleeding. Bone pain caused by metastases is a rare presentation.

SIGNS

The physical findings depend on the stage at which the patient seeks medical advice. Early on, the only abnormality may be a slightly or moderately enlarged liver. Frequently, however, the disease is far advanced when the patient is first seen. The liver is then almost invariably enlarged and may be massively so. The surface is typically rock-hard and may feel irregular. Tenderness is common. A systolic bruit may be heard over the liver in up to 29% of patients and a peritoneal friction rub is occasionally heard.

Ascites occurs in 20–50% of patients. It is usually the result of portal hypertension and is more likely to be present in the early stages in patients with underlying cirrhosis. Ascites may also be caused by malignant invasion of the peritoneum, and it is then likely to be bloodstained. Ascites developing late in the course may be secondary to invasion of the portal or hepatic veins by the tumor. When present, jaundice is usually slight or moderate, although it may deepen in the later stages of the illness. Obstructive jaundice is occasionally seen and may result from compression of the major intrahepatic bile ducts by the primary tumor, obstruction of the common hepatic duct by tumorous glands in the porta hepatis, or tumor invasion of the biliary tree. Hemobilia occurs rarely.

Fever occurs in up to 50% of patients and is usually intermittent or remittent. In black and Far Eastern patients presenting with a short history of severe upper abdominal pain, fever, and an enlarged tender liver, it may be difficult to distinguish between an amebic liver abscess and HCC. A minority of patients are wasted when first seen. Thereafter, however, progressive wasting is the rule and the patients are often emaciated during the latter stages of the disease.

PARANEOPLASTIC PHENOMENA

The depression of genes in the course of malignant transformation may lead to the production of cellular products not normally expressed by mature hepatocytes. Some, such as alpha-fetoprotein, are useful tumor markers. Others are biologically active and may produce recognizable clinical effects. The resultant paraneoplastic phenomena account for many of the deleterious effects of HCC.

Erythrocytosis is one of the most common of the ectopic hormonal syndromes in HCC. Based on hemoglobin and hematocrit values, erythrocytosis has been said to occur in up to 11.7% of patients, but this is likely to be an underestimate because of the expanded plasma volume resulting from the underlying cirrhosis. The probable cause of the syndrome is synthesis and secretion of erythropoietin by the tumor. Hypercalcemia may occur in the absence of skeletal metastases and may be sufficiently severe to be symptomatic. Factors responsible for hypercalcemia in patients with other malignant tumors, including parathyroid hormone-related peptide, transforming growth factor α, epidermal growth factor, and prostaglandin E, have not thus far been incriminated as a cause of this syndrome in HCC. Precocious puberty occurs rarely in young boys with HCC as a consequence of ectopic production of human chronic gonadotropin (this is more common with hepatoblastoma). Feminization due to the tumor acting as trophoblastic tissue and converting dehydrepiandrosterone (sulfate) to estradiol and estrone is also rare.

Metabolic changes include hypoglycemia. This may occur early and may be severe. It results from production by the tumor of abnormal large molecular weight species of IGF II ('big' IGF II) as well as changes in the IGF binding proteins in the serum, resulting in increased amounts of 'free' IGF II causing excessive movement of glucose into the cells. Hypercholesterolemia due to autonomous cholesterol biosynthesis in malignant hepatocytes occurs in up to 16% of patients. The normal feedback inhibition of the rate-limiting enzyme HMG CoA reductase fails because receptors for chylomicron remnants on malignant hepatocyte surfaces are either absent or reduced. Cholesterol is therefore not internalized and does not switch off *de novo* cholesterol biosynthesis by malignant hepatocytes. Dysfibrinogenemias with prolonged prothrombin times may occur as a result of increased sialic acid substitution of fibrinogen synthesized by the tumor. Plasminogen activator inhibitor type 1 is released from malignant hepatocytes *in vitro* and may impair fibrinolysis thus resulting in a hypercoagulable state.

DIFFERENTIAL DIAGNOSIS

The clinical presentation, a high index of suspicion and the availability of sophisticated imaging modalities and other diagnostic facilities direct the investigation of suspected hepatic masses. The major differential diagnoses that need to be considered are hepatic metastases, amebic and pyogenic hepatic abscesses, cholangiocarcinoma, hydatid cysts, chronic hepatic parenchymal disease and benign hepatic tumors.

DIAGNOSIS

LIVER TESTS AND SERUM BIOCHEMISTRY

These are non-specific and reflect, in part, the underlying hepatic parenchymal disease. Space-occupying lesions of the liver are suggested by significantly raised serum alkaline phosphatase levels in the face of normal or near-normal serum levels of bilirubin and the transaminases. Serum cholesterol concentrations may be increased (Chapter 2).

TUMOR MARKERS

Alpha-fetoprotein

Raised serum levels of this alpha-1 globulin may be present in as many as 90% of patients with HCC. However, values are less likely to be raised in populations at low risk of developing HCC. Because various forms of acute and chronic hepatic parenchymal disease can cause slight or moderate elevations of serum alpha-fetoprotein (AFP) levels, a diagnostic level of 500 ng/ml is commonly used in clinical practice. Although the variable affinity of different isoproteins of AFP (attributable to the degree of fucosylation of the sugar chain) for different lectins (lentil and phytohemaglutinin) can be exploited to differentiate HCC from other malignant or benign diseases, most laboratories do not provide this service.

Other markers

Tumor-associated isoenzymes of gamma-glutamyl transferase are present in the serum of 50–60% of patients with HCC. Raised serum levels of des-gamma-carboxy prothrombin have been reported in 60–74% and alpha-L-fucosidase in about 75% of patients. In populations with low or intermediate incidences of HCC these markers may be more useful than AFP, but in high-risk patients, AFP remains the most useful marker.

IMAGING

Chest X-ray

The right hemidiaphragm is raised in about 30% of patients with HCC. This is sometimes associated with a small pleural effusion or basal linear atelectasis. Pulmonary metastases may be evident in up to 20% at the time of diagnosis. Skeletal metastases are infrequent.

Abdominal ultrasound

While routine ultrasound will usually reveal an HCC once a suitable size has been reached, it is important to remember that no ultrasonic features are specific for HCC, and it is unwise to base this diagnosis on the ultrasonic findings alone. Ultrasound is useful in assessing the patency of the inferior vena cava (IVC) and hepatic and portal veins and to differentiate between HCC and amebic liver abscess. However, an abscess may be mistaken for HCC in the early stages, before liquefaction has occurred.

Angiography

Unlike normal hepatic tissue, tumors derive their blood supply from the hepatic artery alone. HCC is usually highly vascular, in contrast with the majority of liver metastases which often have a poor blood supply. Characteristic angiographic features include a tumor blush and neovascularization; the vessels may show an irregular caliber, abnormal tapering, bizarre patterning of the smaller branches, the presence of arteriovenous

(AV) anastomoses and a delay in capillary emptying. Tumor invasion of the portal veins of the IVC may be demonstrated. Angiography is mandatory when considering surgical resection.

Isotopic hepatic scan

This is of limited use in the diagnosis of HCC. For practical purposes it has been superseded by ultrasound, computed tomography (CT) scanning, angiography and magnetic resonance imaging (MRI).

CT scan

The appearances of HCC are non-specific. Lesions usually enhance with contrast. The principal role of CT is to define the extent of the tumor in the liver and to provide evidence of spread beyond its confines.

MRI scan

HCC imaging by MRI is characterized by prolonged T1 and T2 retention times. MRI can demonstrate the tumor architecture and show its relationship to hepatic blood vessels.

Laparoscopy

At laparoscopy, extrahepatic spread of tumor can be sought and needle biopsy of the liver, lymph nodes or peritoneum can be performed under direct vision.

Biopsy

Histological examination of tumor tissue is the definitive diagnostic investigation. There is, however, a risk of promoting the spread of the tumor by allowing the seeding of tumor cells along biopsy needle tracts. This is only of significance in patients who may be suitable for a curative resection. Thus percutaneous biopsy should be avoided in potentially operable lesions and the diagnosis should be confirmed by frozen section at laparotomy (Chapters 5 and 6).

In most other cases, percutaneous or laparoscopic biopsy is appropriate for confirmation of the diagnosis of HCC. Blind biopsy may miss a localized lesion, and the Menghini or Tru-Cut® needle should preferably be guided by ultrasound or CT (Chapter 5). Fine-needle aspiration biopsy yields cells for cytological examination and is less traumatic, but results may be equivocal.

In patients from high incidence areas, clinical and radiographic findings of an inoperable lesion, evidence of an HBV carrier state and a very high AFP concentration are usually considered sufficient to allow the diagnosis of HCC and the patient is spared the potential hazards of a biopsy.

TREATMENT

The success of treatment is largely related to the extent of disease, and the presence of underlying cirrhosis. Surgical resection or liver transplant offer the only hope of 'cure' for HCC, yet most tumors are too far advanced to be resectable. The prognosis of HCC is very poor. The overall 5-year survival is less than 3%. However, in China active screening for HCC is performed and the early detection of asymptomatic tumors has given rise to 5-year survival rates in excess of 60% in some series.

SURGERY

The only cure for HCC at present is surgical resection. Before surgery, the extent of the tumor and its blood supply need to be carefully assessed. Biopsy is withheld until the tumor is resected. Surgery is successful when the tumor is small, has not metastasized, occupies only one lobe of the liver and has arisen in a non-cirrhotic liver. By these criteria, less than 5% of HCCs in Africa are resectable.

With a better understanding of the functional anatomy of the liver and newer techniques of lobectomy and segmentectomy, as well as improved postoperative care, liver surgery is now better tolerated. Surgery following early detection of HCC in the presymptomatic stage by AFP screening and ultrasound yielded a 90% survival at 1 year and 12% at 3 years in one trial. The late mortality reflects the degree to which distant spread has already occurred in HCC, even where present-day imaging modalities have failed to demonstrate it. Such survival figures, however, represent a great improvement on the natural history of the disease. Where both lobes of the liver are affected by HCC, resection is obviously impossible. Where there is no evidence of spread beyond the liver, transplantation may offer improved survival (Chapter 27). Unfortunately, except in the fibrolamellar variant, this is really palliative as tumor recurrence is the rule.

PALLIATIVE TREATMENT

Radiotherapy

The total dose is limited by the risk of radiation hepatitis. In practice this treatment is only used to control pain in symptomatic skeletal metastases.

Systemic chemotherapy

Results have generally been poor though a response of up to 30% has been reported in some series with agents such as doxorubicin. Chemotherapy has no place in the treatment of African HCC.

Hepatic dearterialization

Angiographic embolization of the arterial supply of the tumor may decrease the tumor bulk. This has been employed as a prelude to chemotherapy and may occasionally be considered for palliation where a large tumor causes compressive symptoms.

Hepatic artery chemotherapy infusion

An intellectually appealing approach is the delivery of chemotherapeutic agents direct to the tumor. At angiography, cytotoxics linked to lipiodol are infused directly into the hepatic artery. The lipiodol is taken up by hepatocytes and accumulates in the malignant cells because of their accelerated metabolism and failure to excrete the lipid. Some favorable results have been reported from uncontrolled series abroad; however, this method appears to have little benefit in African patients.

Miscellaneous

Monoclonal antibodies to tumor determinants presently have no place in the management of HCC. Interferons and polyclonal radiolabeled antibodies to ferritin have been used in HCC without benefit. Targeting cytotoxic agents or rescue factors to hepatocytes via the asialoglycoprotein receptor has been utilized in animals models and has potential utility in man.

SUPPORTIVE TREATMENT

Unfortunately the treatment of HCC as seen in southern Africa is highly unsatisfactory. Good supportive care is all that can be offered. This must include adequate analgesia, management of ascites and treatment of paraneoplastic effects such as hypoglycemia and hypercalcemia. Material and spiritual support for both patient and family are crucial.

CONTROL OF HEPATOCELLULAR CARCINOMA

HCC is a scourge in southern Africa. Perhaps the single most important preventive measure could be a drastic reduction in the incidence of chronic hepatitis B virus. Selective immunization of at-risk groups would result in a major decrease in the HBV carrier rate. In the southern African context this would require vaccination not only of traditional risk groups such as male homosexuals, health workers, drug addicts, sexual partners of HBsAg-positive persons and hemodialysis patients, but also large sectors of the black infant population. The cost would be significant, but so too are those of the sequelae of HBV infection, including HCC (Chapter 8).

At the level of the individual patient, the outlook might be improved by regular screening of patients with cirrhosis. Estimations of AFP and serial ultrasound scans at 6-monthly intervals could detect tumors at an earlier stage, allowing resection to be offered to a greater number. This would apply in the first instance to patients with cirrhosis who conform to the north American or European profile of patients at risk of HCC. Ideally one would wish to extend this to all HBV carriers. However, this has enormous implications; most HBV carriers are unrecognized and thus a massive screening campaign to detect these carriers would have to be undertaken, and many of those most at risk live in rural areas far from centers capable of carrying out such surveillance. Indeed, it is not known whether such screening would in fact identify tumors early enough to treat since the disease appears to be so explosively rapid in its development.

RECOMMENDED READING

Beasley, R.P., Lin, C.C., Hwang, L.Y. and Chien C.S. (1981) Hepatocellular carcinomas and hepatitis B virus: a prospective study of 22707 men in Taiwan. *Lancet*, **2**, 1133.

Bova, R., Micheli, M.R. and Nardiello, S. (1991) Molecular biology of hepatocellular carcinoma and hepatitis B virus association. *Int J Clin Laboratory Res*, **21**(2), 190–8.

Brunello, F., Marcarino, C., Pasquero, P. *et al.* (1992) Hepatitis B viruses and hepatocellular carcinoma. *Adv Cancer Res*, **59**, 167–226.

Deugnier, Y.M., Guyader, D., Crantock L. *et al.* (1993) Primary liver cancer in genetic hemochromatosis: a clinical, pathological and pathogenetic study of 54 cases. *Gastroenterology*, **104**, 228–34.

Di Bisceglie, A.M., Order, S.E., Klein J.L. *et al.* The role of chronic viral hepatitis in hepatocellular carcinoma in the United States. *Am J Gastroenterol*, **86**(3), 335–8.

Kew, M.C. (1989) Tumour markers of hepatocellular carcinoma. *J Gastroenterol Hepatol*, **4**(4), 373–84.

Kew, M.C. (1992) Tumours of the liver. *Scand J Gastroenterol*. **192** (suppl), 39–42.

Sato, Y., Nakata, K., Kato Y. *et al.* (1993) Early recognition of hepatocellular carcinoma based on altered profiles of alpha-fetoprotein. *N Engl J Med*, **328**, 1802–6.

Simonetti, R.G., Camma, C., Fiorello, F. *et al.* (1992) Hepatitis C virus infection as a risk factor for hepatocellular carcinoma in patients with cirrhosis. A case-control study. *Ann Intern Med*, **116**(2), 97–102.

21

Iron and the liver

RICHARD HIFT, TOM BOTHWELL and LAWRIE POWELL

INTRODUCTION

Iron, an element essential for life, plays a vital role in processes such as oxygen transport, electron transfer, nitrogen fixation and DNA synthesis. Teleological studies indicate an ancient relationship between iron and the element sulfur. In the most primitive forms of life (and perhaps early in the history of life on this planet) this close relationship may have formed the earliest energy trapping system. Essential primitive electron transfer proteins containing iron and sulfur clusters may have been formed that were able to participate in energy capture and ATP formation. The surfaces of iron sulfide minerals may also have served as catalysts for some reactions, thus functioning as the earliest hydrogenases and dehydratases.

In all higher forms of life, however, the essential energy trapping reactions involve an association of iron with oxygen. Here iron functions in two settings: in non-heme-containing proteins and in hemoproteins, where, incorporated into protoporphyrin, it is involved not only in the coupling of iron and oxygen for electron transport in the mito-chondrial cytochrome chain, but also in the close linking of iron with oxygen to form various iron oxides and hydroxides.

IRON TOXICITY

Iron exists in two oxidation states: ferrous iron (Fe^{2+}) and ferric iron (Fe^{3+}). At physiological pH and oxygen tension the ferrous iron is readily oxidized to ferric iron which is prone to hydrolysis, forming insoluble ferric hydroxide and oxyhydride polymers. In addition, unless appropriately chelated, iron plays a key role in the formation of harmful oxygen radicals which cause peroxidative damage. Because of iron's insolubility and toxicity, specialized mechanisms and molecules have evolved for its transport and storage in soluble non-toxic forms. Iron in excess is toxic to the liver. This is seen after acute iron poisoning and also in states of chronic iron overload such as hemochromatosis. The most likely mechanism of damage is the peroxidative decomposition of membrane phospholipids, which results in damage to cell membranes and to sub-cellular organelles. *In vitro*, the viability of iron-loaded hepatocytes can be prolonged by the addition of either desferrioxamine (an iron chelator) or α-tocopherol (an anti-oxidant). These findings support the hypothesis that iron exerts its deleterious effects via an oxidative pathway; numerous other lines of evidence support the role of lipid peroxidation in this process.

The total body iron content is between 3 and 4 g. The average daily requirement is 1 mg, the amount needed to replace obligatory losses of iron from desquamating epithelial cells of the gut and skin. The daily requirement is increased in premenopausal women because of menstrual blood loss (median 0.45 mg/day), in the latter part of pregnancy (where the daily requirement is 4–6 mg) and in the setting of chronic blood loss.

IRON ABSORPTION

The average Western diet contains about 10 to 15 mg iron per day. Of this, only 50% is processed into a soluble form, just 3 mg is taken up by intestinal mucosal cells and only 0.9 mg is normally transferred to the plasma. In iron deficiency, absorption may rise to 3–4 mg/day whereas in states of iron overload it declines to less than 0.5 mg daily. In the normal state, therefore, the amount of iron absorbed is controlled by the size of the body iron stores.

The amount of iron absorbed from the diet is influenced by the form in which it is present and also by the presence of other dietary substances which promote or retard absorption. Thus the composition of the meal may be more important than the quantity of iron in determining the amount available for absorption. The two major sources of iron are heme and non-heme. The heme iron, which is present as myoglobin and hemoglobin in meat, fish and poultry, forms a relatively small part of total dietary iron but it is well absorbed. The heme molecule is absorbed intact and iron is only released from the porphyrin ring in mucosal cells. The absorption of non-heme iron is variable, being dependent on its degree of ionization within the gut. Ferrous iron is better absorbed than ferric iron. Other ligands present in the diet may enhance or inhibit the absorption of iron. Ascorbic acid is an efficient promoter of iron absorption. It reduces ferric irons to ferrous irons which are better absorbed and also complexes with ferric iron to form a more readily absorbable compound. Other organic acids have similar but less potent promoting effects. In contrast, compounds such as phytates and polyphenols reduce iron absorption. Phytates are present in the bran of cereals, while polyphenols are found in tea, coffee, legumes and sorghum. The absorption of non-heme iron is also dependent on pH and is reduced in achlorhydric subjects.

The first step in iron absorption is the transport of iron from the intestinal lumen into the enterocytes. There is recent evidence that ferrous iron binds to a specific 160-kDa glycoprotein on the brush borders of the mucosal cells in the duodenum and proximal jejunum. Uptake appears to be adjusted according to the need for iron and control may be achieved in part by an increase in the amount of the protein on the mucosal surface in iron deficiency and a decrease when the body is loaded with iron. A variable amount of iron entering the mucosa from the bowel is retained as ferritin within the epithelial cell, while the rest is transferred to the plasma. In iron-deficient subjects, iron is completely transferred into the blood stream, whereas in normals only about 30% reaches the blood, the remainder being lost as sequestered ferritin when the cell is exfoliated. Patients with some forms of iron overload, such as transfusional hemosiderosis, transfer appropriately less to the plasma. In contrast, there is an increased mucosal transfer of iron into the blood in patients with hereditary hemochromatosis, which suggests a breakdown in control at this point.

213

INTERNAL IRON TRANSPORT AND CELLULAR UPTAKE

Very little iron circulates free within the plasma. Most is bound to carrier proteins which serve to keep the iron soluble, to retain it in a non-toxic form, and to transport it from site to site. By far the most important binding protein is transferrin, which belongs to a family of iron-binding proteins that includes lactoferrin and ovotransferrin. Transferrins are monomeric glycoproteins. They consist of two homologous domains, each containing one high affinity ferric iron binding site. *In vitro*, reticulocytes and hepatocytes remove iron equally well from either of the transferrin iron binding sites.

Transferrin has a half-life of 8 days whereas the iron itself normally has a half-life of only 1–2 hours. Each transferrin molecule therefore undergoes about 100 cycles of iron transport during its lifetime. The major destination of transferrin-bound iron is the bone marrow, with small amounts going to the parenchymal cells of the liver and other tissues. Most of the iron is incorporated into hemoproteins in the erythroid marrow, while hepatic iron is stored as ferritin and hemosiderin.

Erythroid precursors receive their iron from transferrin. They express transferrin receptors, which are disulfide-linked transmembrane glycoproteins, on their surfaces. Each receptor can bind one or two molecules of transferrin, and the number of receptors expressed on the cell surface reflects the cell's iron requirement. Diferric transferrin has a much greater affinity for the receptor than monoferric transferrin, thus optimizing the uptake of iron from the former source.

Following binding of transferrin to its receptor, the receptor–transferrin complex is internalized by a process of receptor-mediated endocytosis. Within the endosome, the pH is lowered to less than 5.5 by energy dependent protonation, which allows for the release of the iron from transferrin. The apotransferrin remains bound to the receptor within the endosome and returns to the cell surface where the apotransferrin is released and returns to the circulation.

The uptake of iron by hepatocytes appears to be both more versatile and more complex than that of erythroid cells. Unlike erythroid cells, hepatocytes can take up iron from different iron-bearing compounds, including ferritin, heme, and iron bound to albumin and various chelators. Hepatocytes are also able to release iron back to plasma transferrin.

Under most circumstances the major part of the hepatocyte iron content is derived from transferrin. Hepatocytes possess high affinity transferrin receptors which function in a manner analogous to those of erythroid cells. The transferrin receptor gene has been cloned and sequenced and several sequences have been identified that play an important role in the control of transferrin receptor expression. Since these sequences appear to respond to the cell's need for iron, they are known as iron responsive elements (IREs). The control of iron uptake by the hepatocyte appears to differ from that of erythroid cells. For example, intracellular heme plays an important regulatory role in erythroid cells but appears be less important in the control of hepatocyte iron uptake. Unlike erythroid cells, hepatocytes can continue to take up transferrin even at transferrin concentrations above those needed to saturate the receptors. It appears that they have an additional non-saturable low affinity plasma membrane reduction process which allows for the internalization of transferrin-bound iron without endocytosis or endosomal acidification of transferrin.

Hepatocytes also express specific membrane receptors for ferritin. Circulating plasma ferritin has a very low iron content even in iron overloaded patients and presumably does not constitute an important source of iron for the hepatocyte. However, Kupffer cells found in close proximity to hepatocytes may release large amounts of ferritin from their stores and hepatocytes may accumulate such iron very efficiently using their ferritin receptors. The ingested ferritin is rapidly degraded and the released iron is stored in newly synthesized hepatocyte ferritin. This mechanism may account for the relative resistance of the liver to iron deficiency. In erythroblasts, iron deficiency results in reduced heme synthesis and anemia. In contrast, the synthesis of heme in hepatocytes is not reduced.

Iron may also be taken up by the hepatocyte directly from heme. Both hemoglobin–haptoglobin and heme–hemopexin complexes bind to specific receptors on the hepatocyte and are internalized by endocytosis. Within the cell, iron is released from the heme and enters an intracellular pool.

Other mechanisms of iron uptake are encountered in hepatocytes. When the plasma transferrin is fully saturated, additional iron entering the plasma becomes non-specifically associated with albumin or with low-molecular weight chelators such as citrate, ascorbate, amino acids and carbohydrates. This iron is also available to the hepatocyte and its uptake appears to be carrier-mediated by an electrogenic transport mechanism that is driven by the transmembrane potential difference. This route may be particularly important in subjects with hereditary atransferrinemia. The lack of transferrin limits iron uptake by erythroblasts and, in consequence, affected individuals demonstrate a hypochromic microcytic anemia. However, they also show severe parenchymal iron overload, with massive iron deposition in the liver and pancreas. These findings confirm the presence of mechanisms for iron uptake by hepatocytes which do not involve transferrin.

IRON STORAGE

More than half the storage iron in humans is in the form of ferritin, a compound present in all animal and plant tissues and also in fungi and bacteria. Mammalian ferritin consists of a paracrystalline iron core surrounded by a protein shell. The shell confers solubility to the compound and protects against ferric-mediated oxidative damage to cell constituents. Ferritin can contain up to 4500 iron atoms per molecule. The protein shell is composed of 24 sub-units of two types, heavy (H) and light (L), which give rise to populations of isoferritins. Iron stored as ferritin is readily available for deployment in functional compounds but the exact mechanisms involved in the loading and unloading of iron have not been defined. Assembled ferritin molecules contain eight hydrophilic channels which connect the inner cavity with the exterior. They appear to enable iron and other molecules to enter or leave the shell's interior. Though ferrous iron is more efficiently incorporated into the shell than ferric iron, it is ultimately oxidized to the ferric form and deposited in association with the inner surface of the sub-units in this form. Ferritin is degraded in lysosomes. Such degradation may lead to sequestration of the iron in the insoluble complex hemosiderin, or else to its solubilization for incorporation into functional compounds or for storage again in other ferritin molecules.

The principal regulator of ferritin synthesis is the amount of chelatable intracellular iron. While accelerated synthesis is achieved primarily by an increase in the translation of pre-formed ferritin mRNA, increased transcription of the H and L sub-unit genes also occurs in some cell types. The translational regulation of ferritin synthesis depends on a highly conserved stem loop structure, the iron responsive element (IRE), on the ferritin mRNA. When iron levels are low, translation is prevented by an IRE-binding protein. When intracellular levels of chelatable iron rise, the IRE-binding protein dissociates from the IRE and ferritin synthesis occurs. Identical IREs are present on the mRNA of the transferrin receptor and react with the same IRE-binding protein. In a coupled regulatory mechanism raised chelatable iron levels lead to increased ferritin synthesis and degradation of transferrin receptor mRNA. In this way excess iron is sequestered and less iron is delivered from the plasma into the cell.

Most ferritin is present within the liver, though other ferritin deposits are found in the spleen, bone marrow and muscle. Serum ferritin levels, which mirror body iron stores, rise slowly and progressively with age in men, while they remain constant in women until the menopause, when they start rising to levels similar to those in men.

ASSESSMENT OF STORAGE IRON STATUS

SERUM IRON, TRANSFERRIN SATURATION, AND IRON-BINDING CAPACITY

Traditionally these tests have been used for the detection of both iron overload and deficiency. Iron overload is characterized by a high–normal or raised serum iron concentration, an increased transferrin saturation and a reduced iron-binding capacity, while iron deficiency is accompanied by a low serum iron, a reduced transferrin saturation and an increased iron-binding capacity. The serum iron concentration on its own is a poor indicator of increased body iron stores and is non-specific. A raised serum iron, for instance, may be seen in alcoholics without evidence of iron overload. The transferrin saturation is more sensitive than the serum iron in the diagnosis of iron overload. However, transferrin metabolism is influenced by inflammatory states. Catabolism of transferrin is increased in the acute phase response, with a consequent decrease in serum transferrin. The serum iron declines even further so that the final effect is a reduction in the degree of transferrin saturation as well as a reduced iron-binding capacity. The combination of a low serum iron, transferrin saturation and iron-binding capacity is typical of chronic inflammation.

SERUM FERRITIN

The serum ferritin is the most widely applicable index of iron status. Though the amount of ferritin in the circulation is small in relation to the size of the body iron stores, it mirrors them closely. A low serum ferritin concentration (<12 µg/l) is diagnostic of iron depletion. High serum ferritin levels correlate well with hepatic iron overload. The test is, however, not entirely specific and a raised serum ferritin concentration does not always denote iron overload. Serum ferritin levels may rise as a result of hepatocellular necrosis, malignancy, leukemia, inflammation and active liver disease. Ferritin is an acute phase reactant and may therefore rise to very high levels in inflammatory conditions such as rheumatoid arthritis. The high serum ferritin levels in iron overload may reflect not only excessive iron storage but also a leakage of ferritin from damaged liver tissue. Thus an elevated ferritin is a feature of hepatocyte necrosis, whatever the cause, and its level correlates well with the degree of hepatocellular injury. In one study of the hepatic effects of paracetamol (acetaminophen) toxicity, the ferritin concentration was a more sensitive index of liver damage than the aminotransferase levels. These various points are raised in order to emphasize the caution that must be exercized in interpreting the significance of a raised serum ferritin level.

The relationship between ferritin and the size of the iron stores is not linear. With increasing iron stores, the ferritin : storage iron ratio decreases, so that a high ferritin level does not predict the absolute degree of iron overload with any accuracy. Similarly, during the earlier stages of venesection therapy for hereditary hemochromatosis, considerable variation in serum ferritin levels is seen, making serial determinations a poor marker of successful mobilization of iron until tissue stores have been substantially reduced.

In summary, the serum ferritin on its own is adequate as a definitive marker of iron overload. The diagnosis of hepatic siderosis or hemochromatosis should always be confirmed by liver biopsy.

HEPATIC IMAGING

Both computed tomography (CT) and magnetic resonance imaging (MRI) reflect changes in the hepatic parenchyma in the presence of iron overload. Though there appears to be a good correlation between iron content and image intensity, values overlap widely and a single measurement in an individual patient may not predict iron content accurately. CT scanning is also confounded by such factors as associated fat infiltration which obscures the effects of iron overload on image intensity. Thus, imaging procedures have major limitations. These include insufficient accuracy, lack of specificity and high cost. Currently, they do not replace more established measures such as the determination of serum ferritin levels and transferrin saturation.

Recent studies have suggested that the combination of serum ferritin and CT scanning or MRI has 100% sensitivity in detecting hepatic iron overload more than five-fold above the upper limit of normal. The combined approach does not, however, reliably detect lesser degrees of iron overload. CT and MRI are more specific than the serum ferritin (64% and 92% versus 21%) in the detection of iron excess more than five times the upper limit of normal. However, the correlation between the hepatic iron concentration and the results of non-invasive laboratory or imaging studies is insufficient to permit prediction of hepatic iron content by non-invasive tests alone.

Unfortunately all these non-invasive tests are poor discriminators between the different forms of iron overload; they do not distinguish genetic hemochromatosis reliably from other forms of iron overload, or even from alcoholic liver disease.

OTHER METHODS

Body iron stores may also be quantified by desferrioxamine challenge. Desferrioxamine is injected intramuscularly and mobilizes iron in proportion to the amount present. A proportion of the ferrioxamine formed is passed in the urine where its iron content can be measured. The test, which is of limited sensitivity, is not commonly performed today but may be useful in distinguishing between the high serum ferritin levels of tissue damage, inflammation or malignancy and those found in true iron overload. Quantitative phlebotomy is an accurate measure of iron stores, but is clinically of little use as it is a retrospective measure. When a course of therapeutic venesections is complete, the total amount of iron mobilized can be estimated by multiplying the total volume of blood removed by the estimated iron content of the hemoglobin per unit volume. A new technique, magnetic susceptometry, which is currently under investigation, may provide a reliable estimate of hepatic iron concentration in small areas of the liver. This method is not widely available.

HEPATIC IRON CONCENTRATION

The serum ferritin and transferritin saturation tests remain the preferred screening tests for iron overload. However, no final assessment of the degree of overload can be made without a liver biopsy, since the determination of its iron content biochemically or by atomic absorption spectrophotometry provides an accurate measure of the hepatic iron concentration.

Sections of the biopsy can also be examined histologically to assess the distribution of the iron and associated pathological changes in the liver. In the past, histological scoring systems have been widely applied to assess the degree of iron overload. While the histological grading scale correlates well overall with the true tissue iron content, there are considerable variations in iron concentrations within each histological grade.

IRON OVERLOAD STATES

Hemosiderosis is an imprecise term sometimes used to indicate the presence of hemosiderin in tissues without associated tissue damage. The total body iron content need not be increased, since there is a redistribution of body iron in all anemias except those due to iron defiency or blood loss. Stainable iron may therefore be seen in the liver in subjects with alcoholic liver disease and a variety of chronic diseases even though the total body iron content is normal. The discussion that follows is only concerned with situations in which the total body iron content is markedly raised.

Primary iron overload occurs as a result of a genetically determined increase in iron absorption, while secondary iron overload occurs under several circumstances (Table 21.1). The latter is a feature of several iron-loading anemias, notably thalassemia major, in which there is markedly increased but ineffective erythropoiesis and an inappropriate increase in iron absorption. Secondary iron overload is also found in sub-Saharan Africa, where the local diet contains large amounts of bioavailable iron. Finally, it is a complication of all those anemias where life is sustained over long periods by multiple blood transfusions.

The term 'hemochromatosis' is used when the increased tissue deposits of iron are associated with tissue damage. The degree to which excess iron is deposited in the parenchyma of organs such as the liver is more important

Table 21.1 Classification of iron overload

1. Primary (idiopathic, hereditary, genetic) hemochromatosis

2. Secondary (acquired) hemochromatosis, secondary iron overload
   - iron-loading anemias, i.e. hemolytic diseases with ineffective erythropoiesis and an inappropriate increase in iron absorption (thalassemia major, sideroblastic anemia)
   - dietary iron overload
   - transfusional siderosis

than the total stores in determining the amount of tissue damage. The site of iron storage is dependent in part on the degree of iron overload, but other factors appear to be important. In this context, parenchymal storage with relatively little reticuloendothelial involvement is a feature of hereditary hemochromatosis. It has been postulated that this may be due to impaired reticuloendothelial function. Both parenchymal and reticuloendothelial involvement are present in the iron-loading anemias associated with ineffective erythropoiesis.

HEREDITARY HEMOCHROMATOSIS

Hereditary hemochromatosis (HH), also called idiopathic genetic or familial hemochromatosis, is an autosomal recessive inherited condition characterized by the development of marked parenchymal iron overload. This overload affects many organs, including the liver, the pituitary, testes, heart and pancreas. The build-up of iron occurs gradually over many years and patients do not usually become symptomatic until the 4th or 5th decade of life. Clinical manifestations occur later in female patients, which is due, in part at least, to the protective effect of menstruation in reducing iron stores.

The genetic defect is on chromosome 6 but

the nature of the mutation is not known. The close association of the putative gene for HH and the HLA locus on chromosome 6 accounts for the association noted between HH and the HLA haplotype A3. Since the condition is recessive, it is the homozygote that develops HH. Heterozygotes may absorb a little more iron than normal people, but do not accumulate significant quantities. The gene for HH appears to be common. Studies in white populations suggest that as many as 10% may be heterozygotes, with a calculated homozygote frequency of the order of 1 in 400. With such a high frequency of the gene, pseudodominant inheritance patterns are noted in some families as a result of homozygote/heterozygote matings.

The nature of the pathophysiological defect underlying iron accumulation in HH is unknown. Whatever its nature, it leads to an absorption rate that is inappropriately high in relation to the size of the body stores. The fact that ferritin levels are relatively reduced in both mucosal and reticuloendothelial cells has led to the suggestion that they share a common defect which leads to reduced iron storage in them and the delivery of increased amounts of iron to the plasma. This raises the transferrin saturation and leads to the deposition of iron in the liver and other parenchymal tissues. At the some time, it is clear that both ferritin and transferrin are themselves normal in HH and attention is now focusing on possible abnormalities in more recently discovered intracellular iron-binding proteins.

While HH is primarily a genetic disorder, environmental factors may also play a role in the phenotypic expression of the disorder. Increased availability of iron in the diet (e.g. a high meat intake) accelerates the process of iron accumulation, whereas a lack of available dietary iron retards it. Similarly, regular blood loss (whether via menstruation in females or by voluntary blood donation in either sex) postpones the onset of clinical hemochromatosis.

There appears to be an association between HH and the use of alcohol. This is to be distinguished from the mild degrees of iron overload as well as from the reticuloendothelial hemosiderosis frequently noted in alcoholics. How the use of alcohol accelerates the deposition of iron in hemochromatosis is not known.

Clinical features

The clinical findings in hemochromatosis involve a range of systems. With increasingly early diagnosis, the classic presentation is becoming much less common. Accordingly, many patients now diagnosed by routine screening or because of known hemochromatosis in the family do not show all the classical features described below.

The skin becomes pigmented with a coppery or grayish discoloration. The pigmentation particularly involves exposed areas as well as the genitalia, nipples and oral mucosa. The liver is enlarged and eventually the features of cirrhosis supervene. However, severe portal hypertension, with ascites and varices, is less commonly associated with hemochromatosis than it is with alcoholic cirrhosis. There is evidence that simultaneous alcohol abuse may bring on an earlier and more severe form of liver disease than would be expected with HH alone. Patients with hemochromatosis are prone to primary hepatocellular carcinoma which occurs with a frequency 200-fold that in the general population. It is almost always associated with cirrhosis and may develop long after the excess iron has been successfully removed by phlebotomy.

Pancreatic iron deposition with subsequent diabetes is common. Several factors are involved. Not only is there reduced secretion of iron from the β cells, but insulin resistance also occurs, probably as a result of hepatocyte iron loading and cirrhosis. Hypogonadism is a frequent occurrence and leads to loss of libido, atrophic testes, impotence and amennorhea. Hypogonadism is largely the result of gonadotrophic hormone deficiency secondary to pituitary dysfunction. The secretion of other pituitary hormones is not impaired.

Cardiac involvement is a significant cause of death in untreated patients. The illness may come on acutely with severe cardiac failure, although in older patients a more gradual onset is noted. The clinical presentation is of a congestive cardiomyopathy. Arrhythmias are common and indicate a poor prognosis. Ventricular extrasystoles are common but supraventricular and ventricular tachycardias as well as ventricular fibrillation and heart block are also encountered. Cardiac manifestations are particularly prominent when patients present at a young age, and if untreated the cardiopathy is rapidly fatal.

Another characteristic feature of HH is arthropathy. It typically involves the second and third metacarpophalangeal and proximal interphalangeal joints of the hands, with bony swelling and limitation of movement. Chondrocalcinosis is also often present. Though often asymptomatic, it causes episodes of acute inflammatory synovitis (pseudogout) in some patients. Osteoporosis has also been demonstrated in HH but the mechanisms responsible for it have not been delineated.

Diagnosis of hereditary hemochromatosis

It should be emphasized that the clinical features described in the previous paragraphs represent very late manifestations of HH and are seen today only in patients in whom the diagnosis has been missed for many years. With increasing awareness of the condition and earlier diagnosis, the clinical spectrum is changing. In a recent series, 40% of 56 probands were identified during a periodic health examination. The most common complaints among the remainder were abdominal pain, joint pains, weakness, diabetes and infection. These findings emphasize the need to consider HH in the differential diagnosis of any unexplained liver disease, arthritis or gonadal failure. It is also vital that family members of patients with the disease be screened. Appropriate screening tests, which are both simple and inexpensive, are the transferrin saturation and serum ferritin. The transferrin saturation becomes abnormal before total iron stores are significantly increased. The reason why this should be so is not clear but it may offer a clue to the pathophysiology of HH. A transferrin saturation in excess of 70% is diagnostic; between 50% and 70% on repeated testing is suggestive. The younger the age at which a person is tested, the less likely it is that the transferrin saturation will be unequivocally elevated. It is therefore necessary to test family members at intervals to detect any rise in the transferrin saturation.

The serum ferritin tends to rise later than the transferrin saturation. Since ferritin is not specific for iron overload, the result must be interpreted with care. It is also not entirely sensitive with lesser degrees of iron loading, but is usually very high when severe overload is present. The serum ferritin and transferrin saturation are particularly valuable when assessed together. Tests such as CT scanning, MRI scanning and the desferrioxamine challenge have not yet reached sufficient sensitivity and specificity to be recommended as screening methods. When screening tests suggest the presence of significant iron overload, it is essential that a needle biopsy of the liver be performed. A distinction can then be made between parenchymal and reticuloendothelial iron overload, the amount of iron present can be directly quantitated biochemically or by atomic absorption spectrophotometry and, finally, the presence or absence of cirrhosis (which is important prognostically) can be assessed.

Despite the close association of HH with the HLA type A3, determination of the haplotype is of little importance in the individual patient as the specificity and sensitivity are not sufficiently high. The determination of haplotypes is, however, important in screening families. Family members who share both haplotypes with the affected patient are at high risk of being homozygous and will require investigation. Similar strategems using restriction fragment length polymorphisms at the putative hemochromatosis locus can also be employed. It is, however, simpler and cheaper to screen all family members by determining the transferrin saturation and serum ferritin. Since these tests only become abnormal with the passage of time, repeated testing at intervals of 2–3 years may be necessary.

Approximately one-third of heterozygotes show abnormalities of transferrin saturation or serum ferritin. In such circumstances it is difficult to distinguish between the heterozygote whose tests are unlikely to deteriorate with time and the pre-symptomatic homozygote who will continue to accumulate iron. The most appropriate way to resolve this problem is to estimate iron stores directly, either by liver biopsy or by a programme of venesections with retrospective calculation of the amount of iron mobilized.

Treatment

Removal of iron is essential to prevent the onset of the organ complications of iron overload or to reverse them as far as possible. The method of choice is phlebotomy. About 250 mg iron is removed with each 500 ml blood venesected. By inducing anemia, erythropoiesis is stimulated and iron is mobilized from the tissues to be incorporated into hemoglobin. Prolonged courses of venesections are usually needed, with weekly phle-

botomies for 2 years or more. The progress of venesection is monitored by determining the hemoglobin, transferrin saturation and serum ferritin. Once iron stores are exhausted, re-accumulation of iron can be prevented by quarterly venesections.

Iron can also be mobilized by the use of chelating agents such as desferrioxamine. This approach is, however, slower, much more expensive and more difficult to apply. Work is in progress to assess the place of oral iron chelating agents. It should, however, be stressed that venesection therapy is simple, inexpensive and effective. It has the added advantage that the blood removed can be used for donation purposes.

Once toxic iron concentrations have been reached in the tissues, life expectancy is shortened. Treatment by venesection improves the prognosis and normal life expectancy is possible when venesection is introduced before major complications have arisen. Even where complications such as cirrhosis are present, the prognosis is considerably better with treatment.

IRON LOADING IN ASSOCIATION WITH ANEMIA

Iron loading is a feature in anemias such as thalassemia major that are associated with markedly increased but ineffective erythropoiesis. The reason why this should be so is not clear. While it is true that iron absorption is increased when erythrpoiesis is accelerated acutely, iron absorption is usually normal in chronic hemolytic states with effective erythropoiesis (e.g. hereditary spherocytosis) and those rare individuals in whom iron overload does develop are probably also HH heterozygotes. In contrast, severe iron overload is a major complication in thalassemia major and is a frequent cause of death, with most patients succumbing before the age of 20 years. The iron overload is usually due to a combination of the increased oral absorption of iron and multiple blood transfusions. Clinical manifestations of iron overload usually occur in the teens and include cirrhosis, diabetes, cardiac failure and hypogonadism.

The aims of therapy are two-fold. Firstly, optimal growth and well-being are ensured by maintaining the hemoglobin above 10 g/dl through regular blood transfusions, while excess iron is removed from the body by the use of the chelator desferrioxamine, administered subcutaneously over 12 hours daily. While cumbersome and expensive, chelation therapy has significantly improved the prognosis in thalassemia major. Current research is directed to the development and application of cheap oral chelators.

Severe iron overload is also a feature in a number of chronic anemias in which repeated blood transfusions are necessary to sustain life. Since the body has a very limited capacity to excrete the metal, large amounts of iron derived from the donor blood accumulate in the reticuloendothelial system. The frequency of pathological sequelae depends on the degree to which the iron is relocated from its original location in the reticuloendothelial system. In aplastic anemias there is very little redistribution of the iron and complications are rare. On the other hand, parenchymal loading, with subsequent tissue damage, is much more frequent in anemias associated with enhanced erythropoiesis and an increased turnover of iron within the body.

DIETARY IRON OVERLOAD

There is controversy about whether significant iron overload can result from the prolonged oral intake of increased amounts of iron in normal individuals. Ethiopian subjects have been shown to consume up to 200 mg of inorganic iron in soil daily (200 times the daily requirement) with only a very small increase in reticuloendothelial iron stores. The relevance of these findings is, however, questionable, since iron compounds in soil are of very low bioavailability. Reports of dietary iron overload in European or American populations are rare, though some reports of hemochromatosis occurring in subjects ingesting massive amounts of medicinal iron (over 1000 g) have appeared. The possibility that such individuals may have had HH is, however, not excluded.

The one important exception is the massive iron overload described in southern African blacks previously known as Bantu siderosis. This form of iron overload has been attributed to the consumption of large amounts of beer brewed in iron pots. The iron leached from the pots in the acid environment of the beer is in an ionized, bioavailable form. The condition is clearly distinct from genetic hemochromatosis and shows no association with the HLA haplotype A3. At the same time, there is some recent evidence that it is not only the result of a high intake of bioavailable iron. The results of family studies in Zimbabwe suggest that severe iron loading only occurs in those subjects who are also heterozygous for an iron-loading gene. These interesting findings deserve further investigation.

The clinical and pathological findings in the iron overload occurring in southern African blacks are very different from those in HH. Hepatocytes are loaded with iron but other parenchymal tissues are only modestly affected. In contrast, there is heavy reticuloendothelial involvement through the body. Thus, the bone marrow and spleen are laden with iron and the liver shows massive iron deposition in the portal tracts and Kupffer cells in addition to the hepatocyte involvement. Cirrhosis is an important complication of the condition but the lack of significant parenchymal involvement elsewhere means that diabetes, cardiac involvement and hypogonadism occur only rarely.

Scurvy and osteoporosis are common

sequelae. Affected subjects tend to have a low intake of ascorbic acid but there is also evidence that the large deposits of ferric iron irreversibly oxidize available ascorbic acid to its major breakdown product, oxalic acid. While ascorbic acid is necessary for the synthesis of collagen, the major reason for the osteoporosis appears to be a marked increase in bone resorption. Clinically, the osteoporosis can lead to crippling back pain due to vertebral collapse and to fracture of the femoral neck.

The serum ferritin may be raised to levels as high as 5000 µg/l in black subjects with iron overload. There are, however, factors which complicate the interpretation of individual values. Results may be falsely raised by concomitant alcohol-induced liver damage, while they may be reduced by associated ascorbic acid deficiency. Ascorbic acid deficiency impairs the release of iron from reticuloendothelial cells and, as a result, the serum iron and transferrin saturations may be misleadingly low. There is also experimental evidence that the serum ferritin may be similarly reduced. Ascorbic acid deficiency is also associated with figures for desferrioxamine excretion which are inappropriately low in relation to the size of the body stores. As in HH, the most reliable means of assessing the degree of overload is by liver biopsy, which also provides an opportunity to assess the degree of parenchymal and reticuloendothelial iron loading and to ascertain the degree of associated liver damage.

Very few black patients with iron overload have been subjected to repeated venesections. However, there is every reason to believe that such treatment should be beneficial if continued over long periods. Supplementation with moderate doses of ascorbic acid would also seem to be indicated. Some caution in this regard is, however, necessary since vigorous treatment could theoretically lead to the redistribution of iron from the reticuloendothelial system, where it is relatively innocuous, to parencythymal tissues, such as the heart, where it is toxic.

ALCOHOLIC SIDEROSIS

Iron stores are sometimes moderately increased in alcoholic liver disease. The levels encountered overlap with those found in normals and in persons heterozygous for HH, but are much lower than those occurring in homozygotes. The cause of the overload is not well understood but may be multifactorial. Alcohol increases iron absorption by stimulating gastric acid secretion. In addition, associated folate deficiency and portocaval shunting may also be associated with some increase in iron absorption. Alcoholic siderosis is easily distinguished from HH on liver biopsy.

PORPHYRIA CUTANEA TARDA

This condition, which is associated with both alcohol use and iron overload, is reviewed in Chapter 22.

RECOMMENDED READING

Bomford, A.B., Dymock, I.W. and Hamilton, E.B. (1991) Genetic hemochromatosis. *Gut* (Suppl), S111–15.

Bonkovsky, H.L. (1991) Iron and the liver. *Am J Medl Sci*, **301**(1), 32–43.

Conrad, M.E. (1993) Regulation of iron absorption. *Prog Clin Biol Res*, **380**, 203–19.

Cook, J.D. (1990) Adaptation in iron metabolism. *Am J Clin Nutr*, **51**, 301–8.

Crawford, D.H. and Halliday, J.W. (1991) Current concepts in rational therapy for haemochromatosis. *Drugs*, **41**, 875–82.

De Jong, G., Van Dijk, J.P. and Van Eijk, H.G. (1990) The biology of transferrin. *Clinica Chimica Acta*, **190**, 1–46.

Edwards, C.Q. and Kushner, J.P. (1993) Screening for hemochromatosis. *N Engl J Med*, **328**, 1616–20.

Gordeuk, V.R. (1992) Hereditary and nutritional iron overload. *Baillière's Clin Haematol*, **5**, 169–86.

Hershko, C., Pinson, A. and Link, G. (1990) Iron chelation. *Blood Reviews*, **4**, 1–8.

Kirking, M.H. (1991) Treatment of chronic iron overload. *Clin Pharm*, **10**, 775–83.

Leibold, E.A. and Guo, B. (1992) Iron-dependent regulation of ferritin and transferrin receptor expression by the iron-responsive element binding protein. *Annu Rev Nutr*, **12**, 345–68.

Munro, H. (1993) The ferritin genes: their response to iron status. *Nutr Rev*, **51**, 65–73.

Stremmel, W., Riedel, H.D., Niederau, C. and Strohmeyer, G. (1993) Pathogenesis of genetic haemochromatosis. *Eur J Clin Invest*, **23**, 321–9.

Tavill, A.S., Sharma, B.K. and Bacon, B.R. (1990) Iron and the liver: genetic hemochromatosis and other hepatic iron overload disorders. *Prog Liver Dis*, **9**, 281–305.

Theil, E.C. (1990) The ferritin family of iron storage proteins. *Adv Enzymol*, **63**, 421–49.

Woods, S., DeMarco, T. and Friedland, M. (1990) Iron metabolism. *Am J Gastroenterol*, **85**, 1–8.

22

Porphyria

PETER MEISSNER, RICHARD HIFT and RUDI SCHMID

INTRODUCTION

The porphyrias are a group of metabolic disorders which result from the decreased activity or reduced amount of specific enzymes of the heme synthetic pathway. The diagnosis and management of the porphyrias are critically dependent on an understanding of the biochemistry and enzymology of this pathway: these are reviewed below.

BIOCHEMICAL ASPECTS OF PORPHYRIA

PORPHYRINS AND HEME

Porphyrins are tetrapyrrole macrocycles characterized by their ability to fluoresce a bright red when exposed to ultraviolet light. Various atoms may be incorporated into the center of the porphyrin macrocycle. These include magnesium (giving rise to the chlorophylls), cobalt (leading to vitamin B12 via the corrin intermediates), and iron. The iron–porphyrin complex, heme (Fig. 22.1), plays a central role in biological oxidation reactions and is a vital constituent of hemoglobin, myoglobin, the cytochromes (including the cytochrome P450 family), and some mono- and di-oxygenases, catalases and peroxidases.

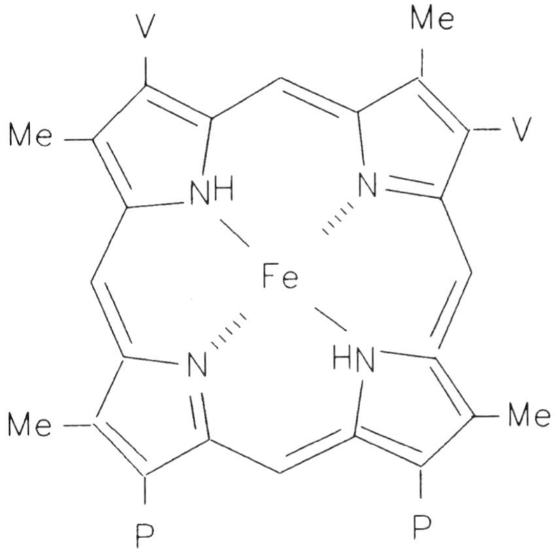

Figure 22.1 Chemical structure of heme.

HEME SYNTHESIS

Heme is produced by a well-defined pathway; it is initiated in the mitochondrion, continued in the cytosol and ultimately returns to the highly reduced environment of the mitochondrion (Fig. 22.2). All cells are able to produce heme. However, in humans most

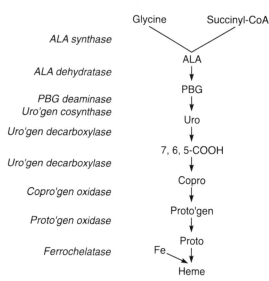

	Glycine	Succinyl-CoA
ALA synthase		
	ALA	
ALA dehydratase	↓	
	PBG	
PBG deaminase	↓	
Uro'gen cosynthase		
	Uro	
Uro'gen decarboxylase	↓	
	7, 6, 5-COOH	
Uro'gen decarboxylase	↓	
	Copro	
Copro'gen oxidase	↓	
	Proto'gen	
Proto'gen oxidase	↓	
	Proto	
Ferrochelatase	Fe ↓	
	Heme	

Figure 22.2 Scheme of mammalian heme biosynthetic pathway showing the corresponding enzymes on the left. ALA, delta-aminolaevulinic acid; PBG, porphobilinogen; uro, uroporphyrinogen-III; 7, 6, 5-COOH, hepta-, hexa- and penta-carboxylic porphyrinogen-III; copro, coproporphyrinogen-III; proto, protoporphyrinogen-IX; uro'gen, uroporphyrinogen-III; copro'gen, coproporphyrinogen-III; proto'gen, protoporphyrinogen-IX.

heme is synthesized in the liver and bone marrow.

Heme synthesis is initiated by the condensation of succinyl-CoA and glycine to delta-aminolaevulinic acid (ALA). Two ALA molecules then form the pyrrole porphobilinogen (PBG). Four molecules of PBG are assembled and then rearranged to form the first tetrapyrrolic porphyrinogen intermediate, uroporphyrinogen-III, which has eight carboxyl groups. Stepwise decarboxylation of uroporphyrinogen-III through hepta-, hexa-, and penta-carboxylic porphyrinogen intermediates to coproporphyrinogen-III is followed by oxidative decarboxylation to yield protoporphyrinogen-IX. Oxidation of this molecule and insertion of ferrous iron (Fe^{2+}) yields heme. Each of these steps is

catalyzed by an enzyme; deficency of a particular enzyme (in most instances inherited) may lead to a specific pattern of porphyrin accumulation and a characteristic clinical syndrome. Collectively these conditions are known as the porphyrias.

REGULATION OF HEME SYNTHESIS

Heme synthesis is normally an extremely efficient, tightly controlled process; efficient because less than 2.5% of the ALA entering the pathway is lost and tightly controlled because the amount of heme produced closely matches the needs of the body. This implies that enzymes involved in heme synthesis are normally able to use all of the substrate presented to them, that they can handle an increased flux through the pathway, and that the pathway may be subject to some form of feedback control. Indeed, there is much evidence to suggest that heme itself modulates its own rate of production, principally at the level of ALA synthase, which is considered the rate-determining enzyme of the pathway. While the precise mechanism of feedback control is not fully understood, it appears to be mediated principally by repression of ALA synthase mRNA transcription. In certain forms of porphyria there is an increased production of ALA, catalyzed by ALA synthase, which exacerbates the accumulation of intermediates immediately proximal to the abnormal enzyme. This is thought by some to represent a response to a diminished 'heme regulatory pool', although there is no direct evidence for the existence of such a pool.

The increase in ALA synthesis seen in this group of porphyrias, where heme synthesis is thought to be compromised, may be aggravated by a variety of circumstances. For example, many drugs induce the synthesis of cytochrome P450 isoenzymes or other hemoproteins. The resultant demand for heme leads to a further increase in ALA synthesis. Other drugs appear to affect ALA synthesis by acting directly on ALA synthase or may act via as yet unknown mechanisms. Apart from drugs, alcohol, hormones, infection, fasting and stress also appear able to increase flux through the heme synthetic pathway.

Under normal circumstances heme synthesis is so well orchestrated that, even under conditions of maximal heme production, the intracellular concentration of the various intermediates and their subsequent excretion are low. However, in porphyria those intermediates proximal to the enzymatic block accumulate to reach clinically relevant concen- trations. While there is still some uncertainty as to the exact mechanism by which heme intermediates affect the body, skin lesions are usually associated with excessive concentrations of porphyrins and acute attacks with accumulation of the porphyrinogen precursors ALA and PBG.

CLASSIFICATION OF THE PORPHYRIAS

The defective enzyme in each of the porphyrias has been identified. Table 22.1 provides a classification based on the primary enzyme defect and summarizes the clinical and biochemical features of each condition. Note that in addition to the inherited porphyrias there are acquired forms which include some forms of porphyria cutanea tarda (PCT) and the 'toxic' porphyrias.

From a clinical point of view it is useful to classify the porphyrias into those associated with acute attacks (acute porphyrias) and those in which acute attacks do not occur (non-acute porphyrias). This information is

Table 22.1 Current classification of the porphyrias

Porphyria	Affected enzyme	Clinical comment	Porphyrin excretion
A. Acute porphyias (mainly hepatic expression)			
1. AIP	PBG deaminase	No cutaneous involvement. Usually manifests postpubertally Degree of clinical expression highly variable and dependent on additional precipating factors. Clinical syndrome more frequent in females. Majority of carriers are clinically latent throughout life. Drug precautions necessary.	Excessive PBG and to a lesser extent ALA and uroporphyrin in urine. PBG, ALA and porphyrin levels very high during the acute attack.
2. VP	Protoporphyrinogen oxidase	Cutaneous involvement and acute attacks. Some carriers clinically latent throughout life. Usually mainfests postpubertally. Drug precautions necessary.	Elevated stool protoporphyrin and, to a lesser extent, coproporphyrin. Urinary PBG, ALA and porphyrins very high in the acute attack. Stool porphyrins raised very high in the acute attack.
3. HCP	Coproporphyrinogen oxidase	Photocutaneous lesions occur but rarely in the absence of acute attacks. Most are clinically latent throughout life. Drug precautions necessary.	Excessive excretion of coproporphyrin in the stool and sometimes in urine. PBG, ALA and porphyrins raised in the acute attack.

Table 22.1 contd

Porphyria	Affected enzyme	Clinical comment	Porphyrin excretion
4. DP	ALA dehydratase	Presents prepubertally. No cutaneous involvement. Acute symptoms only. Similar presentation to lead poisoning. Drug precautions necessary.	Characterized by elevated urinary ALA and coproporphyrin.
B1. Non-acute porphyrias (mainly hepatic expression)			
1. PCT	Uroporphyrinogen decarboxylase	Cutaneous involvement only. No acute attacks. Many forms (see below).	Main feature is elevated urinary and plasma uro- and heptacarboxylic porphyrin. Lesser elevations of hexa, pentacarboxylic and coproporphyrin. Stool porphyrins similarly raised together with elevated isoco-proporphyrin.
(a) Familial PCT		50% decreased uroporphy-rinogen decarboxylase in liver and erythrocytes.	Dominant inheritance. Unresponsive to treatment protocols such as venesec-tion.
(b) Acquired PCT • Sporadic		Appears as an unusual response to alcohol abuse, sex steroids and some forms of iron overload, including 'Bantu' siderosis.	
• Toxic		Appears in response to certain toxic chemicals, particularly poly-halogenated hydrocarbons. Includes 'Turkish' porphyria.	
• Chronic renal failure		Occurs in small number of patients with chronic renal failure on hemodialysis.	
(c) HEP	UROD activity 10%	Probably represents homozygous familial PCT. Severe photosensi-tivity from infancy. Elevated erythrocyte Zn protoporphyrin is a feature.	
B2. Non-acute porphyrias (mainly erythropoietic expression)			
2. EPP	Ferrochelatase	Only cutaneous involvement. Degree of clinical expression highly variable. Potential for liver problems. Mainfests in infancy.	Elevated erythrocyte-free protoporphyrin is the outstanding feature.
3. CEP	Uroporphyrinogen cosynthetase	Severely photomutilating Manifests in infancy. Hemolytic anemia frequent.	Accumulation of uro- and coproporphyrinogen-I in the erythrocytes (and plasma).

AIP, acute intermittent porphyria; VP, variegate porphyria; HCP, hereditary coproporphyria; DP, 'Doss' porphyria ('plumboporphyria'); PCT, porphyria cutanea tarda; HEP, hepato-erythropoietic porphyria; UROD, uroporphyrinogen deaminase; EPP, erythropoietic porphyria; CEP, congenital erythropoietic porphyria; ALA, delta-aminolaevulinic acid; PBG, porphobilinogen.

also given in Table 22.1 which includes an indication of whether the liver or erythron is thought to be the major site of abnormal porphyrin production.

LABORATORY DIAGNOSIS

As with all inherited conditions, knowledge of the mode of transmission and screening of family members is important. However, in the acute porphyrias identification of involved people is vital since, in most cases, patient education will reduce the incidence and the severity of acute attacks.

The diagnosis of porphyria requires accurate, quantitative measurement of porphyrin concentration in an appropriate biological fluid. ALA and PBG and the early porphyrin intermediates are water soluble and are best detected in the urine. Protoporphyrin is much less water soluble and must be assessed in feces. Coproporphyrin is of intermediate solubility and appears in both urine and stool (Fig. 22.3).

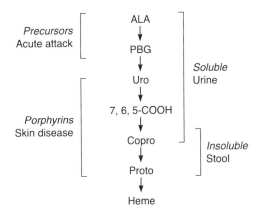

Figure 22.3 Two important principles. Firstly, skin disease of porphyria is associated with porphyrin accumulation while the acute attack is always associated with elevations of delta-aminolaevulinicacid (ALA) and porphobilinogen (PBG). Secondly, the early intermediates are largely water-soluble while the distal intermediates are more hydrophobic. Uro, uroporphyrin-III; copro, coproporphyrin-III; proto, protoporphyrin-III.

In those porphyrias involving the erythron, determination of red cell porphyrin concentrations is essential for diagnosis, while plasma porphyrin concentrations may be helpful in several of the porphyrias (Table 22.1). The choice of biological fluid will thus depend on the clinical picture as well as on the prevalence of the various porphyrias in each geographic region. For example, in South Africa where variegate porphyria is extremely common, fecal porphyrin concentrations form part of the routine investigation of most patients, while in Scandinavia, where intermittent acute porphyria (commonly termed acute intermittent porphyria or AIP) is most common, urine analysis is most important. As the porphyrias cannot be differentiated with certainty from each other on clinical grounds alone, recourse to the laboratory is indispensible.

Unfortunately, several forms of porphyria may clinically be expressed only in the second or third decade of life and many affected patients have a life-threatening latent defect. Thus activity-, immuno- and DNA-assays of specific heme biosynthetic enzymes are becoming more widely used for identification of porphyria and for family screening.

In the absence of specific enzyme assays, equivocal cases may require repeated testing by experienced personnel.

CLINICAL ASPECTS OF PORPHYRIA: ACUTE ATTACKS AND SKIN DISEASE

The porphyrias have two principal clinical manifestations: the acute attack and cutaneous photosensitivity (Table 22.1). Acute intermittent porphyria (AIP) is never accompanied by photosensitivity but is frequently complicated by acute attacks, whereas porphyria cutanea tarda (PCT), congenital erythropoietic porphyria (CEP) and erythropoietic protoporphyria (EPP) present with photosensitivity alone. Variegate porphyria (VP) and hereditary coproporphyria (HCP) may be accompanied by either or both manifestations. With HCP, photosensitivity is usually only described during the acute attack, whereas in VP chronic skin disease is common and may occur during any phase of the disease. Indeed, the combination of skin lesions and acute attacks led to the name variegate being applied to this condition.

ACUTE ATTACKS

The acute attack of porphyria is characterized biochemically by high concentrations of ALA and PBG in the urine and clinically by a neuropathic syndrome consisting of abdominal pain, vomiting, constipation, tachycardia, hypertension, psychiatric symptoms and, in the worst cases, a quadriplegia (Fig. 22.4).

Patients with acute attacks may present as 'surgical abdomen', as the Guillain–Barré syndrome, or even as hysteria. Indeed, the proper diagnosis is too often not considered. Equally dangerous is the tendency to label every episode of abdominal pain in a porphyric person as an acute attack. Exact measurement of urinary ALA and PBG concentrations, or at least qualitative demonstration of increased urinary PBG, are thus mandatory in any patient suspected of having an acute attack.

Pathogenesis of the acute attack

The acute attack consists of a neuropathy which, in the first instance, involves the autonomic nervous system, giving rise to abdominal pain, ileus, tachycardia and hypertension. In more severe cases the motor nervous system is involved with consequent, often asymmetrical, paralysis. Sensory involvement is less common and, if present, gives rise to signs which are subtle and thus often missed.

Although the association with high concentrations of ALA and PBG is well documented, the exact mechanism leading to the neuropathy of acute porphyria is not known. Several hypotheses have been advanced. These include neurotoxicity due to ALA, PBG or a

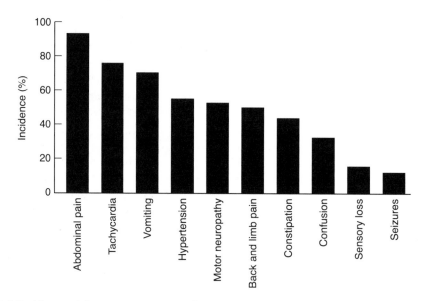

Figure 22.4 Incidence of the main symptoms of the acute attack of variegate porphyria (VP). The incidence of neurological signs is greater in acute intermittent porphyria (AIP). Note: occasionally acute pain in other parts of the body, including limbs, may be a presenting manifestation.

mono- or dipyrrole derived from disordered heme synthesis; deficiencies of other factors such as pyridoxal phosphate; or an intracellular deficiency of heme itself.

Precipitating factors of the acute attack

A precipitating factor responsible for an acute attack can be identified in many instances. The most common cause of an acute attack is the administration of porphyrinogenic medication. Even in the 1990s barbiturates and sulfonamides remain serious offenders. However, many drugs are capable of inducing such an attack, hence the importance of consulting drug lists before prescribing any medication for subjects with the acute porphyrias.

Fluctuations in levels of the female sex hormones are also known to induce acute attacks. In AIP acute attacks are often precipitated by pregnancy and monthly attacks immediately preceding the menses may occur. Patients with VP appear to be much less sensitive to hormonal effects than those with AIP. Hence menses-related acute attacks are extremely uncommon in patients with VP, though they may arise in pregnancy. Some patients with VP will tolerate oral contraceptives, others will not. It appears that the progestogen is more troublesome than the estrogen in this regard.

Other factors which may induce acute attacks include alcohol, fasting, infections and stress. However, it is difficult to assess the importance of these factors since they seldom occur in isolation.

Diagnosis of the acute attack

Acute attacks of porphyria should be suspected in all patients presenting with unexplained severe abdominal pain. The diagnosis must be confirmed in all cases with the Watson–Schwartz test, which requires minimal laboratory skills and only a few minutes to perform.

A positive Watson–Schwartz test indicates the presence of an elevated urinary PBG concentration. In VP, PBG is only significantly elevated during the acute attack; hence a positive test confirms the acute attack. However, in AIP, the PBG often remains elevated in the quiescent phase because of the proximal nature of the enzyme block. Such patients may show a positive test even in remission. However, in a patient with a compatible clinical picture, an acute attack should be assumed to be present and appropriate therapy introduced unless subsequent quantitative ALA and PBG measurements are inconsistent with this diagnosis.

Simple though it is to perform, false-negative test results do occur with the Watson–Schwartz test. In some instances this may be due to extremely dilute urine, but more commonly false-negative results are due to old reagents or to inexperience on the part of the person performing the test. One should not hesitate to repeat the test where strong suspicion exists. Quantitative measurement of the urinary ALA and PBG will provide a definitive answer and help must be sought from an experienced laboratory.

The porphyric patient who presents with atypical abdominal pain constitutes a common problem. If the Watson–Schwartz test is negative it is unlikely that the patient is having an acute attack and another explanation should be sought. Rarely the pain may result from an unassociated condition such as a peptic ulcer. In most instances, it is functional, often falling into the category of irritable bowel syndrome or spastic colon. It is not uncommon for doctors to persist in perpetuating the myth that such patients are suffering from recurrent acute attacks. The condition must be recognized for what it is and handled appropriately. Subjects with VP who regularly complain of atypical pain should have urine submitted to a laboratory during an acute episode. Documentation of low levels of ALA and PBG will exclude an acute porphyric attack as a diagnosis. Quantitation of urinary porphyrins also gives some index of the activity of the porphyria. Where urinary porphyrins (as opposed to fecal porphyrins) are low, it is fair to assume that the VP is exhibiting a low level of activity, and is thus highly unlikely to be responsible for the patient's complaints.

Management of the acute attack

Acute attacks can be divided into three stages of increasing severity. These correspond to those patients who may be treated at home, those who require hospitalization and those who must be admitted to an intensive or high care unit. The transition from the first to the second stage is often marked by the onset of vomiting which prevents oral intake of food and fluids. The transition from the second to the third stage often follows an error of judgment by the attending physician; in particular the continued administration of an unsafe drug, failure to apply adequate therapy in sufficient time, or failure to prevent and treat hyponatremia aggressively.

The symptoms of the acute attack, though unpleasant, are usually easily controlled. It is its complications: hyponatremia (usually secondary to the inappropriate secretion of antidiuretic hormone (ADH) or excessive intravenous administration of fluid) and motor neuropathy which are life-threatening and must be averted.

Treatment at home

Patients with mild attacks, consisting of abdominal pain and nausea alone, may be treated at home provided they are followed-up closely. A precipitating cause, particularly drug exposure, must be identified and removed where possible. Thereafter treat-ment is symptomatic with adequate analgesia and, where indicated, anti-emetics. Oral analgesics such as paracetamol (acetaminophen) or a paracetamol/codeine combination may be adequate. More severe pain will respond to oral dihydrocodeine or parenteral pethidine or morphine. Chlorpromazine, prochlorperazine and metoclopramide given orally, rectally or parenterally may be used as anti-emetics.

Treatment in hospital

Patients with more severe symptoms or with vomiting should be admitted to a hospital. Precipitating causes must be identified and removed. All medication should be stopped and no medication given unless it is reported safe by a specific drug list or its use has been sanctioned by a physician skilled in the management of porphyria. Baseline concentrations of urinary ALA and PBG concentrations should be determined. A common error is to treat symptoms with agents such as hyoscine butylbromide which are unsafe in porphyria and have resulted in aggravation of acute attacks.

Intravenous fluids are given to correct pre-existing dehydration and to maintain fluid balance thereafter. Hyponatremia is common in the severe acute attack. This may lead to convulsions which on occasion have been wrongly treated with barbiturates, leading to further progression of the disease. The cause of the hyponatremia is unclear and may be multifactorial. The syndrome of inappropriate ADH secretion has been invoked, but in some cases a primary salt-losing state has been identified in which saline replacement corrected the hyponatremia whereas fluid restriction did not. No uniform prescription for the treatment of hyponatremia can therefore be given. A decision on the correct response to hyponatremia must be an individual one based on consideration of all factors including the hydration status and urinary and sodium electrolytes.

Though carbohydrates may reduce porphyrin synthesis *in vitro*, the effect has not been shown to be significant either therapeutically or prophylactically. It is our practice to provide supplemental carbohydrates in moderation. A continuous intragastric drip via a fine-bore nasogastric feeding tube can be useful. Milder cases will settle spontaneously. Pain is treated with pethidine or morphine. Beta-blockers may be used to counteract tachycardia and hypertension. Apart from reducing these effects, beta-blockers have also been claimed to reduce porphyrin synthesis.

In those patients with more severe attacks, who do not readily improve, the administration of hematin should be considered. When indicated this should be administered promptly. First introduced into clinical practice in 1971, hematin is the product formed when hemin (obtained from human blood) is dissolved in an alkaline medium. Given intravenously it mimics heme and promptly suppresses ALA synthesis. Two forms of hematin are currently recommended: stabilized lyophilized hematin and heme arginate. Both are efficacious but expensive. The major side effects are a transient coagulopathy or phlebitis at the site of infusion. Heme arginate has a lower incidence of side effects and a longer shelf-life. Both are given in doses of 2–4 mg/kg per day as a simple daily infusion for 3–4 days. A large peripheral vein should be employed because of the danger of phlebitis. It is our practice to dilute the dose in 100 ml of human serum albumin, which appears to reduce the incidence of phlebitis.

In the Cape Town experience, the acute attack of VP tends to settle more easily than the attack of AIP and hematin is not commonly necessary in VP. In both conditions, however, a severe attack or its delayed diagnosis carry the potential to lead to complete paralysis and death, and hematin should not be withheld under such circumstances.

Management in an intensive care unit

Acute attacks accompanied by marked metabolic disturbances, encephalopathy, convulsions or neurological abnormalities are potentially fatal. Such patients should be admitted to an intensive care unit or high care area. Fluid restriction and supplemental feeding are instituted as described above. Therapy with hematin is indicated if the attack does not resolve rapidly.

The patient should be monitored frequently for the onset of a motor neuropathy. The signs include complaints of pain or heaviness in the limbs, progressive loss of reflexes and a decline in vital capacity. In the face of a neuropathy, vital capacity should be followed in a manner similar to that for patients with acute Guillain–Barré syndrome. Respiratory impairment will require intubation and intermittent positive-pressure ventilation. Though a prolonged period of convalescence may be required for full recovery, the porphyric neuropathy is almost always reversible and artificial ventilation may eventually be discontinued.

Hyponatremia should be sought and corrected. Where excessive vomiting has occurred dehydration must be excluded as the cause. In severe hyponatremia, fluid restriction alone may be insufficient and hypertonic saline may be required. This must be administered with great care since its use is hazardous and may result in central pontine myelinolysis. As a general rule, this may be performed safely provided that the correction is slow, i.e. no faster than 1–2 mmol per hour and the serum sodium is not corrected beyond levels of about 130 mmol/l. Several other forms of therapy have been suggested in the past. These include the administration of heavy metal chelators such as EDTA, vitamin therapy, ACTH administration, exchange transfusion, hemodialysis and charcoal hemoperfusion. None is currently advocated.

Management of recurrent acute attacks

Recurrent acute attacks are rare in VP, yet recurring complaints of abdominal pain and ill-health are not uncommon. Accurate and repeated measurement of urinary ALA and PBG concentration is essential in porphyric patients with recurrent episodes of abdominal pain in order to document or refute the diagnosis of porphyria as the cause of the acute pain. If the ALA and PBG levels are indeed elevated, continuing exposure to a porphyrinogenic drug must be ruled out. This may well relate to the injudicious continuation of a drug through misunderstanding or ignorance. In general, patients with AIP are more labile than those with VP and are thus more easily precipitated into acute attacks. Typically such patients are young females. Attacks may occur at monthly intervals, usually immediately preceding menstruation. It is thought that cyclic attacks are provoked by rapid changes in hormone levels occurring at this time. Interruption of this pattern may be extremely difficult. Repeated acute attacks may result in depression, despair and neurotic behavior in the patient and anxiety and doubt in the doctor. Not infrequently, suspicions arise as to the genuineness of the patient's symptoms and psychological dependency on the hospital and even addiction to opiates are invoked as reasons for the repeated complaints. Such labels should, however, be applied to patients only as a last resort since this clinical picture is quite compatible with AIP. As the attacks continue a chronic form of porphyric neuropathy may develop. Initially the features may consist only of feelings of lameness and heaviness in the extremities. However, with time, obvious weakness or loss of musculature becomes evident. Weakness of the dorsiflexors of the wrist is an early sign. Obvious abnormalities of axonal necrosis or muscle denervation can usually be documented by electroneurophysiological studies.

Individual attacks are treated as described above. Milder attacks may be treated at home to reduce the amount of time spent in hospital. Oral analgesia using dihydrocodeine may be complemented by prochlorperazine suppositories to combat vomiting and sedation with chlorpromazine or trifluoperazine. In view of the frequent need for analgesics, a potential for developing opiate dependence exists and their use should be strictly supervised.

Various methods have been employed to suppress menstrual-related attacks. These have included estrogens and progestogens, which are of little benefit and may be dangerous as they themselves can induce an acute attack. Prophylactic infusions of hematin also appear to be of little use, although it may be useful as a last resort. Gonadotrophin-releasing hormone (GnRH) agonists may be used in some patients. They competitively inhibit the GnRH-dependent secretion of follicle stimulating hormone (FSH) and luteinizing hormone (LH) from the pituitary. They may be given by regular daily injection, as a nasal spray or by a depot injection. Treatment is expensive and two principal risks are noted. Firstly, initiation of therapy may result in an acute attack, and secondly, GnRH therapy in effect induces a premature menopause. This is accompanied by accelerated bone loss analogous to that seen in menopausal osteoporosis. Limited experience suggests that such treatment may be very efficacious in about 50% of those in whom it is tried. In general, the more atypical the attacks and presentation, the less likely it is that this treatment will be effective. Experience has also shown that GnRH agonist therapy is only effective for the duration of the treatment. The porphyria remains active as evidenced by high levels of ALA and PBG, and does not appear in any way to be suppressed by the therapy. In effect, GnRH agonist therapy merely removes the hormonal surges that would otherwise constitute the final trigger for the acute attack. Currently it is recommended that treatment be continued for at least 2–3 years.

A novel form of therapy which has a limited place in the management of porphyria is the administration of tin protoporphyrin together with hematin. Tin protoporphyrin is an analog of heme where the central atom of iron is replaced by tin. This interacts with and irreversibly inhibits heme oxygenase, the principal enzyme responsible for the destruction of heme. This will prolong the beneficial effects of hematin, which are otherwise short-lived. Tin protoporphyrin may have a place in the management of some patients with AIP who experience very frequent and severe repetitive attacks, in spite of it inducing photosensitivity.

SKIN DISEASE IN PORPHYRIA

The second clinical presentation of porphyria, photocutaneous sensitivity, is shared by all forms of the disease other than AIP and plumboporphyria. The photosensitivity takes two forms: a rapid phototoxic response seen in erythropoietic protoporphyria (EPP) (and occasionally as a transient phenomenon by patients with VP during a period of accelerated porphyrin synthesis) and a delayed vesicular-erosive (scarring and blistering) form shared by VP, HCP, CEP and PCT.

Pathogenesis of the skin lesions

There are two lines of evidence suggesting that interaction of porphyrins and light in the skin gives rise to cutaneous disease. Firstly, a large amount of porphyrin is present in the skin of porphyric patients, and secondly, only those areas exposed to light are affected. Experimentally, marked photosensitivity indistinguishable from the phototoxic reaction of EPP can be induced in humans and animals by the administration of porphyrins or ALA.

Photobiology of porphyrins

Because porphyrins (and to a lesser extent porphyrinogens) contain extensive double-bond systems, they are photochemically active molecules and absorb both ultraviolet and visible light, particularly in the Soret band around 406 nm. Where accumulated porphyrins come into contact with light of the correct wavelength, there may be photo-stimulation followed by a transfer of energy to surrounding molecules, resulting in photochemical reactions which are thought to generate superoxide and oxygen free radicals. This is thought to be the mechanism of porphyrin-induced skin damage. However, the nature of the energy transfer from porphyrins in the skin to the surrounding structures, and the identity of the accepting molecules, remain unestablished.

The rapid phototoxic response

This form of photosensitivity is typical of EPP; it has been described as a solar urticaria. Following exposure to sunlight, burning, stinging and erythema are felt in exposed skin within a few hours. With continuing exposure, edema of the dermis develops which settles over a few days leaving petechiae in its wake. Photo-onycholysis or light-induced shedding of the nails may accompany this. Such a reaction is largely reversible. Initially, very little chronic destruction results (unlike the vesicular-erosive form of photosensitivity, whose immediate effects are not noticeable, but proceed over months to obvious skin damage). After many years, chronic changes may arise, including coarsening of the skin over the bridge of the nose, the cheeks, forehead and dorsal surfaces of the hands.

The vesicular-erosive scarring pattern

This pattern of photosensitivity is marked by the absence of early symptoms following sun exposure. No immediate discomfort is experienced, and patients often fail to associate their skin disease with exposure to sun. It occurs in PCT, HCP, VP and CEP.

Mechanical fragility of the skin is the most frequent symptom. In response to minimal trauma, the skin abrades easily, leaving painful erosions which occupy the full thickness of the epidermis. These may be accompanied by blisters and vesicles. The lesions are unsightly and heal slowly. Chronic scarring, milia, hypopigmentation and hyperpigmentation result. Such changes are typical of VP, where skin disease develops in the teens and twenties and may lead to an unsightly appearance.

Occasionally more severe disease may involve specialized skin structures giving rise to alopecia, hirsutism, keratoconjunctivitis, osteolysis of the fingers, nail dystrophy, destruction of the nasal and auricular cartilages or scarring of the eyelids and lips. Other features may include scleroderma-like plaques over the upper chest, back and face, and dystrophic calcification of the scalp, neck and pre-auricular skin. Such severe changes are unusual in VP. They are more typical of severe PCT and where a congenital porphyria has been severe and long-standing, particularly with onset in childhood. This is seen in CEP and hepato-erythropoietic porphyria (HEP, or homozygous PCT) and in homozygous VP.

Treatment of skin disease

Prevention of skin damage

Prevention of skin damage may be achieved by reducing exposure to sunlight, blocking its passage to the skin, quenching photoactivation, suppressing the production of porphyrins, or removing excess porphyrins from the skin. All of these have been tried with variable success and are outlined below.

Protection against light: the simplest and perhaps most effective steps to combat skin damage are to avoid exposure to the sun and to wear adequate protection against it. Thus avoiding the mid-day sun, limiting outdoor recreational and work-related pursuits and wearing protective clothing, such as a hat, long sleeves and long trousers, are effective, but are often difficult to implement for social and other reasons.

In severe cases of photosensitivity extreme measures may be required to limit light exposure. Tinted films pasted on windows will reduce the transmission of light of wavelengths below 550 nm. Fluorescent light strips emit strongly in the 405 nm band, which is very detrimental to the skin in porphyria. Replacement of such light strips by incandescent bulbs may be of help. However, such drastic steps are rarely necessary in the more commonly seen porphyrias.

Pharmacological photoprotectants: these have been widely employed to protect the skin in porphyria, but with varying success. They may be divided into two groups, topical sunfilters and systemic photoprotectants.

Topical sunfilters: porphyric subjects do not show an undue sensitivity to ultraviolet light in the sunburn range around 320 nm, against which most suntan preparations offer some protection. It is the wavelengths around the Soret maximum of 406 nm and beyond, against which conventional suntan preparations offer little protection, that are most damaging in porphyria. Thus only those preparations offering significant protection against wavelengths of 400 nm and more are at all likely to influence the degree of skin damage. This excludes nearly all commercially available suntan preparations.

Compounds containing zinc or titanium dioxide, which are opaque and therefore impede the passage of longer wavelengths, are more effective. They tend to be cosmetically unacceptable and have therefore not found wide acceptance among porphyrics. More recently, a few preparations which contain titanium dioxide in a transparent, cosmetically acceptable base combined with a high skin protection factor (SPF) have become available. They may be expected to be more effective, though this remains unproven. Potentially the most effective topical sunfilter is a dermatological preparation (Covermark). Although intended to hide blemishes, its blend of pigments also functions as an extremely effective sun barrier and its use may be recommended in more severe cases.

Systemic photoprotectants: beta-carotene has been widely employed as a systemic photo-protectant. It is very effective in patients with EPP, and over 90% of people with EPP will have their symptoms ameliorated by it. Its mechanism of action is not well understood. Its use is accompanied by a yellowish discoloration of the skin (carotenodermia). This may serve as a barrier to the passage of harmful wavelengths of light through the dermis. Alternatively, or even in addition, carotenoids may act at a molecular level as scavengers of free radicals and singlet-excited oxygen arising from the photoexcitation of porphyrins. Beta-carotene is much less effective in the other porphyrias, including VP.

Vitamin E (alpha-tocopherol) has also been investigated as an agent for limiting photosensitivity in porphyria and has yielded varying results. Its use for prolonged periods is hazardous and its benefit in PCT and VP appears to be negligible. It is thus not recommended.

Sorbent therapy: one study has shown that more than 90% of porphyrins entering the duodenum through the bile duct are reabsorbed over a 15 cm length of the proximal duodenum. This raised the possibility of increasing the fecal loss of porphyrins from the body by administering sorbents such as charcoal or cholestyramine. These would adsorb porphyrins in the bowel thereby interrupting the enterohepatic cycle. As an additional mechanism, binding of bile salts by the sorbent might reduce the competition of bile salts for biliary excretion with porphyrins and thus facilitate their excretion.

Cholestyramine has indeed been shown to bind porphyrins from the duodenal juice of patients with PCT, and to bring about an improvement in their skin disease. Certain brands of activated charcoal have been shown to be even better than cholestyramine. Patients with PCT may well benefit from sorbent therapy. However, they respond so well to venesection and to chloroquine (see below) that charcoal is seldom required in this condition. EPP also responds to charcoal and this treatment may well be of use in the management of the rare patient with severe protoporphyrin deposition in the liver. However, charcoal is probably not indicated in the average patient with EPP since carotenoids are so effective. A single case report showed a dramatic improvement in CEP treated with charcoal, and this has been confirmed in a second patient treated at our clinic. However, compliance is a problem since large doses of an unpleasantly gritty compound must be taken indefinitely. Apart from its taste, the only side effect of long-term treatment appears to be depletion of iron and vitamins. These are easily replaced.

A pilot study with charcoal in the treatment of VP, conducted in Cape Town, showed an unexpected and unexplained deterioration following the introduction therapy. There was an increase in skin disease and a rise in urinary and plasma porphyrin concentrations. Thus, in the short term at least, charcoal would appear to be deleterious in VP. The effects of charcoal taken for a longer period remain unknown.

Suppression of porphyrin synthesis

Though the relationship between ingestion of porphyrinogenic drugs and photosensitivity is not constant, skin disease does appear worse when VP is biochemically active, whether or not symptoms suggestive of an acute attack are present. It therefore seems prudent to avoid porphyrinogenic agents so as to reduce total porphyrin levels

Daily infusion of heme arginate will reduce fecal and plasma porphyrin levels in VP, but when given weekly, lower levels are not maintained and photosensitivity remains unabated. Most patients with CEP have both hemolysis and ineffective erythropoiesis; thus hypertransfusion has been used. By regular 2-weekly or monthly red cell transfusions, the stimulus for further erythropoietic heme production is removed. This results in some lowering of blood porphyrin levels, but in view of the risks of frequent transfusion, such therapy is not practical. Plasmapharesis and charcoal hemoperfusion have both been employed to reduce plasma porphyrin levels. Plasmapharesis has proved effective in treating the skin symptoms of hemodialysis-associated PCT where venesection was contraindicated.

DESCRIPTION OF THE PORPHYRIAS

ACUTE PORPHYRIAS

Acute intermittent porphyria (AIP)

This condition is more accurately termed intermittent acute porphyria. However, the term AIP has become universal and we will thus comply with this convention. AIP is found throughout the world. It is particularly common in northern Europe and Scandinavia. It is an autosomal dominant inherited defect of heme biosynthesis in which the activity of PBG deaminase is reduced by approximately 50%. More than 20 mutations in PBG deaminase have been documented. This results, in most cases, in accumulation of ALA and PBG, which are excreted in the urine. Some subjects with AIP may never manifest abnormal levels of urinary ALA or PBG except during acute attacks. Furthermore, elevated levels of ALA and PBG are not found before puberty and AIP is clinically expressed more often in females than in males. However, the enzyme defect is present in all affected individuals from birth to death and here there is no sex difference. It thus follows that even when PBG and ALA are normal, PBG deaminase activity must be determined before AIP can be excluded. Accurate diagnosis is essential since subjects with AIP may develop acute attacks if exposed to porphyrinogenic agents. Acute symptoms are always associated with elevated concentrations of ALA and PBG in the urine.

PBG deaminase in AIP

Diminished PBG deaminase activity has been shown in a variety of cells. These include hepatocytes, erythrocytes, fibroblasts and amniotic cells. Numerous genetic variants have been found to account for the diminished enzyme activity. Assays for PBG deaminase are fairly simply performed on erythrocytes from samples of fresh heparinized blood and should form part of the service offered by all porphyrin laboratories.

Biochemical profile of AIP

Excessive PBG and, to a lesser extent, ALA and uroporphyrin concentrations in the urine are diagnostic of AIP. PBG and ALA porphyrin levels are very high during the acute attack (20 to 200 times normal). All clinically symptomatic patients and about one-third of clinically asymptomatic carriers show abnormal excretion of PBG.

Variegate porphyria (VP)

VP is an autosomal-dominant inherited defect of heme biosynthesis in which the activity of protoporphyrinogen oxidase is reduced by approximately 50%. VP is also known as South African genetic porphyria because of its high prevalence in the South African population. The gene is thought to have been introduced by an orphan from The Netherlands who married a Dutch settler at the Cape in 1688. For the next two centuries, possibly because of the lack of precipitating pharmacological agents and therefore a low incidence of acute attacks, the disease was relatively benign and the founder effect was sufficient to result in widespread distribution of the trait. Estimates of the incidence of VP based on genealogical data have been as high as 3 per 1000 within the white Afrikaner population. Current estimates put the total figure of affected individuals between 10 000 and 20 000. No accurate figure exists since many subjects with the disease remain asymptomatic and even biochemically latent throughout their lives. Like AIP, VP is only rarely manifest before puberty.

VP is found in other parts of the world but is much less common than in South Africa. Recently, a small population with VP in Western Australia have had their ancestry traced back to the survivors of a Dutch ship, the *Zuytdorp*, which was wrecked off Western Australia in 1712 while under way from the Cape of Good Hope to the East Indies. Historians speculate that the VP gene was transmitted to Australia via a crew member recruited in the Cape.

Biochemical profile of VP

The most striking feature of the porphyrin excretory profile of VP is an elevated fecal concentration of protoporphyrin and, to a lesser extent, of coproporphyrin. This is present both during remission (quiescence) and in the acute attack. During the acute attack, concentrations of protoporphyrin and coproporphyrin are further increased and are accompanied by increases in the more proximal porphyrin intermediates, in particular uroporphyrin. In addition, the acute attack is invariably associated with grossly elevated concentrations of ALA and PBG in the urine.

Heme-synthetic enzymes in VP

Protoporphyrinogen oxidase activity is decreased by approximately 50% in all VP tissues of VP carriers. This explains the accumulation of protoporphyrinogen and coproporphyrinogen which is reflected by increased excretion of these or their derivative porphyrins in the stool.

The mechanism by which PBG and ALA increase in acute attacks has recently been explained by our finding of a small but significant decrease in the activity of PBG deaminase in variegate porphyric subjects. This decreased activity appears to be due to inhibition of PBG deaminase by the protoporphyrinogen and coproporphyrinogen accumulating intracellularly as a result of the primary protoporphyrinogen oxidase defect. When the pathway is relatively quiescent PBG deaminase inhibition is marginal. However, when ALA synthase activity is increased, as occurs during the acute attack, inhibition of PBG deaminase increases to a point where ALA and PBG accumulate in the tissue and are excreted in excess in the urine.

Unusual presentations of VP

A few homozygous cases of VP have been described, including two in South Africa. All of these patients presented as young children, exhibiting severe life-long photosensitivity, variable degrees of growth retardation and neurological involvement; all had increased erythrocyte protoporphyrin in addition to the typical VP fecal porphyrin profile.

Some South African VP patients have so-called 'dual porphyria' in which porphyrin excretory profiles typical of porphyria cutanea tarda are superimposed on those typical of VP. The activities of protoporphyrinogen oxidase and uroporphyrinogen decarboxylase are both decreased in these patients. No clear inheritance pattern for dual porphyria has emerged and the underlying mechanisms are unclear.

Hereditary coproporphyria (HCP)

This rare form of porphyria, inherited as an autosomal-dominant trait, presents with both photocutaneous skin lesions and acute attacks. Diminished coproporphyrinogen oxidase activity has been shown in all tissues obtained from carriers. A homozygous form and a variant form with 10% coproporphyrinogen oxidase activity (harderoporphyria) have been described. The majority of carriers remain clinically latent throughout adult life and photocutaneous skin lesions rarely occur in the absence of acute attacks.

Biochemical profile of HCP

HCP is characterized by increased fecal coproporphyrin (but normal protoporphyrin) concentrations. During acute attacks of HCP, ALA and PBG are found in the urine. HCP is rarely seen before puberty and there is a high percentage of latent carriers of this trait.

ALA dehydratase-deficiency porphyria ('Plumboporphyria'; Doss porphyria)

This, the most recently described porphyria, has an autosomal-recessive pattern of inheritance and is characterized clinically by acute attacks alone. The condition results from a structural mutation in the ALA dehydratase gene. This results in elevated urinary ALA (and coproporphyrin) excretion resembling severe lead poisoning.

NON-ACUTE PORPHYRIAS

Porphyria cutanea tarda (PCT)

PCT (also known as chronic hepatic porphyria or symptomatic porphyria), a syndrome characterized by photocutaneous lesions without acute attacks, is the most common form of porphyria worldwide. PCT may be acquired (sporadic) or more rarely may be inherited as an autosomal-dominant trait. Hepatic uroporphyrinogen decarboxylase activity is decreased in both forms; however, erythrocyte uroporphyrinogen decarboxylase activity is also reduced in familial PCT but is normal in the sporadic form, where the enzyme defect appears to be restricted to the liver.

PCT differs from other porphyrias in several respects. It is the only form of porphyria that may be acquired rather than directly inherited, and usually presents at a later age than the inherited types. There is a strong association with some well-defined medical disorders and, unlike other forms of porphyria, it is clinically reversible although there is uncertainty regarding the normalizing of uroporphyrinogen decarboxylase activity.

Associations

PCT is strongly associated with the moderate to excessive consumption of alcohol. In most cases there is also evidence of hepatic iron overload. In a consecutive series of patients with PCT assessed in Cape Town, 78% had a history of significant alcohol intake and 67% had raised serum ferritin concentrations.

Almost all of the remaining patients had abnormal iron stores on liver biopsy. PCT has also been described in association with estrogen therapy, systemic lupus erythematosus, lymphoma and AIDS (Fig. 22.5). Variants include 'toxic' porphyria, precipitated by the ingestion of substituted hydrocarbons such as hexachlorobenzene, and familial PCT, inherited as an autosomal-dominant trait, presenting at an earlier age and which may be independent of alcohol and iron overload. Hepato-erythropoietic porphyria (HEP), the homozygous form of familial PCT, presents in childhood and is more severe.

Clinical features of PCT

The hallmark of PCT is photocutaneous sensitivity. The vesicular-erosive skin lesions are similar to those seen in VP and CEP. The severity varies. In its most severe form the skin disease may be disfiguring with photomutilation, onycholysis and resorption of digits, and can even mimic scleroderma. Yet many cases are mild and may be unrecognized. Here the manifestations are limited to darkening of the skin over the face and hands, and excess facial hair, particularly over the temples. Indeed, the more PCT is actively sought among hospitalized patients, the more frequently it is found. Mild liver disease usually accompanies PCT and probably reflects alcohol use or iron overload. Liver disease must be sought and treated as it may ultimately give rise to serious illness.

Biochemical profile of PCT

The main biochemical features are elevated urinary and plasma uro- and hepta-carboxylic porphyrin while lesser elevations of hexa-, penta-carboxylic and coproporphyrin also occur. Stool porphyrins are similarly raised in addition to a striking elevation of isocoproporphyrin.

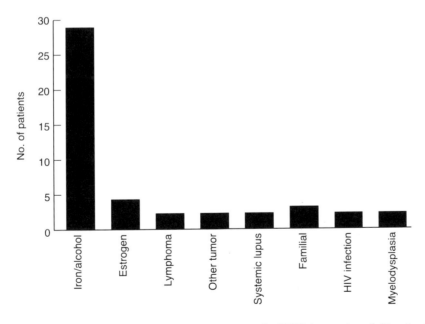

Figure 22.5 Conditions associated with porphyria cutanea tarda (PCT) in a series of 45 patients evaluated at Groote Schuur Hospital.

Investigation of PCT

Once a diagnosis of PCT has been confirmed, liver disease and evidence of iron overload must be sought. The serum ferritin concentration is a more sensitive and reliable predictor of hepatic iron overload than serum iron, transferrin saturation and total iron-binding capacity. However, ferritin is an acute-phase reactant and may be elevated in the absence of iron overload where other illness is present. Liver biopsy yields useful diagnostic and prognostic information and is a valuable guide to iron stores. In our series of patients, the liver biopsy was abnormal in every case and 95% had raised serum transaminases, whereas only 33% had clinically apparent liver disease.

Therapy of PCT

Patients with PCT should be urged to abstain from alcohol consumption, to cease estrogen therapy or to avoid iron supplements. General principles of treatment for the skin are as previously described. However, therapy with venesection or chloroquine is so uniformly effective in improving the disease that it is often unnecessary to maintain these measures for long.

Reduction of iron stores is nearly always accompanied by a marked improvement in clinical and biochemical features of PCT. Excellent results have been obtained using venesection or desferrioxamine infusion. Desferrioxamine is much more expensive and is associated with a slower response. It is thus used only where venesection is contraindicated because of coexistence of anemia. Venesection is easy to perform, has minimal side effects and is cheap. Treatment is by removal of 500 ml of blood on a flexible schedule, usually at 2–4-weekly intervals. On each occasion blood samples are sent for liver chemistry, full blood count, plasma porphyrins and ferritin and a urine sample is

obtained for estimation of urine porphyrins. An improvement in photosensitivity is often noted after 3–4 venesections and the plasma and urine porphyrin concentrations tend to fall to lower levels after 3–8 venesections.

Venesection can be discontinued once the serum ferritin is in the low normal range, the plasma is clear of porphyrins and urine porphyrins are reduced. Conventional iron studies, with a rise in the total iron-binding capacity, may be more sensitive than the ferritin level in detecting the onset of iron deficiency. After remission has been induced, patients should be encouraged to become regular blood donors as bleeding every 2–3 months will maintain remission as a state of moderate iron deficiency should be maintained.

Apart from its ability to ameliorate photosensitivity by a poorly understood mechanism, a property employed in the treatment of skin conditions such as systemic lupus erythematosus, chloroquine has an additional and more important action in PCT. It greatly enhances the clearance of porphyrin from the liver by complexing with hepatic porphyrins to form water-soluble compounds which are then released and excreted in the urine. Such a release, if not carefully controlled, may result in lysis of hepatocytes. Thus, where standard anti-malarial or photoprotective doses of chloroquine are used in PCT, an acute hepatotoxic reaction marked by fever, malaise, pain, nausea, vomiting and elevated transaminases is common. Chloroquine should therefore be used in a low dose such as 125 mg twice to thrice weekly. Initiation of therapy is often followed by a massive outpouring of porphyrins, with a reddish urine, an elevation of urinary porphyrin concentrations and sometimes a transient deterioration in the skin disease. With continued administration, porphyrin concentrations decrease and remission occurs after 2 or 3 months. This low-dose regimen has the added advantage of minimizing the risk of chloroquine retinal toxicity. Chloroquine therapy will not reverse the iron overload; a plausible reason for favoring venesection as initial therapy. In cases where the response to venesection is tardy, the simultaneous administration of chloroquine appears to accelerate improvement. It is now our standard practice to employ venesection and chloroquine simultaneously.

Erythropoietic protoporphyria (EPP)

EPP is characterized by diminished activity of ferrochelatase, inherited as a dominant trait with partial penetrance. Clinical expression is variable and results in life-long cutaneous photosensitivity and a predisposition to cholelithiasis and to hepatic protoporphyrin deposition with liver failure. The outstanding biochemical feature of EPP is elevated free protoporphyrin in erythrocytes.

The skin disease of EPP manifests as a prompt phototoxic response, and is discussed in more detail below. It arises in infancy and may give rise to chronic skin changes in the course of years.

Liver disease in EPP

The most feared complication of EPP is excessive protoporphyrin accumulation in the liver leading to hepatic failure. All patients with EPP should be monitored yearly. Any abnormality of liver function tests, particularly the transaminases, should be regarded as an indication for liver biopsy. If this shows accumulation of protoporphyrin, easily demonstrated by intense red fluorescence of the biopsy under ultraviolet light or detection of protoporphyrin crystals, the use of oral charcoal to reduce these abnormal stores should be considered. For advanced liver disease accompanying protoporphyrin deposition, liver transplant may be unavoidable.

Management of the skin disease of EPP

Avoidance of exposure to the sun is pivotal in the management of skin disease in EPP. Patients will usually comply with these measures because of the discomfort they experience during exposure. Indeed the burning, stinging and itching after sun exposure is usually sufficient to bring about a voluntary modification of behavior.

The administration of beta-carotene, the precursor of vitamin A, is extremely effective in ameliorating EPP photosensitivity. Over 90% of patients placed on this therapy will have a beneficial response, and in many of these the protection is such that they will be able to live normal lives. Sufficient beta-carotene must be taken for carotenodermia (a yellowish discoloration of the skin, initially of the palms of the hands) to develop. Beta-carotene should be taken in doses of 50–150 mg daily. Several months' therapy are required for the carotenodermia to become apparent, following which amelioration of the disease is noted. Unfortunately, the preparations which contain adequate amounts of beta-carotene have been withdrawn from the market in some countries because of a fear of their abuse by those seeking an easy tan. The raw material is still available from the manufacturers and can be made up by a pharmacist.

Canthaxanthine is a synthetic carotenoid similar in its efficacy to beta-carotene. When taken in combination, the skin pigmentation takes a more acceptable form, looking more like a natural tan than the yellowish color of beta-carotene alone. The two agents have been combined in the ratio 2 : 3. This combination is often cosmetically more acceptable to subjects with EPP but carries the risk of deposition of canthaxanthine crystals in the retina. This has not been shown to be deleterious, yet one would advise caution. People taking beta-carotene and canthaxanthine should undergo regular ophthalmological examination. Should deposits become apparent, consideration should be given to reducing or stopping the canthaxanthine and continuing with beta-carotene alone.

In vivo, beta-carotene serves as a precursor of vitamin A. Yet vitamin A, *per se*, is of no benefit in protecting against the photosensitivity of EPP. Vitamin A in large amounts is toxic. Carotene is very much less toxic as the body is relatively inefficient at converting it to vitamin A. Our current practice is to treat our patients with beta-carotene and canthaxanthine in combination. Once a response is noted, the dose may be reduced. Combination therapy may also be given in reduced doses during winter and increased doses in the early spring and summer.

Congenital erythropoietic porphyria (CEP)

CEP, an extremely rare condition, is thought to have been responsible for the first published case of porphyria, probably because of its dramatic clinical signs. These are characterized by life-long acute cutaneous photosensitivity and severe photomutilation. Biochemically CEP is characterized by decreased uroporphyrinogen cosynthase activity. This results in accumulation of the uroporphyrin-I isomer. CEP is inherited as an autosomal-recessive trait and is diagnosed by the presence of increased uro- and coproporphyrinogen-I isomers in the erythrocytes (and plasma). Increased hemolysis is almost always present, yet splenectomy is of little benefit.

CONCLUSION

The medical care of patients and, indeed, families with porphyria requires a balanced and holistic approach. A knowledge of applied biochemistry translates into more reliable diagnosis and monitoring; genetic counseling is essential in view of the familial nature of most of these conditions. Indeed in

the case of an acute porphyric it is essential to conduct family studies in order to detect latency in other family members. Education of patients, their families, doctors and pharmacists in the safe use of drugs will minimize the risks of the acute attack. Skilled and knowledgeable treatment of these attacks and of the skin disease of porphyria will allow many to lead essentially normal lives, and will minimize discomfort for the remainder.

RECOMMENDED READING

Bissel, D.M. and Schmid, R. (1987) Hepatic Porphyrias, in *Diseases of the Liver*, 6th edn (eds L. Schiff and E.R. Schiff), J.B. Lippincott, Philadelphia, pp. 1975–2092.

Dailey, H.A. (ed.) (1990) *Biosynthesis of Heme and Chlorophylls*, McGraw Hill, New York.

Disler, P.B. and Moore, M.R. (eds) (1985) *Porphyria, Clinics in Dermatology*, J.B. Lippincott, Philadelphia, pp. 1–163.

Eales, L., Day, R.S. and Blekkenhorst, G.H. (1980) The clinical and biochemical features of variegate porphyria: an analysis of 300 cases studied at Groote Schuur Hospital, Cape Town. *Int J Biochem*, **12**, 837–53.

Eales, L. (1979) Clinical Chemistry of the Porphyrins, in *The Porphyrins*, vol. 6 (ed. D. Dolphin), Academic Press, New York, pp. 663–804.

Hift, R.J., Meissner, P.N. and Meissner, D.M. (1991) *Porphyria: A Guide for People with Porphyria and their Doctors*, MRC/UCT, Cape Town.

Meissner, P.N., Meissner, D.M., Sturrock, E.D. *et al.* (1986) Porphyria – The UCT experience. *S Afr Med J*, **72**, 755–61.

Moore, M.R., McColl, K.E.L., Rimington, C. and Goldberg, A. (Eds) (1987) *Disorders of Haem Metabolism*, Plenum Medical, New York.

Sassa, S. and Kappas, A. (1981) Genetic, metabolic and biochemical aspects of the porphyrias, in *Advances in Human Genetics*, vol 2 (eds H. Harris and K. Herschorn), Plenum Medical, New York, pp. 121–231.

23

Pregnancy and the liver

ERIC LEMMER, SIMON ROBSON and CAROLINE RIELY

INTRODUCTION

Severe liver disease occurs in less than 0.1% of pregnancies. Clinically, the appearance of spider nevi and palmar erythema are common manifestations of normal pregnancy. In contrast, the liver and spleen should remain impalpable. Thus clinical enlargement of these viscera suggests disease.

Certain tests used in assessing liver function are influenced by pregnancy (Table 23.1). The serum alkaline phosphatase (ALP) concentration increases slowly to the seventh month, after which it rises more rapidly to reach a peak at term. The serum albumin concentration decreases by 5–8 g/l. This is largely a dilution effect due to the increased plasma volume.

Liver disease in pregnancy can be classified into three categories:

- liver disease unique to pregnancy;
- liver disease concomitant with pregnancy;
- the effects of pregnancy on pre-existing liver disease.

LIVER DISEASE UNIQUE TO PREGNANCY

INTRAHEPATIC CHOLESTASIS OF PREGNANCY (ICP)

ICP is a disorder characterized by generalized pruritus and biochemical evidence of cholestasis, with or without clinical jaundice. This condition occurs during the second half of pregnancy, resolves rapidly after delivery, and tends to recur in subsequent pregnancies. ICP is 10 to 100 times more prevalent in Chile and in Sweden than in other countries. Although the cause is unknown, the syndrome appears to represent an exaggerated reaction of the maternal liver to the high circulating levels of estrogens and progesterone attained during pregnancy. This reaction appears to be due in part to an inherited predisposition and in part to environmental factors.

Pruritus is the initial symptom. It usually develops in the third trimester and dominates the symptomatology. About 3–4 weeks after the onset of pruritus the patient may notice that her urine has become dark and her stools light. Physical examination is generally

Table 23.1 Changes in liver function related to normal pregnancy (from Schorr-Lesnick *et al.*, 1991)

Test	Usual range during pregnancy
Plasma volume	Increased greater than 50%
Blood volume	Increased 40–50%
Alkaline phosphatase	1.5 to 4-fold increase
Transpeptidase II (GGT)	Either increased, slightly decreased, or unchanged
5'-Nucleotidase	Either increased or unchanged
Lactic dehydrogenase	Slightly increased
Transaminases (AST, ALT)	Unchanged or slightly increased to upper limits of normal
Bilirubin	Unchanged
Prothrombin time	Unchanged
Coagulation Factors VII–X	Increased
Fibrinogen	Increased
Albumin	Decreased 10–20% below level in non-pregnant women
Globulins	Alpha and beta increased, gamma decreased
Cholesterol	2-fold increase
Triglycerides	Increased

AST, aspartate aminotransferase; ALT, alanine aminotransferase.

normal except for excoriations due to pruritus. Jaundice is present in a minority of patients. Liver function tests show a cholestatic pattern. Serum alkaline phosphatase, 5'-nucleotidase, bile acids, cholesterol, and lipids are increased and lipoprotein-X is present. The serum conjugated bilirubin concentration may be raised. Vitamin K deficiency may lead to hypoprothrombinemia, especially in patients on cholestyramine. Liver biopsy reveals mild cholestasis with intracellular bile pigment and canalicular bile plugs.

The pruritus usually responds to cholestyramine 12–24 g/day in three divided doses. Parental vitamin K1 may be required, especially at the time of delivery. The pruritus diminishes in intensity within 2 days post-partum and disappears in 10–14 days. Jaundice resolves within 1–2 weeks. Persistence of symptoms beyond this period should suggest another cause.

ACUTE FATTY LIVER OF PREGNANCY (AFLP)

AFLP is a rare, potentially fatal condition which complicates the latter half of approximately 1 in 13 000 pregnancies. AFLP usually presents after week 35, resolves completely in those patients who recover and usually does not recur in subsequent pregnancies.

Presenting symptoms include anorexia, nausea, vomiting, malaise, epigastric pain, headache and progressive jaundice. In severe cases gastrointestinal bleeding, hepatic encephalopathy and oliguria may occur. Physical examination reveals jaundice and tenderness in the right upper quadrant. The liver is shrunken. Signs of associated pre-eclampsia are present in 20–40% of cases. Laboratory tests confirm severe hepatic failure, acute renal failure and, in severe cases, evidence of disseminated intravascular coagulation. The serum transaminases are generally in the range of 300–500 units/l. Neutrophilia, thrombocytopenia ($<150 \times 10^9/l$) and the presence of normoblasts in the peripheral blood smear are early uniform findings. The differential diagnosis includes fulminant viral hepatitis and pre-eclamptic liver disease. Liver biopsy is diagnostic and reveals swollen pale pericentral hepatocytes with microvesicular fatty infiltration. Special stains such as oil red-O may be necessary to demonstrate the latter (Chapter 6). Where liver biopsy is contraindicated by the presence of severe coagulopathy the diagnosis may be made on clinical and laboratory criteria.

The only specific therapy for AFLP is rapid delivery. Expert, supportive care for hepatic failure and its complications is vital. Special consideration must be given to the prevention of hypoglycemia. Fetal and maternal mortality rates have been reduced from about 85% in the 1970s to less than 25%, mainly due to earlier recognition and more rapid termination of pregnancy. Although unusual, recent reports have documented the recurrence of this syndrome in a subsequent pregnancy. In some of these individuals evidence points to an underlying defect in mitochondrial fatty acid oxidation.

PRE-ECLAMPTIC TOXEMIA

The liver is not primarily involved in patients with pre-eclampsia, but may be damaged as the disease progresses. Most patients do not have complaints referable to the liver, and the disease is detected by abnormal liver biochemistry in a patient with pre-eclampsia.

The other end of the spectrum of liver involvement associated with pre-eclamptic toxemia is the HELLP syndrome (hemolysis, elevated liver enzymes, low platelets). This life-threatening condition is most common in older, white patients and most often presents at about 32 weeks, particularly where the diagnosis of pre-eclampsia has been delayed. However, an important minority of patients present during the postpartum period and a small number of these may have no antepartum evidence of pre-eclampsia.

The etiology of the hepatic damage in toxemia is not known. Segmental vasospasm and vasodilatation may cause a vasculopathy with disruption of endothelial cells and subsequent platelet deposition and fibrin precipitation.

Patients present with right upper quadrant pain, headache, nausea and vomiting in addition to features of toxemia. Laboratory tests show microangiopathic hemolytic anemia, thrombocytopenia and elevated transaminases. Some may develop hepatic failure, presumably due to microemboli in the hepatic vasculature causing ischemia and tissue damage. Maternal mortality is about 3% and fetal mortality around 35%.

Hematoma and rupture of the liver, severe complications of pre-eclampsia and HELLP usually involve the right lobe of the liver. Patients generally present with severe right upper quadrant pain and sudden hypotension. The mortality rate for mother and fetus is about 60%. Hepatic rupture is preceded by parenchymal and sub-capsular hematoma, which can be demonstrated by ultrasound and computed tomography of the liver. Therapy is angiographic immobilization or laparotomy with prompt control of hemorrhage (Chapter 4).

Liver biopsy is not required to make the diagnosis of HELLP but reveals periportal fibrin deposition and/or hemorrhage, and hepatocellular necrosis (Chapter 6).

Treatment of patients with mild hepatic involvement is that of the underlying toxemia and aims at control of hypertension and seizures. Prompt delivery is usual where the fetus is mature. Where toxemia occurs in early pregnancy expectant management is adopted. This includes bed rest and anti-hypertensive therapy. Where toxemia is complicated by the HELLP syndrome, rapid delivery and intensive supportive therapy are important. Patients developing the syndrome in the postpartum period have a higher incidence of pulmonary edema and renal failure and usually require intensive supportive care.

HYPEREMESIS GRAVIDARUM

Hyperemesis gravidarum is characterized by intractable vomiting during early gestation resulting in dehydration, electrolyte abnormalities and nutritional deficiencies with weight loss. Abnormalities of liver function are uncommon in hyperemesis gravidarum, unless it is severe enough to require admission to hospital. The etiology of deranged liver function tests is probably multifactorial, and contributing factors include metabolic acidosis, dehydration and weight loss. The jaundice in hyperemesis has no prognostic significance and requires no specific therapy.

LIVER DISEASE CONCOMITANT WITH PREGNANCY

VIRAL HEPATITIS

Viral hepatitis (Chapter 8) is the commonest cause of liver disease in pregnancy throughout the world although there is a marked geographical variation in the viruses responsible for this disorder. Hepatitis may occur at any time during pregnancy and symptoms may resemble those of normal pregnancy. e.g. nausea, vomiting, fatigue and malaise. The presentation, clinical features and course are similar to that in non-pregnant patients. However, hepatitis E virus (HEV) may be associated with a 20% mortality rate in pregnant women particularly during the third trimester.

The hepatitis B virus (HBV) is by far the most important cause of viral hepatitis in pregnancy worldwide. Vertical transmission from mother to child may occur during the perinatal period. The virus rarely crosses the placenta, and vertical transmission is thought to occur during the passage of the neonate through the birth canal, perhaps via abrasions or swallowed blood. Vertical transmission from asymptomatic mothers is much commoner in Asian countries (30–70%) than in the USA (5–20%), Europe and Africa. In the latter areas vertical transmission is more likely to occur when HBV infection occurs during the third trimester of pregnancy. Finally, more than 80% of mothers who are HBeAg positive transmit HBV to their offspring whereas the figure is 25% if the mothers are anti-HBe positive. Approximately 90% of neonates infected become chronic HBV carriers and are at greatly increased risk of developing hepatocellular carcinoma (HCC) in later life.

Perinatal transmission of HBV is prevented by a combination of passive and active immunization. Passive immunization involves the intramuscular administration of hyperimmune hepatitis B immunoglobulin (HBIG). HBIG should be administered within 48 hours (dosage 100 units) of birth, and preferably within 12 hours, to prevent perinatal transmission. A second dose of HBIG should be given 30 days after initial administration. Active vaccination, with either a plasma-derived or a recombinant yeast-produced vaccine, involves an intramuscular injection into the deltoid muscle at 0, 1 and 6 months (dosage 10 μg for neonates). Universal infant immunization is the ideal in areas where endemic HBV infection occurs, such as sub-Saharan Africa. In Africa, the peak occurrence of HBV infection occurs in children between the ages of 2 and 11 years. The mechanism of this horizontal transmission of HBV in the first decade of life is unclear.

EFFECTS OF PREGNANCY ON PRE-EXISTING LIVER DISEASE

CIRRHOSIS AND PORTAL HYPERTENSION

Fertility is reduced in patients with chronic liver disease and pregnancy is thus rare. Fetal outcome is adversely affected by the presence of cirrhosis (Chapter 14). Pregnant cirrhotic patients have an increased risk of variceal bleeding. The pathogenesis is probably multifactorial; increased plasma volume and cardiac output, raised intra-abdominal pressure, and repeated Valsalva maneuvers during labor are all thought to play a role. Portal pressures are greatly increased during vaginal delivery, and assisted vaginal delivery or Caesarean section has thus been advocated for these patients. Sclerotherapy is regarded as the treatment of choice both for acutely bleeding varices and for documented variceal bleeding after initial stabilization. Intravenous vasopressin should be avoided in pregnancy as it may induce labor. Ascites and hepatic encephalopathy do not occur with greater frequency in pregnancy, despite the overall tendency to increased fluid accumulation.

HEPATIC TUMORS

Focal nodular hyperplasia (FNH) and liver cell adenoma (LCA) are two benign liver tumors associated with both oral contraceptive use and pregnancy. FNH is a hypervascular lesion whereas LCA (a true neoplasm) is poorly vascularized. This distinction in vascular pattern allows differentiation of the two lesions (Chapter 4). Adenomas may enlarge during pregnancy and become symptomatic. The most significant complication of LCA during pregnancy is acute rupture which is associated with a high maternal and fetal mortality. Management of a liver mass lesion may necessitate arteriography or exploration to establish the correct diagnosis.

Hepatocellular carcinoma (HCC) is rare in pregnancy, but may occur in patients with chronic HBV infection since infancy. When present during pregnancy HCC may be complicated by intraperitoneal hemorrhage. HCC is almost uniformly fatal. However, the fibrolamellar variant, which occurs almost uniformly in young women, may be suitable for resection and have a more favorable prognosis (Chapter 20).

AN APPROACH TO THE PREGNANT PATIENT WITH LIVER DISEASE

Pregnant women with liver disease should be managed jointly by an obstetrician and a hepatologist. Accurate diagnosis of the underlying cause of liver dysfunction is critical. Diagnostic pointers include the time of presentation during pregnancy, a history of similar illness during previous pregnancies or with oral contraceptive use, and a family history of liver disease during pregnancy. Presenting symptoms, signs and the pattern of laboratory abnormalities may provide further clues. The most important diagnostic possibilities are shown in Table 23.2. Where indicated, viral hepatitis or biliary tract disease may be excluded using standard diagnostic procedures. Presentation with bleeding esophageal varices suggests underlying chronic liver disease. Liver biopsy may be required if the cause of liver disease is unclear. Hopefully, increased recognition and understanding of liver disease during pregnancy will diminish maternal and fetal mortality.

Table 23.2 Pregnancy-associated liver disease (adapted from Schorr-Lesnick *et al.*, 1991)

Characteristic	ICP	AFLP	Hepatic toxemia (HELLP syndrome)	Viral hepatitis
Trimester	3rd	3rd	3rd	All
Recurrence	Yes	Unusual	No	No
Familial	Yes	No	No	No
Association	Contraceptive-induced cholestasis	Toxemia 20–40% primiparas, male babies, twins	Hepatic rupture, nulliparas, twins, extremes of age	Rare vertical transmission
Major symptoms	Pruritus, increased bilirubin	RUQ pain, vomiting, jaundice, liver failure	RUQ epigastric pain or none	Nausea, vomiting
Laboratory abnormalities	Bile acids, ALP, cholesterol, transaminases, cholestasis	Abnormal coagulation, thrombocytopenia, hypoglycemia, neutrophilia	Thrombocytopenia raised transaminases, hemolysis	Transaminases >40 times normal upper limit, hepatitis viral serology
Liver biopsy	Cholestyramine	Microvesicular steatosis	Fibrin deposition, hemorrhage	Typical
Therapy	Disappears after delivery	Early delivery	Early delivery	Immuno-globulin HBV vaccination of newborn

ICP, intrahepatic cholestasis of pregnancy ; AFLP, acute fatty liver of pregnancy; HELLP, hemolysis, elevated liver enzymes, low platelets; RUQ, right upper quadrant; TBR, total bilirubin; ALP, alkaline phosphatase

RECOMMENDED READING

Abell, T.L. and Riely, C.A. (1992) Hyperemesis gravidarum. *Gastroenterol Clin North Am*, 21, 835–49.

Barron, W.M. (1992) The syndrome of preeclampsia. *Gastroenterol Clin North Am*, 21, 851–72.

Barton, J.R. and Sibai, B.M. (1992) Care of the pregnancy complicated by HELLP syndrome. *Gastroenterol Clin North Am*, 21, 937–50.

Gitlin, N. (1992) Liver disease in pregnancy, in *Wright's Liver and Biliary Disease*, 3rd edn (eds G.H. Millward-Sadler, R. Wright and M.J.P. Arthur), W.B. Saunders, Philadelphia, pp. 1155–69.

Kaplan, M.M. (1985) Acute fatty liver of pregnancy. *N Engl J Med*, **313**, 367–70.

Lee, W.M. (1992) Pregnancy in patients with chronic liver disease. *Gastroenterol Clin North Am*, **21**, 889-903.

Mabie, W.C. (1992) Acute fatty liver of pregnancy. *Gastroenterol Clin North Am*, **21**, 951–60.

Mabie, W.C. (1992) Obstetric management of gastroenterologic complications of pregnancy. *Gastroenterol Clin North Am*, **21**, 923–35.

Mishra, L. and Seeff, L.B. (1992) Viral hepatitis, A through E, complicating pregnancy. *Gastroenterol Clin North Am*, **21**, 873–87.

Reyes, H. (1992) The spectrum of liver and gastrointestinal disease seen in cholestasis of pregnancy. *Gastroenterol Clin North Am*, **21**, 905–21.

Rolfes, D.B. and Ishak, K.G. (1985) Acute fatty liver of pregnancy: a study of 35 cases. *Hepatology*, **5**, 1149–58.

Schorr-Lesnick, B., Lebovics, E., Dworkin, B. *et al.* (1991) Liver diseases unique to pregnancy. *Am J Gastroenterol*, **86**, 659–68.

Steven, M.M. (1981) Pregnancy and liver disease. *Gut*, **22**, 592-614.

24

Pediatric liver disease

WENDY SPEARMAN and CAROLINE RIELY

INTRODUCTION

Pediatric liver diseases which differ from those seen in adult patients, consist largely of disorders of early infancy and of genetic traits which manifest in the first decade of life. Their pattern varies geographically. In poor regions infectious diseases – viral, bacterial, spirochetal and protozoal – dominate, while in richer areas pediatric liver disease largely comprises genetic disorders (metabolic and structural) and a variety of conditions of unknown etiology usually presenting in early infancy.

Hepatobiliary disease in childhood differs from adult liver disease not only in its causes but also in its tempo and effects. Thus liver disease in the young may influence growth, neurological and intellectual development. The consequences of inadequate supply of protein, energy and micronutrients such as the fat-soluble vitamins are also most marked during periods of rapid growth.

JAUNDICE

The approach to jaundice at all ages is greatly simplified by knowing whether the accumu-lated bilirubin is unconjugated or conjugated. This distinction is of even greater importance in the neonate where unconjugated hyper-bilirubinemia may result in bilirubin encephalopathy.

UNCONJUGATED HYPERBILIRUBINEMIA

Physiological jaundice

Transient, so-called physiological jaundice, occurs in 90% of healthy newborn infants. This jaundice, due to accummulation of unconjugated bilirubin, is believed to result from the relative inability of neonatal livers to remove and/or to conjugate a slightly increased load of bilirubin. The latter is thought to arise from increased turnover of red blood cells and other heme proteins normally observed during the neonatal period, from increased absorption of bilirubin released from bilirubin glucuronide in the gut.

The serum bilirubin concentration reaches a maximum of less than 100 µmol/l (almost all unconjugated) between the second and fourth day of life, and the jaundice usually clears by the seventh day in full-term infants.

In premature infants, maximum serum bilirubin concentrations are between 200–250 μmol/l and occur between the fifth and 10th day of life, with the jaundice usually clearing by the 14th day. Serum bilirubin levels may only return to normal between the 21st and 28th day of life.

Physiological jaundice is, strictly speaking, not a disease of the liver. However, it may be aggravated by sepsis, breast feeding, hemolysis, hypoxia, hypoglycemia, hypothyroidism and various drugs and may mask true liver disease during the first week of life.

Pathological unconjugated hyperbilirubinemia

The presence of jaundice during the first 24 hours of life or any deviation from the norm for physiological jaundice strongly suggests the presence of disease. Hemolysis should be excluded. Hypoxia, dehydration, hypoglycemia, intestinal obstruction and bacterial infections must be identified and treated. Drugs sharing excretory pathways with bilirubin should be withdrawn and less common conditions associated with jaundice such as galactosemia, fructosemia and hypothyroidism should be considered.

Apart from good antenatal and intranatal care and the early diagnosis of conditions requiring special treatment, management consists of phototherapy and exchange transfusion.

Prolonged neonatal unconjugated hyperbilirubinemia

Jaundice persisting beyond 10–14 days of age, and in which the causes listed above have been excluded, is most often due to breast feeding. This condition, which is not known to be associated with kernicterus, usually also occurs in three-quarters of siblings of affected infants and may persist for up to 4 months.

The jaundice usually settles within 7 days if breast feeding is discontinued and may not recur if breast feeding is re-introduced. Where bilirubin levels exceed 290 μmol/l, it is prudent to discontinue breast feeding for 1–2 days.

CONJUGATED HYPERBILIRUBINEMIA

Conjugated hyperbilirubinemia is always pathological and may be hepatocellular or biliary in origin. The rapid progression of some of the disorders demands an urgent but rational diagnostic approach which aims to identify those conditions requiring immediate, special management and those requiring surgical intervention.

Hepatitis syndrome of infancy

This syndrome, caused by a large number of hepatobiliary disorders, is characterized by jaundice (usually commencing within the first week of life but occasionally as late as 4 months), dark urine and pale-colored stools. Failure to thrive is common. Hepatomegaly is usual and splenomegaly is present in about one-half of patients.

Serum biochemistry reveals a hyperbilirubinemia of which a significant portion, 40% or more, is conjugated. The serum transaminase and alkaline phosphatase activities are usually increased at between 1.5–6 times the upper limit of normal.

Investigations

The clinical history, examination and biochemistry are seldom helpful in establishing the diagnosis. It is thus important to diagnose the specific and potentially treatable causes of cholestasis. These include bacterial infections, viral infections (cytomegalovirus (CMV), herpes), endocrinopathies (hypothyroidism, hypopituitarism), nutritional hepatoxicity (galactosemia, fructosemia) and specific metabolic disorders (tyrosinemia, alpha-1 antitrypsin deficiency and cystic fibrosis). If infectious causes are suspected, viral and bacterial cultures (blood, urine), specific viral serology and Venereal Disease Research Laboratory (VDRL) titers should be performed. Other important screening tests include serum ferritin levels, sweat chloride test for cystic fibrosis, thyroxine (T4) and thyroid stimulating hormone (TSH) levels and metabolic screens (urine reducing substances, urine and serum amino acid profiles).

Intrahepatic causes of cholestasis should be distinguished from their extrahepatic counterparts. Certain features on history and clinical examination may be helpful. Infants with intrahepatic cholestasis tend to have a low birth weight, splenomegaly and general features of liver disease. Infants with extrahepatic cholestasis tend to have a normal birth weight, a higher incidence and earlier onset of acholic stools and firm, enlarged livers.

Abdominal ultrasonography should be performed as soon as possible as it may demonstrate biliary tract dilatation or a choledochal cyst. Percutaneous transhepatic cholangiography (PTC) and endoscopic retrograde pancreatocholangiography (ERCP) are difficult in small infants and not generally used. Hepatobiliary scintigraphy (technetium-labeled iminodiacetic acid analogs usually administered after 3 days of phenobarbitone) may help to distinguish between extra- and intrahepatic cholestasis. In biliary atresia, hepatocyte function is intact and thus uptake of iminodiacetic acid analogs is normal but excretion into the intestine is absent.

Liver biopsy is important as distinctive histological features are seen in intra- and extrahepatic cholestasis (Chapter 6).

Management

Unfortunately, specific treatment is available for only a few disorders. Fructose and galac-tose are omitted from the diet until fructosemia and galactosemia have been excluded. It is important to pay attention to the nutritional deficiencies associated with cholestasis, particularly fat-soluble vitamin deficiencies. A formula rich in medium-chain triglycerides may be beneficial. Phenobarbitone or rifampin is useful in the treatment of pruritus. It is important to maintain an optimal nutritional status. Orthotopic liver transplantation is often the only therapeutic option in children with progressive disease.

SPECIFIC DISORDERS

INFECTIONS

Urinary tract infections, septicemia and gastroenteritis with associated endotoxemia may manifest with conjugated hyperbilirubinemia and elevated transaminases. Many viral infections present with a hepatitic picture. Generalized infections such as CMV, herpes simplex, rubella, coxsackie, enteric cytopathic human orphan (ECHO) virus and adenovirus may be acquired *in utero*, during delivery, or during the neonatal period.

Other infections such as syphilis, tuberculosis, toxoplasmosis and malaria must always be considered as they are amenable to treatment.

Histologically cholestasis, portal inflammation and variable fibrosis, hepatocyte necrosis and extramedullary hematopoiesis is seen. Viral inclusions, except in CMV and herpes, are rarely present. Spirochaetes and micro-abscesses containing listeria and toxoplasma cysts are also rare. Thus serology and positive cultures are important in confirming these diagnoses.

TOTAL PARENTERAL NUTRITION (TPN)

In infants the prolonged use of TPN (in the absence of oral intake), may result in cholestasis and hepatocellular damage which can progress to cirrhosis. There is an increased risk in premature infants. Aggravating factors include sepsis, surgery, blood transfusions, hypoxia and hepatotoxic drugs. Jaundice usually resolves within 4 weeks of stopping TPN.

Histologically, cholestasis, portal fibrosis and inflammation, extramedullary hematopoiesis and eosinophilic bodies are seen.

'IDIOPATHIC' NEONATAL HEPATITIS

In many infants the cause of jaundice remains obscure despite adequate investigation. This heterogeneous group, termed 'idiopathic' neonatal hepatitis, is characterized by prolonged jaundice, which usually starts in the first week of life but may present at any stage between (often premature) birth and 4 months.

Liver biopsy typically shows a diffuse giant cell hepatitis, hepatocellular and canalicular cholestasis, extramedullary hematopoiesis and eosinophilic bodies. A mild inflammatory infiltrate consisting mostly of lymphocytes is seen in the portal tracts and parenchyma. Portal tracts are usually small and ductular proliferation and portal fibrosis are not prominent.

At least three possible sub-sets with a poor prognosis have been identified. These include patients with a family history of liver disease, the development of sclerosing cholangitis, and those with marked portal fibrosis on biopsy. In the remaining patients the prognosis is usually good.

Familial cholestatic jaundice

This group of distinct but rare familial syndromes includes arteriohepatic dysplasia (Alagille's syndrome), progressive familial cholestasis (Byler disease), familial recurrent cholestasis and hereditary cholestasis with lymphedema.

METABOLIC DISORDERS

These are usually divided into those that may respond to therapy and those for which there is currently no treatment. Early diagnosis of galactosemia, fructosemia and tyrosinemia is essential since their consequences may be significantly lessened by the immediate introduction of an appropriate diet.

Clinical features may be helpful but in each instance specific biochemical tests (urine and blood) are necessary for diagnosis. Histology usually only broadly categorizes the metabolic disorder. Giant cell transformation is usually absent and portal inflammation is minimal. Metabolic disease should be considered in the presence of hepatocyte fat vacuoles and intralobular sinusoidal fibrosis. Ductular proliferation and portal fibrosis is variable.

DISORDERS OF CARBOHYDRATE METABOLISM

Galactosemia

This autosomal-recessive condition is characterized by decreased activity of galactose-1-phosphate uridyl transferase in the liver, erythrocytes and leukocytes. This results in an accumulation of galactose, galactitol and galactose-1-phosphate throughout the body. As most milks contain high concentrations of lactose, anorexia, vomiting, diarrhea, jaundice, hepatomegaly and evidence of a bleeding tendency usually occur soon after birth. In severely affected infants, a septicemic shock-like state plus a profound coagulopathy lead to death within 48 hours of delivery. Occasionally infants merely fail to thrive and present with cirrhosis by the age of 6 months.

The presence of decreased or absent erythrocyte galactose-1-phosphate activity is the only reliable way to confirm the diagnosis. Galactosuria is often used as a

255

screening test but is not diagnostic as it may also occur in gastroenteritis and other forms of hepatobiliary disease and may be absent in proven cases of galactosemia.

Treatment with a galactose-free diet usually results in clinical improvement and stabilization of organ damage. Cataracts may regress, but brain damage is usually irreversible. Despite adequate treatment, mental development is impaired and learning difficulties occur in up to 50% of patients.

Female galactosemia carriers should have a lactose-restricted diet. Antenatal diagnosis by amniocentesis and chorionic villus biopsy is possible.

Fructosemia

Three forms of this condition have been described: benign fructosemia, hereditary fructose intolerance and fructose-1,6- diphosphatase deficiency.

Benign fructosemia occurs as a result of fructose kinase deficiency and has no harmful effects.

Hereditary fructose intolerance, due to a deficiency of fructose-1-phosphate aldolase, an enzyme normally found in liver, gut and kidney, is inherited as an autosomal-recessive trait. Fructose uptake by hepatocytes is impaired and there is an accumulation of fructose-1-phosphate and depletion of ATP, GTP and inorganic phosphate. Glycogen breakdown and gluconeogenesis are impaired. This accounts for the severe hypoglycemia which is commonly seen in this condition.

Vomiting, anorexia, failure to thrive and hepatomegaly are found at the time that fructose or sucrose are first introduced into the diet. Drowsiness, coma, convulsions, pallor and a hemorrhagic diathesis should suggest the diagnosis. Profound hypoglycemia often occurs. An acute fructose load may be followed by fulminant liver failure. In older children chronic low-grade fructose ingestion may result in cirrhosis which may be complicated by the development of hepatocellular carcinoma.

Diagnosis is confirmed by demonstrating fructose-1-phosphate aldolase deficiency in small intestine or liver biopsies. Treatment involves a fructose- and sucrose-free diet with resulting clinical improvement and gradual improvement in hepatic synthetic and renal tubular function. Hepatomegaly decreases but histologically steatosis persists and progression to cirrhosis may continue.

Fructose-1,6- diphosphatase deficiency, is inherited as an autosomal-recessive trait. Gluconeogenesis is impaired resulting in hypoglycemia and the accumulation of amino acids, alanine and glutamine. Impaired metabolism of amino acids and glycerol results in marked hepatic steatosis. Serum lactic acid and pyruvic acid levels are increased.

Symptoms, less severe but otherwise similar to those seen in hereditary fructose intolerance, follow fructose ingestion. Hepatomegaly is marked. Lactic acidosis and hypoglycemia occur and may be aggravated by sepsis. Jaundice does not occur and liver and renal function tests are normal. Ketoacidosis may be marked, even in the absence of hypoglycemia.

The diagnosis is confirmed by demonstrating fructose-1,6-diphosphate deficiency on liver biopsy.

Treatment with a fructose- and sucrose-free diet and frequent carbohydrate-rich meals usually results in regression of symptoms and signs.

DISORDERS OF AMINO ACID METABOLISM

Hereditary tyrosinemia

This deficiency of hepatic fumaryl acetoacetate hydrolase, inherited as an autosomal-recessive trait, results in hepatocellular damage, renal tubular defects and hypophosphatemic rickets. The deficiency of hepatic fumaryl acetoacetate hydrolase results in a characteristic plasma amino acid profile in which tyrosine, phenylalanine, methionine and the tyrosine metabolite *p*-hydroxyphenyl-lactic acid are markedly elevated. Serum alpha-fetoprotein concentrations may be increased 10–100-fold. High urinary concentrations of succinyl acetoacetate are diagnostic.

In the more severe, acute form, vomiting, failure to thrive, diarrhea, edema, ascites and hepatomegaly occur in the first few weeks of life. Few of these infants survive beyond one year of age.

The chronic form presents with rickets, cirrhosis and renal tubular dysfunction. Most die within the first decade. Hepatocellular carcinoma complicates the majority of cases.

Liver biopsy demonstrates cholestasis, fatty infiltration, giant cell hepatitis and progression to cirrhosis.

Treatment involves dietary restriction of tyrosine, phenylalanine and methionine. Vitamin D and phosphate supplements are important in the prevention of rickets. Although treatment improves the general condition of the infant, it does not prevent or delay the development of liver failure and hepatocellular carcinoma. Thus, liver transplantation is recommended before the age of 3 years.

DISORDERS OF LIPID METABOLISM

Niemann–Pick disease

This condition is characterized by an abnormal accumulation of sphingomyelin in tissues. Widespread sphingomyelinase deficiency is found in types A and B, but in type C hepatic and leukocyte sphingomyelinase activity is preserved while fibroblast sphingomyelinase activity is decreased.

Niemann–Pick type C is the second most common genetic cause of liver disease in infancy in the UK. There is an increase in liver sphingomyelin. Some 80% of affected individuals present with hepatitis in infancy or with the development, *in utero*, of ascites; 30% of infants die by the age of 6 months. In the remainder, the liver disease regresses to an inactive cirrhosis. However, after the age of 2 years, progressive neurological damage occurs which eventually leads to the patient's death.

The diagnosis is suggested by the finding of sphingomyelin storage deposits in bone marrow and in neurones on rectal biopsy. The presence of defective cholesterol esterification in fibroblasts confirms the diagnosis. Liver transplantation does not prevent the development of neurological disease. Genetic counseling is important and prenatal diagnosis by amniocentesis is possible.

Gaucher's disease

This is due to a deficiency of lysomal enzyme glucocerebridase and is inherited as an autosomal-dominant trait. Symptoms usually present within the first year of life. Hepatosplenomegaly and portal hypertension with hypersplenism occur as a result of severe derangement of the liver architecture.

Liver biopsy shows abnormal lipid storage cells and the diagnosis is confirmed by demonstrating the specific enzyme deficiency.

Bone marrow transplantation offers biochemical correction but long-term results are not known. Pre-natal diagnosis is possible.

Glycogen storage diseases

Twelve forms of glycogen storage disease are currently recognized. Although each has a distinct enzyme defect, all are associated with abnormal accumulation of glycogen in various tissues, and most with defective release of glucose. All but one, a variant of type III, have an autosomal-recessive mode of inheritance. The defect usually involves glycogen catabolism and the resultant hypoglycemia leads to compensatory changes in amino acid, lipid and purine metabolism. Each form involves a particular group of organs. These include the liver, skeletal muscle, heart, kidney and brain.

Clinically these disorders are characterized by recurrent hypoglycemia, a failure to thrive, and massive hepatomegaly. Other features include a bleeding tendency (due to platelet dysfunction), recurrent leukopenia and susceptibility to infection, xanthomata and gouty tophi. The severity of the clinical and biochemical features varies with each type. Symptoms frequently regress during childhood.

Histologically, hepatocytes are distended with pale cytoplasm containing glycogen and lipid vacuoles. Sinusoidal compression occurs. Periportal fibrosis occurs in type III and may progress to cirrhosis. Cirrhosis is almost always present in type IV.

The diagnosis is confirmed by demonstrating the specific enzyme defect in leukocytes, erythrocytes, muscle or liver. Treatment involves dietary management; allopurinol is occasionally required for hyperuricacidemia and bicarbonate for acidosis. The aim of dietary management is to prevent hypoglycemia and this may involve frequent carbohydrate-rich feeds. Galactose and fructose should be restricted as they aggravate lactic acidosis.

Although clinical features improve with dietary management, the beneficial effect on the development of hepatic fibrosis, adenoma formation and hepatocellular carcinoma is not certain. Liver transplantation is a therapeutic option but it is uncertain whether this prevents the development of neurological disease in the majority of cases.

MUCOPOLYSACCHARIDOSES

These disorders are characterized by the deposition of abnormal polysaccharides (complexes containing amino acids, amino sugars, uronic acids and sulfates) in tissues. This results in progressive skeletal damage, mental impairment, cataracts and visceral enlargement, particularly hepatosplenomegaly. Inheritance is usually autosomal-recessive except for Hunter's syndrome which is X-linked.

Symptoms usually start at about 6 months with death occurring within 10 years. The diagnosis is confirmed by detecting the excretion of mucopolysaccharides in urine or demonstrating the specific enzyme deficiency in leukocytes.

Bone marrow transplantation may arrest progression of these diseases, but long-term follow-up is not available.

METABOLIC DISEASE WITH PARTIALLY UNCHARACTERIZED DEFECTS

Alpha-1 antitrypsin deficiency

Some 25% of individuals with homozygous alpha-1 antitrypsin deficiency present with liver disease in infancy. Indeed, alpha-1 antitrypsin deficiency phenotype Z is one of the major causes of the 'hepatitis syndrome' in infancy where it accounts for 15–20% of cases.

Affected infants usually present with profound, often complete, cholestasis, which may be indistinguishable from biliary atresia, in the first weeks to months of life. The prognosis is worse than for idiopathic neonatal hepatitis. Roughly a quarter of infants presenting with cholestasis will die from cirrhosis by the age of 10 years. While liver disease may resolve in approximately 25% of patients others may develop an initially compensated cirrhosis.

Histologically, severe intrahepatic cholestasis is seen but prominent giant cell transformation and portal tract inflammation are unusual. Portal tracts may be prominent due to bile duct proliferation and fibrosis or bile duct paucity may occur. Alpha-1 antitrypsin cytoplasmic granules are usually not seen in children below the age of 3 years. Intrahepatic cholestasis makes interpretation of periodic acid–Schiff (PAS) and immunoperoxidase stains difficult, as cytoplasmic bile is variably PAS-positive and is brown, the color of a positive immunoperoxidase stain. Electron microscopy may detect alpha-1 antitrypsin granules but sampling may be a problem. Thus it is important to measure serum alpha-1 antitrypsin levels, and to confirm the diagnosis by phenotyping.

All patients with cirrhosis should be considered for liver transplantation. Antenatal diagnosis through villus sampling is possible at 10–11 weeks.

Cystic fibrosis

A small number of affected individuals present with cholestasis in infancy. This may be due to prolonged conjugated hyperbilirubinemia presenting as a hepatitis syndrome, due to intrahepatic disease or due to extrahepatic bile duct obstruction by inspissated bile secretions. Biliary lavage may be necessary to clear these inspissated secretions.

Marked hepatic steatosis with protein malabsorption may also occur. These infants present with edema, ascites and hypoalbuminemia and usually respond to the administration of pancreatic supplements. Neither of these syndromes progresses to cirrhosis.

ANATOMIC ABNORMALITIES

CONGENITAL HEPATIC FIBROSIS

Congenital hepatic fibrosis is characterized histologically by bands of fibrous tissue, containing spaces lined by biliary epithelium, which link the portal tracts.

Clinically, affected individuals usually present at 1–2 years with hepatomegaly and features of portal hypertension and occasionally with cholangitis. Liver function is normal

and hepatic encephalopathy is rare. Biochemical tests tend to be normal, except for the alkaline phosphatase which may be elevated in the presence of cholangitis. Variceal bleeding is managed with injection sclerotherapy.

INFANTILE POLYCYSTIC DISEASE OF LIVER AND KIDNEYS

This autosomal-recessive trait is dominated in severe cases by renal failure. In milder forms there is minimal renal involvement and these patients present, usually between the age of 3 months and 5 years, with hepatomegaly and features of portal hypertension.

Liver function tests, besides alkaline phosphatase, which may be elevated, are normal. Ultrasound confirms the presence of renal cysts but those in the liver are too small to be seen. Liver biopsy demonstrates portal tracts distended by fibrous tissue containing dilated channels lined by biliary epithelium. The hepatic parenchyma is normal. The main complication is variceal bleeding which is well controlled with injection sclerotherapy.

CAROLI'S DISEASE

This congenital abnormality is characterized by segmental dilatation and stenosis of the intrahepatic bile ducts. Recurrent cholangitis and intrahepatic calculi occur.

There are two types of Caroli's disease; a rare form, not associated with cirrhosis and portal hypertension, which is characterized by recurrent episodes of cholangitis and the more common form which is associated with congenital hepatic fibrosis and presents with hepatosplenomegaly and esophageal varices.

The diagnosis can be made on liver biopsy and cholangiography. There is an increased risk of cholangiocarcinoma.

EXTRAHEPATIC DISORDERS

EXTRAHEPATIC BILIARY ATRESIA

This condition, which has an incidence of 0.8–1.0 per 10 000 births, is characterized by a progressive segmental or diffuse obliteration of the common bile duct, common hepatic duct or the right and left hepatic ducts. The small intrahepatic ducts are patent. The extrahepatic ducts are not congenitally absent but are obliterated by inflammation and fibrosis postnatally. This destructive sclerosing inflammatory process rapidly extends to the major intrahepatic ducts. This has important therapeutic implications since, to be effective, surgery must be performed as soon as possible as occlusion of the main bile ducts at the porta hepatis usually occurs at about 60 days.

The etiology of extrahepatic biliary atresia remains unknown. A number of viruses, including rubella, CMV, hepatitis B and reovirus type III have been implicated but the evidence for any of these remains inconclusive. Landing (1974) has suggested that neonatal hepatitis, biliary atresia and choledochal cyst are different manifestations of a single disease process which he termed infantile obstructive cholangiopathy. According to this the etiological agent causes both hepatitis (neonatal hepatitis) and inflammation of the extrahepatic ducts. In some individuals, the extrahepatic ducts are more severely affected by the sclerosing inflammatory process resulting in extrahepatic biliary atresia, while in others, the inflammatory process results in the weakening of duct walls leading to dilatation (choledochal cyst). This would explain the clinical and histological similarities between the three conditions and the finding that some patients with biliary atresia develop progressive hepatic fibrosis and liver failure despite corrective surgery.

Clinically, the condition presents as jaundice which persists beyond the first week of life. The stools are usually acholic. However, 30% of patients may have pigmented stools for the first few weeks of life. The liver is enlarged and firm due to development of fibrosis and splenomegaly may be found. Affected neonates fail to thrive and develop complications relating to malabsorption of fat-soluble vitamins; 10% have associated congenital anomalies including intestinal rotation, situs inversus, polysplenia, congenital heart disease and abnormalities of the inferior vena cava and hepatic artery.

Liver biopsy at 6 weeks of age shows intrahepatic cholestasis, focal hepatocellular necrosis (eosinophilic bodies), extramedullary hemopoiesis and a mild portal lymphocytic infiltrate. Ballooning of hepatocytes and focal hepatocyte giant cell transformation cause lobular disarray. All these findings are non-specific and are found in many cholestatic diseases of infancy. However, the portal tracts show ductular proliferation (5–6 ducts/tract) and portal fibrosis which suggest extrahepatic obstruction. Portal fibrosis may extend into the parenchyma and ductular cholestasis in the portal tracts is prominent.

At exploratory laparotomy, cord-like extrahepatic ducts are seen. The gallbladder is usually small and empty. Cholangiography frequently shows a small, patent common bile duct with a cord-like common hepatic duct, right and left hepatic ducts. Occasionally, the extrahepatic biliary system cannot be demonstrated cholangiographically.

Surgery involves excision of the entire extrahepatic biliary system plus the wedge of fibrous tissue usually present at the porta hepatis followed by a portoenterostomy (Kasai operation). The porta hepatis usually only contains small biliary ducts 3 mm diameter) with epithelial pyknosis, sloughing, inflammation and extensive periductular fibrosis.

Good bile flow with resolution of jaundice after 1–3 months occurs in up to 80% of infants operated on before 60 days of age. Results are much less successful with later surgery (only 20% will have bile flow).

Complications following the Kasai operation include recurrent cholangitis which occurs in up to 50% of infants in the first 2 years. Age is thought to be an important factor in determining the outcome of the Kasai operation. Some 80% of infants operated on before the age of 8 weeks became jaundice-free compared with only 40% of infants operated on between 8–12 weeks of age. Long-term survival also appears to be improved if surgery is performed early. Surgical expertise is another important factor determining outcome of the Kasai procedure. Re-operation after a failed Kasai procedure is usually not successful.

Liver transplantation should be considered for those infants who present too late for corrective surgery, who have a failed Kasai procedure or who present with progressive disease despite an initially successful Kasai procedure. Biliary atresia is the commonest indication for liver transplantation in most pediatric programmes.

CHOLEDOCHAL CYST

This is a diffuse or segmental enlargement or dilatation of the extrahepatic biliary system. The intrahepatic bile ducts may be dilated and biliary cirrhosis eventually develops. Complications include cholangitis, bile duct rupture, pancreatitis, liver abscesses and carcinoma of the cyst wall.

There tends to be a female predominence. Infants present with cholestasis; older children may present with recurrent upper abdominal pain and a palpable cystic mass. Diagnosis is confirmed on cholangiography and treatment is surgical with biliary drainage via a Roux-en-Y loop.

SPONTANEOUS PERFORATION OF THE BILE DUCT

This condition should be suspected when a previously healthy child develops jaundice. Perforation most often occurs at the junction of the cystic and common hepatic ducts. Infants usually present with mild jaundice, acholic stools and ascites. Occasionally the scrotum may be bile-stained. Serum transaminases and alkaline phosphatase are usually normal. At laparotomy a distal obstruction of the bile duct due to inspissated bile may be present. Treatment is surgical with biliary drainage via the gallbladder into a Roux-en-Y loop.

MISCELLANEOUS DISORDERS

REYE'S SYNDROME

This is an acute disorder characterized by severe encephalopathy, cerebral edema and diffuse fatty infiltration of organs. The syndrome, which usually follows a viral illness, appears to result from a self-limiting, 2–6-day abnormality of mitochondrial function and structure.

Children present with profuse vomiting, become encephalopathic and there may be rapid progression to brain death within 40–60 hours. Infants are frequently tachypneic but may present with respiratory failure and become apneic. Seizures are common. Biochemical abnormalities include hypoglycemia, raised transaminases, acidosis and a coagulopathy. Jaundice is not prominent.

Diagnosis is confirmed on liver biopsy with electron microscopy. Swollen, pleomorphic mitochondria with reduced mitochondrial enzyme activity are found during the first 2–5 days after the onset of encephalopathy. Microvesicular fatty infiltration of the liver is prominent but not diagnostic.

Death may occur in up to 40% and survivors may be left with permanent brain damage. Treatment is supportive. Patients should be managed in an intensive care unit experienced in controlling raised intracranial pressure and maintaining cerebral perfusion (Chapter 12).

AUTOIMMUNE CHRONIC LIVER DISEASE IN CHILDREN

AUTOIMMUNE CHRONIC ACTIVE HEPATITIS

This disorder tends to present acutely in children. Like adults, there is a female predominance. These children appear to have an increased incidence of HLA-A1, B8, DR3 haplotype, complement component C4 deficiency and decreased suppressor/cytotoxic T lymphocytes with increased IL-2 receptor expression on activated lymphocytes.

Three sub-types of autoimmune chronic active hepatitis are described according to the type of non-organ specific auto-antibody detected.

Anti-nuclear antibody positive chronic active hepatitis

These children tend to have a better prognosis. They usually do not have evidence of chronic liver disease at the time of presentation and are frequently able to be weaned off immunosuppression without relapse.

Anti-smooth muscle antibody-positive chronic active hepatitis

This group in which the anti-nuclear factor (ANF) may be positive or negative appears to have an intermediate prognosis.

Anti-liver–kidney microsomal antibody-positive chronic active hepatitis

These children have the worst prognosis, are frequently cirrhotic at the time of presentation and tend to be steroid-dependent.

Liver-specific auto-antibodies such as anti-liver specific protein (LSP) and anti-asialoglycoprotein receptors are present in all three groups and antibody titers are useful markers of disease activity. It is important to assess the need for immunosuppression in the form of prednisone and azathioprine as soon as the children present in order to prevent the progression to cirrhosis.

PRIMARY SCLEROSING CHOLANGITIS

This has a very similar clinical, biochemical and histological presentation to autoimmune chronic active hepatitis. IgG, antinuclear, anti-smooth and anti-LSP antibody levels are elevated. However, the number and function of suppressor T cells are normal and the IL-2 receptor expression on activated T-cells is not increased.

Children tend to have evidence of colitis prior to the development of sclerosing cholangitis. The prognosis is variable with the disease being stable for many years in some children and rapidly progressive in others.

Steroids should be considered in the treatment of these children as many respond with a fall in transaminases and often with histological improvement.

RECOMMENDED READING

Akader, H.H. and Balistreri, W.F. (1989) Neonatal cholestasis, in *Current therapy in Gastroenterology and Liver Disease*, 3rd edn, Mosby Yearbook, St Louis, pp. 493–6.

Balistreri, W.F. (1990) Interrelationship between the infantile cholangiopathies and paucity of the intrahepatic bile ducts, in *Paediatric Hepatology* (eds W.F. Balistreri and J.T. Stocker), Hemisphere Publishing Corp., Washington, pp. 1–18.

Balistreri, W.F. (1991) Fetal and neonatal bile acid synthesis and metabolism – clinical implications. *J Inher Metab Dis*, **14**, 95–111.

Desmet, V.J. (1987) Cholangiopathies: past, present and future. *Semin Liver Dis*, **7**, 67–76.

Heubi, J.E., Partin, J.C. and Partin, J.S. (1987) Reye's syndrome: current concepts. *Hepatology*, **7**, 155–64.

Landing, B.H. (1974) Considerations of the pathogenesis of neonatal hepatitis, biliary atresia and choledochal cyst: the concept of infantile obstructive choliangopathy. *Prog Pediatr Surg*, **6**, 113–19.

Montgomery, C.K. and Ruebner, B.H. (1976) Neonatal hepatocellular giant cell transformation. A review. *Perspect Paediat Pathol*, **3**, 85–101.

Mowat, A.P. (1987) *Liver disorders of childhood*, 2nd edn, Butterworths, London, pp. 1–408.

Riely, C.A. (1987) Familial intrahepatic cholestatic syndromes. *Semin Liver Dis*, **7**(2), 119–33.

Ryckman, F.C. and Noseworthy, J. (1987) Neonatal cholestatic conditions requiring surgical reconstruction. *Semin Liver Dis*, **7**, 134–54.

Scriver, C.R., Beautt, A.L., Sly, W.S. and Valle, D. (eds) (1989) *The Metabolic Basis of Inherited Disease*, 6th edn, McGraw–Hill, New York.

Sisto, A., Feldman, P., Garel, L. *et al.* (1987) Primary sclerosing cholangitis in children: study of 5 cases, review of the literature. *Pediatrics*, **80**(6), 918–23.

Sokol, R.J. (1990) Medical management of neonatal cholestasis, in *Paediatric Hepatology* (eds W.F. Balistreri and J.T. Stocker), Hemisphere Publishing Corp., Washington, pp. 41–76.

Vegnente, A., Larcher, V..F, Mowat, A.P. *et al.* (1984) Duration of chronic active hepatitis with development of cirrhosis. *Arch Dis Child*, **59**, 294–8.

Whitington, P.F. and Balistreri, W.F. (1991) Liver transplantation in pediatrics: indications, contraindications and pretransplant management. *J Pediatr*, **118**(2), 169–77.

25

Nutrition in liver disease

STEPHEN O'KEEFE, COLETTE CYWES and NEIL McINTYRE

INTRODUCTION

The provision of adequate and appropriate nutrition is essential for the well being and support of patients with acute or chronic liver disease. This, in the vast majority of cases, can be accomplished simply by encouraging patients to consume normal diets. The recommendation of archaic dietary restrictions, such as the avoidance of fat in acute hepatitis, is unscientific, inconvenient for the patient and may itself lead to malnutrition, failure to thrive, vitamin and trace element deficiencies, encephalopathy, steatorrhea and infections in these patients. This review will detail present-day guidelines for nutritional support of patients with liver disease and the practical difficulties often encountered in their implementation.

EFFECT OF LIVER DISEASE ON NUTRIENT METABOLISM

Patients with chronic liver disease have increased energy expenditure. This may be due in part to decreased hepatic glycogen stores so that the response to normal overnight fasting is mainly via gluconeogenesis, an energy-requiring process.

In fulminant liver failure, hypoglycemia due to a combination of increased insulin production, impaired gluconeogenesis and an inability to mobilize glycogen stores, is present in up to 50% of patients. In chronic non-alcoholic liver disease hypoglycemia is rare. Here, mild, predominantly postprandial, glucose intolerance, due to insulin resistance, is often seen.

Patients with chronic liver disease have increased plasma concentrations of cholesterol, triglycerides and certain fatty acids. The former is due in part to reflux from the liver and in part to a deficiency of lecithin–cholesterol acyltransferase (LCAT) resulting from decreased hepatic synthesis. Although fat absorption is largely dependent on hepatic secretion of bile acids, clinically significant steatorrhea is surprisingly rare and most patients tolerate normal fat intake.

Whole-body turnover of protein is increased in patients with chronic liver disease. Protein catabolism is thought to increase in order to compensate for the body's unmet energy requirements. Most patients with chronic liver disease require at least 0.75 g protein/kg body-weight per day in order to maintain nitrogen balance and

1.5 g/kg is considered optimal. The liver plays a vital role in processing amino acids absorbed from the gut or produced as a result of extrahepatic protein catabolism. As such it is an important site of plasma protein synthesis and gluconeogenesis, it regulates the supply of amino acids to peripheral tissues and converts ammonia arising from deamination of amino acids or from bacterial synthesis in the gut to urea. Thus liver disease may be associated with low levels of certain plasma proteins, an abnormal plasma amino acid profile and the accumulation of nitrogenous metabolites such as ammonia in the bloodstream. The influence of liver disease on the synthesis of plasma proteins and urea is dealt with in Chapter 2. However, it is important to stress that hepatic protein synthetic ability is relatively well maintained and is often impaired by a lack of dietary essential amino acids rather than by liver disease *per se*.

Liver disease, and in particular cholestasis, has a profound influence on the absorption of fat-soluble vitamins. Vitamin K deficiency is almost invariable in patients with cholestasis and is not uncommon in patients with acute and chronic parenchymal liver disease. In the former it is largely due to decreased absorption while in the latter it is thought to be due to a combination of decreased absorption and an increased demand due to sub-clinical disseminated intravascular coagulation (Chapter 3). Vitamin D deficiency is also common and probably occurs as a result of a combination of poor intake, decreased absorption and decreased exposure to sunlight. Vitamin A deficiency is present in most patients with cholestasis and may also occur in patients with alcoholic liver disease. Finally, vitamin E deficiency is thought to be frequent and may be clinically relevant in children.

Changes in the water-soluble vitamins are less clear-cut. This is often due to a discrepancy between biochemical and clinical evidence of vitamin deficiency. Thus, patients with alcoholic liver disease rarely exhibit clinical signs of thiamine deficiency despite biochemical evidence suggesting that such deficiency is common. Tests also suggest that pyridoxine deficiency is present in many patients with alcoholic liver disease. In contrast, there is good clinical and biochemical evidence of folic acid deficiency in a high percentage of patients with alcoholic liver disease. Pellagra is rarely seen in developed countries but the few cases described are almost all associated with chronic alcohol abuse.

Minerals are also affected by liver disease. Poor intake of calcium, coupled with decreased active vitamin D may result in changes in bone density. Iron deficiency has been reported in roughly a quarter of patients with cirrhosis, and zinc and magnesium deficiencies have also been described.

Against this background it is not surprising that a high proportion of patients with chronic liver disease are malnourished.

PATIENT EVALUATION

It is important that each patient is evaluated individually. Where nutrition is obviously not a problem a normal, thorough history and examination should suffice. However, where relevant, it is essential that a detailed dietary history is obtained. Apart from enquiring about appetite, anorexia, nausea, vomiting and weight loss, attention should be paid to the patient's food preferences, eating habits and alcohol consumption. Similarly a detailed assessment of nutrition should form part of the physical examination of these patients. This should be accompanied by appropriate anthropometric measurements. Many anthropometric parameters such as skinfold thickness and creatinine height index may be influenced by fluid overload and ascites. However, they are still useful in identifying those patients at risk for malnutrition. Of these, the body mass index (weight (kg)/ height (m)²) is useful in the early stages of liver disease. Despite its obvious limitations, recent weight change correlates well with morbidity and mortality, especially in end-stage liver disease. A decrease of more than 10% in body weight (allowing for fluid status) requires aggressive nutritional support. Perhaps the most practical anthropometric means of identifying chronic malnutrition is a combination of triceps skin fold thickness (TSF) and the measurement of mid-arm circumference. Together, these relatively simple and inexpensive measurements provide an objective assessment of arm muscle area, while TSF correlates well with body fat content.

BIOCHEMICAL INDICES

Although plasma albumin is commonly used as an index of protein nutritional status, its value as such is limited in patients with liver disease. Plasma albumin concentration may be influenced by several factors other than nutrition. These include a dilutional effect due to fluid retention; maldistribution (as evidenced by the fact that in cirrhosis up to 80% of newly synthesized albumin may be delivered into the ascitic fluid compartment); and, in severe liver disease, decreased albumin synthesis. Retinol binding protein and transferrin are subject to the same limitations.

Blood tests are also useful for detecting mineral and trace element deficiencies (e.g. zinc, magnesium, iron, calcium) and vitamin deficiencies (vitamins A, D, E and C, prothrombin time, nicotinic acid, transketolase, folic acid, pyridoxine).

NUTRITIONAL REQUIREMENTS

The aim of supporting the patient is to facilitate hepatocyte regeneration, so as to improve liver metabolism and thus nutritional status. Table 25.1 outlines the energy requirements while Tables 25.2 and 25.3 list nutrient requirements.

TREATMENT STRATEGIES

Inadequate dietary intake is a major factor in malnutrition associated with chronic liver disease. This is usually due to anorexia and is often compounded by poor dietary advice.

Dietary regimens should depend on the nature, duration and severity of the liver disease, the nutritional status of the patient, and the presence of complications. Thus, although the principles are constant, management needs to be individualized.

Patients with uncomplicated mild liver disease need a normal, appetizing, balanced diet. Where disease is more severe, supplementation will be needed to maintain intake levels (Table 25.2).

ACUTE LIVER DISEASE

Dietary restrictions have no place in the management of mild or moderate acute parenchymal liver disease. These patients usually experience a relatively short-lived period of anorexia, nausea and weight loss.

Table 25.1 Energy requirements

- 35–45 kCal / kg* / day
- Basal energy expenditure (BEE) × (1.5–1.75) or resting energy expenditure (REE) + 500 kCal
- BEE (males) = 66.4 + (13.75 × weight) + (5 × height) – (6.75 × age)
- BEE (females) = 655.09 + (9.56 × weight) + (1.85 × height) – (4.67 × age)

* Estimated dry weight.
REE, indirect calorimetry using a metabolic monitor; BEE, Harris Benedict equation. Physical data are given as weight (kg), height (m) and age (years).

Table 25.2 Nutrient requirements

Carbohydrate requirement

- The maintenance of normal blood glucose levels is imperative for normal body function.
- 200–250 g glucose/day should not exceed insulin reserves
- Respiratory complications: increase fat to approximately 40% of non-nitrogen calories

Fat requirement

- 25–40% of non-nitrogen calories but less than 100 g fat/day
- 45 g fat/day is sufficient for immune function and essential fatty acid synthesis
- Fat should be provided as polyunsaturated fats with <<50% as long-chain TG to prevent impaired bacterial clearance

Protein requirement

- No hepatic encephalopathy: use 1.5 g protein/kg/day
- Hepatic encephalopathy present: use 0.8 g protein/kg/day
- With improvement, increase protein by 10 g/day to limit of tolerance
- End-stage liver disease: no less than 0.8 g protein/kg/day with adequate calorie coverage (100 kCal /g nitrogen); up to 45% of protein may be branched-chain amino acids

Table 25.3 Fluid, electrolyte and micronutrient requirements

Fluid and electrolytes

- 1–1.5 l/day
- Sodium restriction, not less than 2 g sodium/day

Vitamins and minerals

- A minimum of the reccomended daily allowance (RDA) is required daily.
- The following supplementation is suggested:

Enteral

- Vit A   5000 i.u./week
- Vit D   500 i.u./week
- Vit E   10.0 mg alpha-tocopherol/day
- Vit K   10 mg/week
- Vit C   500 mg/day
- Folate   5 mg/day
- Zinc   1.3–3.0 µg/kg/day
- Copper 2–4 mg $CuSO_4$/day

Parenteral*

- Vit A   3300 i.u./day
- Vit D   200 i.u./day
- Vit E   10 i.u./day
- Vit C   100 mg/day
- Folate   400 µg/day
- Niacin   40 mg/day
- Vit B_2 3.6 mg/day
- Vit B_1 3.0 mg/day
- Vit B_6 4.0 mg/day
- Vit B_{12} 5.0 µg/day
- Biotin   60 µg/day

* Parenteral is the optimal route for fat-soluble vitamins; i.u., international unit.

Adequate intake should be encouraged and patients should be advised to take nutrients in the form most appealing or least offensive to them.

Patients with severe disease require admission to units experienced in the care of acute liver failure and should be managed as described in Chapter 12.

Patients with acute biliary obstruction usually require immediate surgical or endoscopic relief and therefore do not need special nutritional care, apart from vitamin K, unless there are pre-existing disorders.

CHRONIC LIVER DISEASE

General principles

Patients with well-compensated chronic parenchymal liver disease should be encouraged to take a well-balanced normal diet supplemented, where necessary, with water- and fat-soluble vitamins.

Patients with decompensated chronic liver disease should avoid excessive salt intake and should be encouraged to maintain adequate energy consumption. These patients often do better on multiple small meals which have been shown to reduce the need for gluconeogenesis and thus to conserve body proteins and nitrogen balance.

In addition to the above, patients with chronic cholestasis usually require monthly injections of the fat-soluble vitamins. Patients with steatorrhea should be advised to decrease fat intake and may be given medium-chain triglycerides.

Oral diets

Most patients with cirrhosis resulting from whatever cause will be able to maintain adequate nutritional status with a modified oral diet. Modifications should be made to the frequency, volume and caloric density of meals so that they meet the patient's taste and needs.

Patients with hepatic encephalopathy in whom precipitating factors have been managed or excluded and who fail to respond to lactulose (Chapter 13) will need advice on dietary protein consumption. In the first instance the type of protein consumed should be examined. A number of studies have shown that vegetable proteins are better tolerated than animal proteins by patients with chronic encephalopathy. Where possible, 75% of dietary protein should be of vegetable origin. The mechanism for the improved tolerance is unclear, but maybe related to differences in amino acid, fiber, or carbohydrate content of the diet or alternatively increased fecal nitrogen loss, improved nitrogen balance or changes in hormonal response. The help of a dietitian should be sought to evaluate the patient's normal dietary intake and advise on the avoidance of foods such as salami and blue cheese, which have a high aromatic

amino acid content. Vegetables are preferable to milk, which in turn is better than meat. Unfortunately, tolerance of and compliance with vegetable protein diets is often poor because of their bland taste, bulky nature and increased flatus production. Only where lactulose and dietary adjustment fails should protein restriction be considered. Where restricted, protein intake should be at the highest level compatible with normal mental function. This level will not be constant and should be re-assessed at each visit.

SUPPLEMENTS

Caloric intake gradually decreases with increasing severity of liver disease. When this occurs commercial liquid formula supplements may be useful when taken as drinks between normal meals.

Patients with end-stage chronic liver disease, in particular those with alcoholic or cholestatic liver disease, require vitamin supplementation. The absorptive defect can often be overcome by giving oral supplements of commercial mixtures containing water- and fat-soluble vitamins. If deficiencies persist, monthly parenteral injections will be necessary.

NASO-ENTERIC FEEDING

With advancing liver disease, anorexia worsens. Furthermore, secondary disturbances in intestinal function develop which further compromise nutrient uptake and utilization. Nutrition can, however, be maintained by the use of naso-enteric feeding which involves the infusion of a complete, balanced, liquid formula diet via a fine-bore nasogastric feeding tube over a 24-hour period. In this way nutritional intake can be maintained and gut absorptive capacity maximized. An alternative approach in less severe cases is to supplement a normal daily dietary intake with an 8-hour nocturnal infusion of the liquid formula to provide an additional intake of approximately 1000 kCal. The tube can then be flushed and sealed during daytime to permit ambulation and normal eating.

TOTAL PARENTERAL NUTRITION (TPN)

Parenteral feeding is the only way that nutrition can be maintained when gut failure occurs. In practical terms, gut failure can be defined as the failure of enteral feeding. Metabolic control is not as efficient with TPN as the route of infusion is into the systemic circulation rather than into the hepatic portal bloodstream. In addition, the risk of catheter sepsis is increased in patients with chronic liver disease due to reduced host–defense mechanisms. One advantage is that total nutrient requirements can be given in only one liter of fluid per day and salt restriction is now possible, facilitating management of ascites. 'Liver-specific' amino acid (branched-chain amino acid-enriched, aromatic amino acid-depleted) formulations may have beneficial effects on encephalopathy and protein synthesis, but unfortunately are expensive. Blood glucose control is facilitated by the use of single 24-hour solutions containing up to 250 g/day glucose. However excessive glucose use should be avoided as it will exacerbate cholestasis. Additional calories should be given in the form of fat. Lipid emulsion clearance is only mildly impaired and up to 50g/day as a continuous infusion is well tolerated.

POSSIBLE COMPLICATIONS

Patients with chronic liver disease, tend to retain salt and water, resulting in ascites and peripheral edema. Despite increased body salt content, plasma sodium levels are often low. The mainstay of treatment is to restrict fluid intake. Increasing dietary salt will exacerbate the situation (Chapter 16). Only those patients with end-stage liver disease who are clearly volume depleted should receive intravenous saline.

Fluid balance must be carefully monitored in all patients receiving nutritional support. Remember that the metabolic abnormalities associated with liver failure produce an inability to withstand overfeeding as well as underfeeding. Therefore, infusion rates must be carefully regulated and blood tested regularly for blood glucose and triglycerides as well as for electrolytes, urea and creatinine concentrations.

DRUG–NUTRIENT INTERACTIONS

Most diuretics lead to a loss of potassium, magnesium and zinc. However, spironolactone should conserve potassium and thus should not be given with potassium supplements. Cholestyramine results in the loss of vitamin A, D, E and K by binding bile salts. The use of neomycin may cause villous atrophy leading to a loss of zinc and an increased incidence of diarrhea. Lactulose may cause diarrhea leading to sodium, zinc and fluid loss. Glucocorticoids frequently cause loss of vitamin D and calcium due to selective blocking of nutrient transport. Antibiotics such as amikacin and gentamicin result in increased losses of potassium, magnesium and calcium due to altered excretion. Cephalosporins cause decreased gastrointestinal bacterial synthesis of vitamin K. These losses should be monitored and corrected where necessary.

TRANSPLANTATION

As cirrhosis progresses to end-stage liver disease, it becomes increasingly difficult to match dietary intake to changing metabolic requirements and the only solution becomes

269

liver transplantation. Every effort must be made to optimize nutritional status prior to surgery since poor nutrition is associated with a bad outcome after transplantation. Nutritional support should continue postoperatively. However, recent studies have shown that nutritional requirements rapidly return to normal following successful transplantation.

RECOMMENDED READING

Bianchi, G.P., Marchesini, G., Fabbri, A. *et al.* (1993) Vegetable versus animal protein diet in cirrhotic patients with chronic encephalopathy: a randomized cross-over comparison. *J Int Med*, **233**, 385–92.

Blackburn, G.L. and O'Keefe, S.J.D. (1989) Nutrition in liver failure (editorial). *Gastroenterology*, **97**, 1049–51.

Morgan, M.Y. (1991) Nutritional aspects of liver and biliary disease, in *Oxford Textbook of Clinical Hepatology* (eds N. McIntyre, J.-P. Benhamou, J. Bircher *et al.*), Oxford University Press, Oxford, pp. 1339–88.

O'Keefe, S.J.D. (1993) Parenteral Nutrition and Liver Disease, in *Clinical Nutrition: Parenteral Nutrition*, 2nd edn (eds J.L. Rombeau and M.D. Caldwell), W.B. Saunders, Philadelphia, pp. 676–95.

Swart, G.R., Zillikens, M.C., Vuuve, J.K. *et al.* (1989) Effect of a late evening meal on nitrogen balance in patients with cirrhosis of the liver. *Br Med J*, **299**, 1202–3.

26

Anesthesia for patients with liver disease

MICHAEL JAMES, JAY KAMBAM and JACK FRANKS

INTRODUCTION

Anesthesia and surgery in patients with advanced liver disease represents a major clinical problem. Not only does the presence of liver disease present a number of serious physiological problems to both anesthetist and surgeon, but also both anesthesia and surgery are likely to exacerbate any pre-existing liver dysfunction. The mortality associated with anesthesia and surgery in patients with unsuspected liver disease (especially viral hepatitis) is extremely high. In view of the fact that liver disease is frequently asymptomatic, the importance of a careful pre-operative evaluation of patients who might be at risk from liver disease becomes apparent.

PHYSIOLOGICAL CONSEQUENCES OF LIVER DISEASE

Liver disease has widespread effects on various organ systems and metabolic processes. Liver disease will also alter the handling of anesthetic drugs in various ways.

CARDIOVASCULAR FUNCTION IN LIVER DISEASE

Patients with liver disease frequently have a hyperdynamic cardiovascular state which includes a significantly increased cardiac index and a low systemic vascular resistance (Chapter 14). Sympathetic nervous system modulation is abnormal, blood flow through many vascular beds is altered and increased concentrations of noradrenaline (norepinephrine) are frequently found. Patients often have a resting tachycardia and bounding pulse; blood volume may be increased as a result of sodium and water retention but perfusion of various organs including the liver and the kidneys may be reduced; the increase in noradrenaline concentrations may result in down-regulation of catecholamine receptors in the heart with a consequent blunting of the response to catecholamines. Ascites may further compromise cardiovascular function by increasing intra-abdominal pressure resulting in aortocaval compression, thereby reducing venous return to the heart. In addition, chronic ethanol abuse may lead to an alcohol-induced cardiomyopathy.

RESPIRATORY SYSTEM IN LIVER DISEASE

The arteriovenous shunting seen in the peripheral circulation may also occur in the lungs and in addition there is a perfusion–diffusion defect. Consequently arterial hypoxemia is seen frequently in patients with disordered liver function. Between 12% and 28% of patients with cirrhosis will demonstrate moderate hypoxemia and a small percentage will have gross hypoxia. Unlike other forms of respiratory disease, dyspnea in this condition may be worsened on standing, presumably due to increased shunting through the basal areas of the lung. In addition to shunting, other factors such as ascites and pleural effusions may limit diaphragmatic excursion and decrease functional residual capacity (FRC), resulting in basal atelectasis. Patients with spider nevi may represent a sub-group at increased risk of the hepatic pulmonary syndrome. In this sub-group of patients a true shunt may be present and hypoxemia may not respond to oxygen administration.

In addition, several liver disorders are associated with specific lung pathologies. In primary biliary cirrhosis there is an association with lymphocytic interstitial pneumonitis, and severe emphysema may develop in patients with alpha-1 antitrypsin deficiency. It is of interest that the somatostatin analog octreotide has been associated with a rapid improvement in oxygenation in patients with the hepatopulmonary syndrome. The mechanism is not known but may involve inhibition of the release, or direct antagonism of the action, of vasodilator neuropeptides. The hypoxemia associated with liver disease appears to be functional in nature as it tends to resolve following successful liver transplantation. Hypoxemia is, therefore, only a relative contraindication to liver transplantation.

RENAL FUNCTION IN LIVER DISEASE

Renal function is frequently abnormal in patients with liver disease. Renal handling of sodium and water is profoundly disturbed in patients with ascites. In addition to the sodium overload there is an impaired ability to handle water loads which may result in dilutional hyponatremia. Hypokalemia, which is multifactorial in origin, may also develop. The avid sodium retention results in potassium loss, and this can be exacerbated by a respiratory alkalosis secondary to hyperventilation which is in turn consequent on the hypoxemia. The use of loop diuretics in the management of ascites will result in further potassium loss and, in addition, water retention may produce a dilutional hypokalemia.

In patients with advanced liver disease progressive oliguric renal failure is frequently seen and this is termed the hepatorenal syndrome. This may be distinguished from acute tubular necrosis by a low urinary sodium and a high urine : plasma creatinine ratio. In general, renal function is salvageable if the liver pathology is corrected, for example, by liver transplantation. Patients with liver failure, especially those with significant cholestasis, are at increased risk for acute tubular necrosis.

HEMOSTATIC FUNCTION

Liver disease may result in major disruptions of the coagulation mechanism which will depend on the nature of the hepatic dysfunction (Chapter 3). In cholestatic disorders where the absence of bile in the gut results in poor vitamin K absorption, the vitamin K-dependent Factors II, VII, IX and X will all be deficient. Provided hepatocellular function remains at an adequate level, the coagulation defect resulting from vitamin K deficiency will respond rapidly to parenteral administration of this vitamin given 1–2 days before surgery. In hepatocellular disease, in addition to the vitamin K dependent factors, many other substances involved in normal coagulation will be diminished as most of these are totally or partially synthesized by the liver. These include Factors V, XI, XII, XIII and fibrinogen. Fibrinolytic proteins and protease inhibitors such as protein C, anti-thrombin III and heparin co-factor 2 may also be decreased. In addition, leukopenia, thrombocytopenia and abnormal platelet function may be present due to hypersplenism, and disseminated intravascular coagulopathy may occur.

CENTRAL NERVOUS SYSTEM IN LIVER DISEASE

Hepatic encephalopathy is a reversible functional change in which the patient's level of consciousness can vary from lethargy and confusion to stupor and coma (Chapter 13). The signs and symptoms of hepatic encephalopathy are well known and will not be reviewed in this chapter, but it is important to realize that the development of hepatic encephalopathy may be associated with an increase in intracranial pressure and that this will require careful attention from the anesthetist during operations on such patients. This will apply, in particular, to patients with fulminant hepatic failure undergoing orthotopic liver transplantation where intracranial pressure monitoring has been recommended, with the epidural placement of monitors being favored.

ANESTHETIC PHARMACOLOGY AND THE LIVER

There are two aspects to liver function and anesthetic drugs. The first is that the drugs may, themselves, impair hepatic function; the second is the impact that disordered hepatic function will have on the pharmacokinetics and pharmacodynamics of many of the drugs used in anesthesia.

EFFECT OF ANESTHETIC DRUGS ON THE LIVER

Most anesthetic agents will produce a reduction in enteric blood flow and consequently a decrease in hepatic perfusion. Of the inhalational agents, halothane probably causes the greatest reduction in hepatic blood flow and isoflurane the least. Recent investigations suggest that sevoflurane may be similar to isoflurane but desflurane does not appear to have been studied in this regard at the present time. Of the inhalational agents, halothane also appears to cause the greatest disruption in liver function and elevated liver enzymes are seen frequently after halothane anesthesia. There is no evidence, however, that halothane is more likely to produce a worsening of the hepatic state of the patient than any of the other inhalational agents. A major controversy centers around the role of halothane-induced liver damage, particularly in terms of the rare fulminant hepatic failure which can follow halothane anesthesia ('halothane hepatitis'). This condition is thought to be related to the metabolites of halothane and is, therefore, much less common with the more modern inhalational agents which are metabolized to a far lesser degree. However, a similar form of hepatic failure has been reported, although much less frequently, with enflurane and even isoflurane has been associated with this kind of fulminant hepatic destruction. There is one recent report of fulminant hepatic failure in association with sevoflurane anesthesia. Guidelines placing restrictions on the frequency of halothane administrations in an attempt to avoid the condition are weakly based and of dubious significance. A full review of the topic is beyond the scope of the present discussion, but, on balance, halothane is best avoided in patients with significant liver disease.

Other agents used in anesthesia can adversely affect hepatic function primarily through mechanisms involving alterations in hepatic blood flow. Isoflurane may preserve hepatic blood flow better than other agents by maintaining hepatic arterial blood flow, since portal flow with this agent is reduced in the same manner as with the other inhalational agents.

Pharmacokinetics

Of more relevance to the patient with liver disease is the effect that severe hepatic dysfunction can have on drug disposition and elimination and on the patient's pharmacological responsiveness.

Liver disease may affect pharmacokinetic and pharmacodynamic profiles of drugs in various ways. The volume of distribution (V_d) of a drug is influenced by many factors including protein binding, lipid solubility and the size of fluid compartments, all of which are likely to be altered in patients with advanced liver disease. Consequently, V_d of various drugs may vary widely in patients with hepatic dysfunction, with the greatest effect being seen on compounds which are normally highly protein-bound and have a small V_d. Thus unpredictable changes in the unbound drug concentration available for pharmacodynamic responses and for metabolism may occur.

The rate of removal of a drug from the body is measured by its clearance (Cl), which is the volume of the central compartment which is cleared of drug in unit time. Clearance is the net result of all the processes which result in drug elimination and may involve the sum of several processes, including both hepatic and extra-hepatic removal mechanisms. The half-life of a drug is related to the clearance and the volume of distribution in the following manner:

$$t\frac{1}{2} = 0.693.V_d/Cl$$

Thus the half-life of a drug may be prolonged

by increases in V_d without any change in hepatic clearance, and a reduction in hepatic clearance, together with an increased V_d will cause markedly delayed elimination of drugs, although the relationships may be complex. For poorly extracted drugs a decrease in volume of distribution will necessitate reductions in loading dosages. However, increased volumes of distribution are frequently accompanied by reductions in serum proteins, resulting in higher concentrations of the unbound free fraction of highly protein-bound drugs and such agents do not necessarily require increased initial dosage to compensate for the increased volumes of distribution. Less highly bound drugs, such as muscle relaxants, may require a larger than normal initial dose where V_d is increased; consequently, prolonged action of these drugs can be anticipated.

Alterations in hepatic blood flow will alter the rate at which drugs are presented to the hepatocytes for metabolism. Hepatic blood flow is generally reduced in liver disease and portosystemic shunting may result in significant quantities of drug bypassing the hepatic sinusoids. Hence, drugs with high extraction ratios, for which small decreases in the total mass of drug extracted will result in large increases in plasma concentration, will be markedly affected by changes in hepatic blood flow. Drugs with low extraction ratios will be relatively unaffected by changes in hepatic blood flow and reduced hepatic metabolic capacity. This has resulted in drugs being categorized into three main groups with reference to their hepatic metabolism:

● high-risk;
● limited-risk;
● low-risk drugs.

High-risk drugs are those which have high hepatic extraction ratios, usually in excess of 70% on their first pass through the liver. These include drugs such as glyceryl trini-

274

trate, labetalol, lignocaine, morphine and verapamil. Drugs with low or limited risk of altered pharmacokinetics include the benzodiazepines, theophylline and warfarin.

ANESTHETIC MANAGEMENT

PRE-OPERATIVE ASSESSMENT

Given the large increases in morbidity and mortality associated with anesthesia and surgery in patients with significant liver disease, good pre-operative evaluation of hepatic function is clearly important. However, it should be appreciated that tests of liver function are generally fairly insensitive and that advanced disorders of liver performance are required before significant abnormalities in function occur. Nevertheless, it is appropriate that pre-operative assessment of the degree of liver dysfunction be conducted before subjecting a patient to exploratory laparotomy. In addition, a careful systemic review with appropriate investigations should be conducted by the anesthetist to evaluate the effect that the liver disease may have had on other organ systems.

Pre-operative evaluation should include a consideration of possible cardiovascular, renal and pulmonary function in addition to assessment of the extent and severity of the liver dysfunction. Appropriate history and clinical examination should be conducted supported by the investigations indicated in Table 26.1.

Evaluation of the extent of hepatic dysfunction should include a clinical examination for the stigmata of chronic liver disease together with biochemical testing. Enzyme testing generally reflects the extent of acute liver injury rather than hepatic function, and tests of synthetic function are a better indicator of the liver capacity (Chapter 2). In particular, the ability of the liver to produce albumin and clotting factors is quite a sensitive indicator of disordered liver function, and coagu-

Table 26.1 Pre-operative investigations

Cardiorespiratory
    Chest X-ray
    Exercise ECG
    Pulmonary function tests
    Blood gases

Metabolic
    Serum glucose
    Serum electrolytes
    Serum urea
    Serum creatinine
    Urinary electrolytes
    Urinary urea
    Urinary creatinine
    Creatinine clearance

Hematological
    Hemoglobin
    White blood cell count
    Platelet count
    Coagulation tests

Liver function
    Serum albumin/globulin
    Serum bilirubin
    Liver enzymes

Hepatic imaging
    Ultrasound, computed tomography, angiography

Microbiological
    Cultures
    Hepatitis markers
    Viral antibodies

lation tests may usefully predict hemorrhagic tendency. There have been a number of attempts to evaluate the extent of the surgical risk in patients with liver disease according to a number of factors. The basis for this evaluation remains some variant of Child's classification, and although this has not been fully evaluated for its predictive accuracy in all types of liver disease, it remains a useful guide. The degree to which individual disorders of hepatic function can affect perioperative risk in cirrhotic patients has been

Table 26.2 Risk factors for patients with cirrhosis (adapted from Conn, 1991)

Factor	Mortality Absent (%)	Mortality Present (%)
Serum albumin <3 g/dl	12	58
Pre-operative infection	21	64
Prothrombin time > 1.5 sec over control	18	63
Bilirubin > 50 mmol/l	15	44–62
Ascites	11–53	37–83
Abdominal surgery	10	35
Emergency surgery	10–40	45–86

examined by several authors, and these are summarized in Table 26.2.

Pre-operative management should consist of correction of coagulopathy and electrolyte abnormalities, control of ascites and encephalopathy, and elimination of infection. Prothrombin time should be corrected to within 3 seconds of control values either with vitamin K or fresh-frozen plasma. Failure of response to vitamin K demonstrates severe intrinsic hepatic dysfunction and implies a poor prognosis. The use of pre-operative administration of oral bile salts in an attempt to reduce the risks of endotoxemia and consequent reduction of renal function is controversial and not universally accepted.

CONDUCT OF ANESTHESIA

Once the condition of the patient has been optimized, consideration should be given to the site and nature of the surgery, and planning of the anesthetic should include consideration of the likelihood of massive hemorrhage and the extent of monitoring appropriate to the medical condition of the patient and the extent of the surgical procedure. Pharmacological considerations will include the likely effects that agents used will have on liver function and the effect that the disordered function will have on the behavior of any agent used. Generally, drugs selected should be those with relatively short half-lives which have minimal dependence on hepatic function for their removal. Reduced gastric motility and the presence of ascites will both predispose to vomiting on induction of anesthesia, and precautions against regurgitation should be adopted in the majority of cases.

Pre-operative preparation should include an analysis of the likelihood and probable magnitude of blood loss, and the availability of appropriate volumes of blood and blood products arranged in advance. The use of devices which reprocess the patient's own shed blood as washed red cells for re-infusion have been shown to reduce requirements for transfused blood in major liver surgery. Washing of the cells is important to remove excess potassium and bilirubin, but patients with abdominal malignancy or infective processes should not receive salvaged blood.

Premedication

Sedative drugs should not be used in patients with advanced liver disease (Child's B or C), but otherwise a short-acting benzodiazepine such as temazepam is appropriate. However, other benzodiazepines such as diazepam or midazolam should be avoided unless restoration of liver function by transplantation is being envisaged. If regurgitation is a potential risk, reduction of gastric pH by the use of a drug such as ranitidine may be considered. Metoclopramide and sodium citrate may also be used. Intramuscular injections should be avoided in patients whose coagulation status is impaired.

Induction of anesthesia

For most patients with advanced liver disease, a rapid sequence induction is the most appropriate technique, but the choice of induction agent is not crucial. As induction agents depend more on redistribution than on elimination for termination of their action, the route of elimination of the agent chosen is of relatively little importance and considerations of pharmacodynamics are of more relevance than those of kinetics, unless infusions are being considered. Propofol elimination is relatively unaffected by deteriorating liver function until the degree of impairment is marked. Etomidate elimination may be significantly prolonged as it is particularly sensitive to increases in its volume of distribution. Some patients with alcoholic liver disease may exhibit marked cross-tolerance between anesthetic agents and ethanol.

Suxamethonium is the relaxant of choice for rapid sequence induction, but impaired synthetic hepatic function will result in a decreased formation of plasma cholinesterase and consequent prolongation of the action of this agent. This is generally not a clinical problem as the duration of action is extended by no more than 20 minutes unless multiple doses are given. At least in theory, a nerve stimulator should be used to establish that the action of suxamethonium has been terminated before a non-depolarizing agent is used.

Maintenance of anesthesia

Hemodynamic considerations are paramount during surgery on patients with disordered liver function, and particular attention must be paid to the effects that anesthetic techniques may have on the circulation in general and on splanchnic and hepatic blood flow in particular. A balanced technique using combinations of opiates and inhaled anesthetics is generally favored for this reason.

Alterations in protein binding and changes in volume of distribution result in larger than normal doses of both *d*-tubocurarine and pancuronium being needed to establish neuromuscular blockade, but the duration of action of both drugs will be prolonged. Vecuronium is less affected in terms of the initial dose, but its elimination is mainly hepatic and its duration of action can be greatly prolonged. Mivacurium is unpredictably and extensively affected by hepatic dysfunction, and both of these latter two drugs should probably be avoided in patients with liver disease. Atracurium, which is independent of the liver for much of its elimination, is probably the drug of choice. Ideally, neuromuscular transmission should be monitored and relaxant dosage titrated to effect, although if postoperative ventilation is planned, this may be a less important consideration.

The synthetic opiates fentanyl and sufentanil have been shown to exhibit virtually unchanged kinetics in cirrhotic patients although the duration of action can become unpredictable in end-stage liver disease. Both drugs have been used successfully in liver disease and during orthotopic liver transplantation. Alfentanil, however, has a volume of distribution four times that of fentanyl and is thus more likely to be affected by liver disease.

For reasons discussed above, isoflurane is currently the volatile anesthetic agent of choice, and for reasons of economy is generally administered using a circle system and low fresh gas flows. It is also advisable to include an airway warming device to diminish heat loss in these patients. Heat loss can be a major problem, and attempts to prevent this complication should include the use of leg and arm wrapping, avoidance of patient contact with cold solutions wherever possible, and possibly the use of hot air devices on non-exposed body areas.

Good fluid management is crucial to the prevention of renal complications, and most authorities advocate some form of renal protection in the form of mannitol infusions. The place of dopamine in the prevention of the hepatorenal syndrome is less well established, but it is, nonetheless, widely used. A system capable of delivering very large volumes of intravenous fluids, particularly blood, should be made available and there are many commercial devices which can be used for this purpose. The sodium overload which many of these patients will have may make the use of crystalloid solutions less advisable, and frequent analysis of plasma electrolytes should be undertaken. Hypokalemia should be scrupulously avoided, and rapidly corrected should it occur. The avoidance of hyperventilation and maintenance of a normal Pa_{CO_2} is important in preventing the worsening of hypokalemia through respiratory alkalosis, and is also of value in maintaining gastrointestinal perfusion. Hyper- ventilation may worsen hepatic blood flow by increasing intrathoracic pressure and thus reducing abdominal venous return, and hypocarbia fosters the conversion of ammonium to ammonia. Thus, although a high inspired oxygen partial pressure is advisable, positive pressure ventilation should be carefully controlled to produce a normal, or even slightly increased, arterial carbon dioxide partial pressure.

Monitoring

The degree of monitoring necessary for each case will depend on the severity of the underlying disease and the extent of the surgery to be performed. The majority of patients with advanced disease and those undergoing major hepatic surgery will require extensive monitoring in addition to the routine anesthetic monitoring of ECG, pulse oximetry and capnography.

Direct intra-arterial pressure monitoring is advisable for the majority of these patients. The placement of small radial artery catheters has been shown to be associated with a lower morbidity than the placement of simple intravenous cannulae and there should be no hesitation about placing radial arterial lines in these patients.

Hemostatic considerations may demand that the arterial puncture is performed by an expert to reduce the risk of multiple artery damage. The advantages of arterial pressure monitoring are not only related to the hemodynamic variability which these patients frequently exhibit, but also to the ease of obtaining arterial blood samples for blood gas analysis and for biochemical determinations. It should be remembered that many of the commercially available pulse oximeters give erroneous readings in severely jaundiced patients, and arterial PaO_2 monitoring may be the only reliable guide to oxygenation of the patient in these circumstances. In major cases such as liver transplantation many units adopt the practice of inserting bilateral radial arterial lines so that hemodynamic monitoring is not interrupted by the need to sample arterial blood frequently.

Central venous cannulation, particularly when the lines are placed through the internal jugular route, is more invasive and carries a higher risk of complications, particularly of hemorrhage, and great care should be exercised during placement. The subclavian route, which may result in occult bleeding, is less advisable for this reason. Nevertheless, the hemodynamic and fluid balance disturbances which are frequently seen in these patients means that central venous pressure monitoring is advisable in many cases and should be regarded as mandatory in patients with either severe liver disease or those undergoing major hepatic surgery.

Monitoring of neuromuscular transmission is advisable in most patients and should preferably be conducted using a device which contains a printout so that a constant observation of the state of neuromuscular transmission can be made and drugs titrated accordingly.

Heat loss is frequently a problem in patients undergoing major hepatic surgery, in particular during orthotopic liver transplantation, and core temperature must be monitored. If a pulmonary artery catheter with thermodilution cardiac output capabilities is used this will obviously provide a suitable form of monitoring.

Fluid balance must be monitored meticulously. A urinary catheter is mandatory for all but the most minor of procedures so that urine output can be accurately monitored and any decline in renal function rapidly corrected. In major liver surgery, particularly in orthotopic liver transplantation, blood loss may be massive and extremely rapid. A system should be in place to keep track of administered fluids in situations in which very large quantities of infused fluids may be administered and fluid packs should be retained so that a postoperative check that the records are indeed accurate may be performed.

Monitoring of coagulation parameters is extremely important. Routine laboratory coagulation tests which include measurements of the platelet count, fibrin degradation products, the prothrombin time, partial thromboplastin time and the activated clotting time are generally time-consuming and the results are frequently not available until 60 minutes after the taking of the sample. Hence their relevance in a rapidly changing environment may be minimal. Alternative forms of assessment of coagulation status of the patient are now available and include the thromboelastograph (TEG) and sonoclot systems. Both of these devices measure the whole process of coagulation including the rapidity with which clot formation commences, the quality of the clot formed and the presence of fibrinolysis. Although a full TEG trace may take an hour, in general an answer regarding the development of clot can be obtained within 15 or 20 minutes, and if significant fibrinolysis is present it is frequently evident within half an hour. The use of the thromboelastograph can be very useful in judging the use of drugs such as aprotonin which can have a marked effect on the need for donor blood transfusion in patients undergoing liver surgery.

Biochemical monitoring should be conducted in all patients receiving massive fluid or blood transfusions as rapid changes in electrolyte status may occur. In our own practice, regular blood gas analysis and estimation of sodium potassium and ionized calcium is performed within the operating theater complex so that results are available within minutes. Blood sugar monitoring is conducted at regular intervals throughout the procedure.

Vascular access

In patients undergoing hepatic surgery, particularly orthotopic liver transplantation, placement of appropriate vascular access is crucial. Large-diameter intravenous cannulae are placed in the largest available veins in the arms. For liver transplantation these cannulae are placed only in the right arm so that the veins in the left arm are undisturbed should they be needed for venovenous bypass. Bilateral 8FG sheath introducers are placed in each internal jugular vein and for liver transplant patients a Swan–Ganz catheter is inserted via the right internal jugular introducing sheath. If liver transplantation is not being performed, or venovenous bypass is not going to be used, then both arms can be used for line placement. Fluid administration sets should be of the high capacity type to allow for rapid infusion, but care must be exerted when these devices are used as overtransfusion can readily occur in a very short space of time.

POSTOPERATIVE MANAGEMENT

The post-surgical management of the patient will in many ways be simply an extension of the anesthetic management. The severity of the liver disease and the extent of surgery will determine the need for postoperative care, but in general, patients with advanced liver disease, or those with major hepatic surgery, will benefit from an initial period in the intensive care unit. Many patients will require postoperative ventilation, but this should again be conducted with a view to maintaining as near normal blood gases as possible. Pleural effusions and right basal atelectasis are likely to develop, and good pain management together with physiotherapy are essential. Pain relief is difficult to provide as many patients will be unable to metabolize opiates in the normal manner, and regional techniques such as thoracic epidural analgesia will be precluded by the presence of coagulopathies. Continuous infusions of opiates are thought to be less appropriate than small bolus injections because of the difficulty of predicting adequate elimination and the consequent risk of accumulation. Despite good intraoperative care, a number of these patients will require rewarming in the postoperative period, and this may require very careful fluid balance management. Close monitoring of sodium and water loads and the concentration of other electrolytes remains vital; great care must be taken to avoid sodium and water overload. Renal function must be closely monitored and maintained at above 0.5 ml/kg per hour using mannitol and/or frusemide.

CONCLUSIONS

The anesthetic management of a patient scheduled to undergo major surgery who has serious liver disease requires a team approach. Co-operation between physician, anesthetist, surgeon and intensivist will produce the best results. A good working knowledge of the likely problems and possible solutions is essential if a good clinical outcome is to be achieved in this very high risk group of patients.

RECOMMENDED READING

Browne, D.R.G. (1990) Anaesthesia in impaired liver function. *Curr Anaesth Crit Care*, **1**, 220–7.

Carton, E.G., Rettke, S.R., Plevak, D.J. *et al.* (1994) Perioperative care of the liver transplant patient: Part 1. *Anesth Analg*, **78**, 120–33.

Conn, M. (1991) Preoperative evaluation of the patient with liver disease. *Mt Sinai J Med* (NY), **58**, 75–80.

Eagle, C.J. and Strunin, L. (1990) Drug metabolism in liver disease. *Curr Anaesth Crit Care*, **1**, 204–12.

Farman, J. (1986) Anaesthesia and perioperative care for patients with liver disease. *Br J Hosp Med*, **36**, 448–52.

Friedman, L.S. and Maddrey, W.C. (1987) Surgery in the patient with liver disease. *Med Clin North Am*, **71**, 453–76.

Gholson, C.F., Provenza, J.M. and Bacon, B.R. (1990) Hepatologic considerations in patients with parenchymal liver disease undergoing surgery. *Am J Gastroenterol*, **85**, 487–96.

Gordon, P.C., James, M.F.M., Lopez, J.T. *et al.* (1992) Anaesthesia for liver transplantation. *S Afr Med J*, **82**, 82–5.

McEvedy, B.A., Shelly, M.P. and Park, G.R. (1986) Anaesthesia and liver disease. *Br J Hosp Med*, **36**, 26–34.

27

Liver transplantation

DELAWIR KAHN and THOMAS STARZL

INTRODUCTION

Liver transplantation, the ultimate therapeutic option in liver disease, has ceased to be an experimental procedure. Indeed, transplantation, which is currently the treatment of choice for patients with chronic end-stage liver disease, should now be part of the therapeutic armamentarium of all practicing hepatologists.

The first human liver transplant was performed in Denver in 1963. The early years were difficult and the overall results poor, with only the minority of patients surviving for any significant period of time. However, it is noteworthy that nearly 20% of patients treated before 1979 are still alive 14 to 24 years later. The introduction of the new immunosuppressive drug cyclosporine in the late 1970s saw a dramatic improvement in the results of liver transplantation. This led to the important NIH Consensus Development Conference in 1983, where it was decided that liver transplantation should no longer be regarded as an experimental procedure but one that merited widespread clinical application. The late 1980s saw a phenomenal increase in the number of transplant centers and the number of patients being transplanted, not only in the USA and Europe but throughout the world. Indeed, over 2000 liver transplants were undertaken in the USA in 1989.

Several factors contributed to the dramatic improvement in the results of liver transplantation during the 1980s. The surgical procedure became standardized and can now be performed by any competent hepatobiliary surgeon. Refinements in the surgical technique include the introduction of the venovenous bypass, the use of a 'growth factor' for the vascular anastomoses, standardization of the biliary anastomosis and modifications in the donor technique. Better patient selection, the introduction of new immunosuppression regimens, and improvements in organ preservation have also contributed to the improved results.

Many centers are now able to achieve 1-year survival figures in excess of 90% providing only good risk patients are treated. Patients who survive the first year after the transplant may expect a favorable long-term outcome with a low rate of attrition.

INDICATIONS FOR LIVER TRANSPLANTATION

The indications for orthotopic liver transplantation include chronic advanced liver disease, hepatic malignancy, fulminant hepatic failure and metabolic liver disease (Table 27.1).

Table 27.1 Indications for orthotopic liver transplantation

Chronic liver disease
    Cholestatic liver disease
      ● primary biliary cirrhosis
      ● primary sclerosing cholangitis
      ● biliary atresia
    Hepatocellular liver disease
      ● viral hepatitis
      ● alcoholic liver disease
      ● drug-induced liver disease
      ● autoimmune liver disease
      ● cryptogenic cirrhosis
    Vascular disease
      ● Budd–Chiari syndrome

Hepatic malignancy
    Hepatocellular carcinoma
    Cholangiocarcinoma
    Carcinoid

Fulminant hepatic failure
    Viral hepatitis
    Drug-induced

Metabolic liver disease
    Wilson's disease
    Tyrosinemia
    Alpha-1 antitrypsin deficiency

The chronic liver diseases can be divided into those which are predominantly cholestatic in nature and include primary biliary cirrhosis, primary sclerosing cholangitis and biliary atresia, and those diseases which predominantly affect the hepatocytes and include chronic viral liver disease, chronic drug-induced liver disease, alcoholic liver disease and autoimmune liver disease. Some patients with the Budd–Chiari syndrome may also benefit from a liver transplant. Liver transplantation for hepatic malignancy is a controversial area since many of these patients die from recurrence of the tumor soon after the transplant. On the other hand, patients with chronic liver disease with an incidental small hepatoma noted in the resected liver do well after liver transplantation and have much the same prognosis as patients who are transplanted for end-stage liver disease. Some tumors appear to behave less aggressively. Indeed, patients with fibrolamellar tumors and hemangioendotheliomas do relatively well after transplantation. In addition, better survival and lower rates of recurrence have been reported after liver transplantation in patients with cirrhosis of the liver and a small (<5 cm) histologically non-invasive hepatocellular carcinoma when compared with liver resection. In contrast, cholangiocarcinoma is regarded as a relative contraindication to liver transplantation because of the high rate of recurrence and poor survival figures.

Liver transplantation for fulminant hepatic failure is another controversial area. Because of the unpredictable natural history of the disease, many patients with fulminant hepatic failure die before a suitable donor becomes available. Although a small number of patients in stage 4 coma may recover with medical support only, over 80% are likely to die as a result of their disease (Chapter 12). Thus transplantation should be considered in these patients.

Of great interest to some physicians are the various inborn errors of metabolism that are now potentially treatable by liver transplantation. These patients can be divided into those where the liver is severely damaged by cirrhosis, such as in cases of Wilson's disease, alpha-1 antitrypsin deficiency and tyrosinosis, and the liver transplant is indicated because of chronic liver disease, and those patients where the liver is morphologically normal although it contains a metabolic defect which is damaging another system. For example, patients with familial hypercholesterolemia have normal lipid levels after liver transplantation.

CONTRAINDICATIONS TO LIVER TRANSPLANTATION

The contraindications to liver transplantation (Table 27.2) are being continually revised. Certain diseases in which transplantation might have previously been precluded or strongly discouraged are no longer absolute contraindications for transplantation.

Table 27.2 Contraindications to liver transplantation

Absolute contraindications
  Sepsis outside the biliary tree
  Advanced cardiopulmonary disease
  Metastatic hepatic malignancy
  AIDS

Relative contraindications
  Portal vein thrombosis
  Age >60 years
  Advanced dialysis-dependent renal disease
  HBsAg positivity
  HIV-positive
  Previous upper abdominal surgery
  Cholangiocarcinoma
  Hypoxemia with right to left shunts

Patients who have active sepsis outside of the liver and patients who have severe cardiac or respiratory disease are not considered as transplant candidates. Metastatic malignancy and AIDS are also regarded as absolute contraindications. A few centers have transplanted patients who are HIV-positive but without clinical AIDS. Various techniques have been devised to circumvent the problem of portal vein thrombosis and this is no longer a contraindication. Neither is age. Indeed, many patients over the age of 60 years have undergone successful orthotopic liver transplantation. Patients with advanced chronic renal disease can be subjected to

kidney transplantation in addition to the liver transplant. Liver transplantation in patients who are hepatitis B surface antigen-positive remains controversial because of the high rate of recurrent disease after transplantation. However, many patients do survive long-term. Those patients who are HBV-DNA negative and those who receive immunoprophylaxis after liver transplantation have a more favorable prognosis. Upper abdominal surgery, in the form of portacaval shunts or major hepatobiliary surgery, add to the complexity of the transplant procedure. Cholangiocarcinoma is a relative contraindication because of the high incidence of recurrence of the tumor. Hypoxemia with right to left shunts is also regarded as a relative contraindication.

TIMING OF LIVER TRANSPLANTATION

One of the most difficult aspects of liver transplantation is the optimal timing of the transplant procedure. Many patients with chronic advanced liver disease die while awaiting liver transplantation. Furthermore, if one waits too long before referring patients for liver transplantation their general condition may deteriorate to a point where the outcome of the transplant procedure may be compromised. Thus early referral has to be balanced against operative mortality as well as long-term benefit. Guidelines have been devised to help in determining the best time for referring patients for transplantation (Table 27.3). Any patient with chronic advanced liver disease who has a major complication such as a major variceal bleed, intractable ascites, recurrent bacterial peritonitis or the development of the hepatorenal syndrome should be given the option of a liver transplant.

OPERATIVE PROCEDURE

In orthotopic liver transplantation, the

283

Table 27.3 Indications for liver transplantation

Acute liver failure
- Bilirubin >20 mg/l (400 μmol/l)
- Prothrombin time > 30 sec above control
- Progressive encephalopathy ≥ grade 3

Chronic liver disease
    Cholestatic liver disease:
- Bilirubin > 12 mg/l (200 μmol/l)
- Intractable pruritus
- Advanced bone disease

    Hepatocellular liver disease:
- Albumin < 2.5 g/l
- Hepatic encephalopathy worst grade ≥ 3
- Prolonged prothrombin time

    Factors common to both
- Hepatorenal syndrome
- Recurrent bacterial peritonitis
- Refractory ascites
- Recurrent biliary sepsis
- Development of hepatoma
- Major variceal bleeding

diseased native organ is removed and replaced with a new liver in the most anatomically normal way possible. The technical aspects of the transplant procedure have undergone major refinements over the years, and have been described in detail elsewhere. Various techniques have been devised to circumvent anomalies of donor or recipient blood vessels. The introduction of the extracorporeal venovenous bypass in 1983 to decompress the splanchnic and systemic venous circulations during the anhepatic phase has been one of the most important refinements in the surgical technique. The venovenous bypass is used either routinely or selectively in patients with severe portal hypertension and compromised renal function or in those who fail a trial of cross-clamping. Reconstruction of the biliary tract has also become standardized and can be done either by connecting the donor and recipient common ducts end-to-end over a T-tube or the common duct of the donor to a jejunal limb in a Roux anastomosis.

IMMUNOSUPPRESSION

The introduction of the new immunosuppressant agent cyclosporine in the late 1970s led to a significant improvement in the results of solid organ transplantation. The search for new and more potent immunosuppressive drugs continues. Currently most patients receive a combination of cyclosporine, steroids and azathioprine after liver transplantation. Some centers have used a sequential immunosuppression regimen where a monoclonal or a polyclonal antibody is used for the first 7–10 days and cyclosporine introduced thereafter. This is done to minimize the nephrotoxic effects of cyclosporine. The new immunosuppressant agent FK506 was discovered in 1984 in the northern regions of Japan and has been shown, *in vitro*, to be many times more potent than cyclosporine. These initial findings were confirmed, *in vivo*, in heart, liver and kidney transplants in dogs, rats and primates. FK506 has been shown to be effective as a form of salvage or rescue therapy in patients who continue to reject the liver grafts despite conventional treatment of acute rejection. The initial multicenter trials comparing FK506 against cyclosporine showed better patient and graft survival in Europe but no difference in the USA compilations. However, in both series there was a different spectrum of side effects, less steroid-resistant rejection and lower steroid usage with FK506. Other immunosuppressive agents under investigation include brequinar sodium, dyspergaulin and RS61443.

LIVER PRESERVATION

The major advance in liver transplantation in the 1980s was the introduction of a new preservation medium, the Wisconsin solution. Although livers can be stored for longer than 24 hours, recent studies have indicated that ischemic times of longer than 12–15 hours are associated with a greater incidence of primary non-function as well as delayed intrahepatic biliary strictures. However, liver transplants can now be performed as an elective procedure. It has also made it possible to increase the size of the donor pool and therefore increase the number of liver transplants being performed.

REDUCED-SIZE LIVER TRANSPLANTATION

The lack of organ donors continues to be a major limiting factor in transplantation. This is especially true for pediatric patients awaiting liver transplantation. To overcome this critical shortage of suitable-sized pediatric donors, a lobe or segments of an adult liver can be transplanted into a pediatric recipient. Mortality rates for children awaiting liver transplantation are now almost negligible. The results of reduced-size liver transplantation are as good as intact livers. In contrast, the results of split liver transplantation are poorer.

LIVING RELATED LIVER TRANSPLANTATION

The number of live related liver transplants and the number of centers performing this procedure have increased significantly in recent years. Graft and patient survival have been as good as intact liver transplantation. The risk to the donor has been acceptable with only one mortality documented thus far. The major advantage is that the transplant can be undertaken electively with the patient in optimal condition.

RECOMMENDED READING

Scharschmidt, B.F. (1984) Human liver transplantation: analysis of data on 540 patients from four centers. *Hepatology*, **4**(suppl 1), S95–101.

Starzl, T.E., Iwatsuki, S., Esquivel, C.O. *et al.* (1985) Refinements in the surgical technique of liver transplantation. *Semin Liver Dis*, **5**, 349–56.

Starzl, T.E., Iwatsuki, S., Shaw, B.W. *et al.* (1984) Analysis of liver transplantation. *Hepatology*, **4**, 50.

Starzl, T.E., Iwatsuki, S., Shaw, B.W. *et al.* (1985) Immunosuppression and other nonsurgical factors in the improved results of liver transplantation. *Semin Liv Dis*, **5**, 334–43.

Starzl, T.E., Todo, S., Gordon, R. *et al.* (1987) Liver transplantation on older patients. *N Engl J Med*, **316**, 484–5.

28

An overview of basic immunology

SIMON ROBSON, MARIO EHLERS and DAVID SHAFRITZ

INTRODUCTION

Immunology is the study of protective (immune) responses and the mechanisms responsible for these. An interesting parallel can be drawn between the immune system and the nervous system as both have protective and identification functions. Both systems are able to recognize and to discriminate between self and non-self. Both systems must recognize the difference between innocent and dangerous signals and respond accordingly. Both neurons and immune cells appear to have been derived from a common ancestral cell, and both have similar, unique membrane proteins which are acted on by similar hormones or peptide messengers.

The major function of the immune system is to protect the host against foreign organisms and cells by recognizing foreign proteins and mobilizing host defenses against these intrusions. Once the threat has been contained, the host must then be able to reduce its response while preserving immunological 'memory' of the invasion to allow for more rapid mobilization on repeat exposure.

The immune system may be conveniently sub-divided into an **innate** or **natural immunity** and an **acquired immunity** with specific memory responses. Innate immune mechanisms can be compared to reflex activity. They are always present, do not need to be learnt, and are not augmented by repeat exposure. Acquired immune responses may be likened to cognition in that the host has been exposed to the stimuli for these responses, has learnt how to deal with such stimulation, and is able to respond more effectively on repeat exposure. As with neurological function, immunological memory may diminish over time and repeated exposures may be necessary to maintain adequate immunological responses.

INNATE IMMUNITY

EXTERIOR HOST DEFENSES

These are designed to prevent bacterial or viral invasion of the host and comprise the skin with a layer of keratin and sebaceous gland secretions that are anti-bacterial and anti-fungal. The skin acts as a protective barrier to prevent bacterial colonization. Unlike the skin, the oral, vaginal and colonic mucosae are colonized by specific non-pathogenic bacteria. Treatment with antibiotics may disturb this natural bacterial flora and, for example, lead to stomal ulcers or diarrhea. Similarly, oral contraceptives may, by altering vaginal pH, predispose to vaginal fungal infections. Moreover, the lining of the respiratory and gastrointestinal tracts is covered with mucus that entraps bacteria and foreign material, which is then expelled by specialized cells with cilia that move the mucus towards the exterior. The mucus from the respiratory tract may be swallowed or coughed up and expectorated. Bacteria entering the stomach are neutralized by the presence of acid in the digestive juices. Lysozyme in many secretions is directly antibacterial. These exterior host defenses markedly reduce bacterial, viral and fungal invasion of the host.

PHAGOCYTES AND NATURAL KILLER CELLS

Once pathogenic organisms enter the host, they are immediately subjected to natural immune responses comprising phagocytes and, in the case of viruses, natural killer cells. Phagocytosis is the process whereby foreign organisms and/or particulate matter are ingested by specialized immune cells and digested intracellularly. Certain cells are able to re-express fragments of bacteria or foreign proteins on their cell membranes ('antigen presentation') and thereafter to specifically activate other cells in the immune response. This triggers specific immunity and increases immune responses against invading microorganisms (see below).

The primary phagocytes of the host are monocyte macrophages and polymorphonuclear leukocytes (neutrophils). These cells are also able to use oxygen to make hydrogen

peroxide (H_2O_2) which is toxic to bacteria (and tissues).

Natural killer cells are innate immune response cells that are able to control viral infection in the early stages. They are activated by interferon which is released from virally infected cells. Interferon is responsible for fever and myalgia/backache in many viremic illnesses ('flu').

ACUTE PHASE RESPONSE

During acute immunological reactions, certain proteins released by the liver are able to influence immune responses. These proteins may coat bacteria and improve phagocytosis. They are called acute-phase reactants and are usually secreted in response to host inflammation. Complement comprises a series of proteins that 'complement' normal host responses. These proteins are activated in a cascade by bacterial products and antibodies produced by cells that mediate acquired immunity against bacteria. Complement is able to kill bacteria directly by creating defects in their cell walls. Complement is also able to coat bacteria, allowing for more efficient binding to phagocytes by specific complement receptors on these cells. Coagulation factors are also activated by host immunity and may lead to deposition of clotting proteins (particularly fibrin) on bacteria. Thrombosis of vessels in the area of inflammation tends to limit the spread of bacteria throughout the body.

ACQUIRED IMMUNITY

Host responses improve after repeated exposure to infective organisms or following vaccination. This implies that the immune response is able to 'learn' from prior exposure to foreign protein (antigen), and devise specific memory functions that allow the host to deal with infection more efficiently on repeat exposure. The cells orchestrating this learned response are called lymphocytes and they make up the lymphoid organs of the host. These lymphoid organs are predominantly the lymph nodes, thymus, the mucosa-associated lymphoid tissue (MALT) and, in humans, the bone marrow.

CELLS OF THE IMMUNE RESPONSE

All cells responsible for immunity derive from common progenitor cells in the bone marrow. These cells divide and eventually form cells of the myeloid and lymphoid systems. Myeloid cells are predominantly those cells concerned with phagocytosis, generation of hydrogen peroxide and superoxide radicals, and presentation of bacterial products to the lymphoid system. The myeloid series comprises those with oval or kidney-shaped nuclei (the mononuclear phagocytes which comprise monocytes and macrophages) and those that have segmented nuclei (the poly-morphonuclear series or neutrophils, eosinophils and basophils). The lymphoid series comprise B cells which are responsible for humoral immunity (antibodies), T cells which are responsible for cellular immunity, and the null cell, or natural killer cell, which is responsible for early innate responses against virally infected cells (see earlier). Other cells involved in the immune response are platelets, endothelial cells and mast cells.

HUMORAL AND CELLULAR IMMUNE RESPONSES

When antigens enter the body, two different types of immunological reaction may occur:

1. In the **humoral response**, antigens bind to B cells and activate these cells, leading to the development of plasma cells and release of free antibody into body fluids and blood. This is often under the direction of T cells. These antibodies act by binding to and neutralizing bacterial proteins and toxins, or by coating bacteria to enhance phagocytosis.

2. In the **cellular immune response**, sensitized T lymphocytes participate in reactions such as delayed hypersensitivity and specific killing of virally infected cells. Here processed antigens are bound by mononuclear phagocytes and presented to T cells.

HUMORAL IMMUNE RESPONSES AND ANTIBODIES

Antibody activity is associated with the classic gamma-globulin fraction of serum. Antibodies are also termed immunoglobulins, and may be sub-divided into different classes on the basis of the structure of their backbone. In the human there are five major structural types or classes: immunoglobulins G (IgG), IgM, IgA, IgD and IgE.

Immunoglobulin G (IgG)

IgG comprises two heavy and two light chains linked together by inter-chain bonds. Purified IgG appears to be a Y-shaped molecule with a common core structure, the Fc region, which directs the biological activity of the antibody molecule. The two arms of the Y section of the antibody molecule dictate antibody specificity. All classes of antibody have been shown to have binding affinity for antigen associated with this so-called Fab region.

IgG is the major immunoglobulin synthesized during the humoral response. Through its ability to cross the human placenta, it provides the neonate with a major line of defense against infection for the first few weeks of life. This antibody is also found in early mother's milk or colostrum. IgG diffuses more readily than other immunoglobulins into the extravascular body spaces, and is responsible for neutralizing bacterial toxins and binding bacteria to enhance phagocytosis.

Complexes of bacteria and antibody attract phagocytic cells by positive chemotaxis. These phagocytes adhere to bacteria through surface receptors for complement (which is activated by antibody) and the Fc portion of IgG. Binding to the Fc receptor on phagocytes then stimulates ingestion of microorganisms through phagocytosis.

Immunoglobulin A (IgA)

IgA appears selectively in serous or mucus secretions such as saliva, tears, nasal fluids, sweat, colostrum and secretions of lung and gastrointestinal tract. This protein is secreted as a dimer (two molecules of IgA). IgA acts like an antiseptic paint that inhibits adherence and invasion of bacteria.

Immunoglobulin M (IgM)

IgM is often referred to as the macroglobulin antibody because it is made up of five antibody units. The free molecule looks almost like a star. IgM antibodies are efficient at agglutinating and killing bacteria. They appear early in the response to infection. These antibodies are largely confined to the bloodstream and play an important role in controlling septicemia. IgM precedes IgG in host responses and is known as the antibody of the primary response.

Immunoglobulin D (IgD)

IgD occurs on the surface of a proportion of blood lymphocytes and interacts early with antigen in the regulation of B cell activation.

Immunoglobulin E (IgE)

IgE is present in low concentrations in serum and only a very small proportion of plasma cells in the body synthesize IgE. These antibodies are responsible for allergy and are able to bind to mast cells, leading to specific allergic responses such as hay fever and asthma. IgE is also linked to resistance to infection with endo- and ectoparasites. This antibody is able to bind eosinophils which are able to directly damage parasites invading the host.

ANTIGENS AND ANTIBODIES

Antigenic determinants (epitopes) must be of consistent shape and charge in order to be recognized by specific antibodies. All biological molecules will induce an antibody response. Antigens range from protein molecules, carbohydrates, synthetic peptides, and chemically modified proteins to entirely unnatural substances such as certain drugs. Natural antigens are usually multivalent (i.e. they will bind multiple different antibodies). Antigenic stimulation resulting in antibody responses is characterized by a lag phase followed by the appearance of IgM in the serum. If the same antigen is re-injected at a later point, the lag phase is much shorter and IgM is noted to switch to IgG which then persists in the serum.

The initial specific recognition of antigen is mediated by B lymphocytes which may be able to recognize antigen without intermediary cells. When B lymphocytes bind antigen they become activated and start dividing rapidly. This is associated with a small degree of specific mutation. The antibodies made gradually become better-fitting for the specific antigen. B cells that mutate in this positive way are favored by binding more antigen. B lymphocytes differentiate into both primed (memory) cells and activated (or effector) cells which give rise to plasma cells. The memory cells persist in the host. Humoral B-cell responses are usually dependent upon signals received from the T helper lymphocyte population, which in turn is activated by monocyte-macrophages or dendritic cells that act as presenters of antigen and intermediary cells. The successful cooperation between B and T cells and macrophages to effect the production of antibody is dependent upon the physical and functional integrity of these populations.

CELL-MEDIATED IMMUNITY

T lymphocytes are important in protection against intracellular organisms such as various bacteria, protozoa and viruses. They are also responsible for reaction against foreign tissue grafts, tumor cells and for delayed hypersensitivity. T cells are processed in the thymus following their release from bone marrow during their maturation process. Various T-cell surface receptors and cell membrane antigens appear during the course of development on different sub-populations. Most important are the T-cell receptors and T-cell markers, such as CD1, CD2 and CD3, the T-helper cell marker (CD4) and the T suppressor and cytotoxic cell marker (CD8). These are referred to as cluster determinant markers.

The T-cell antigen receptor specifically recognizes antigen in association with specific host histocompatibility proteins expressed on dendritic cells or monocyte-macrophages and other antigen-presenting cells. The T-cell receptor is similar to the antibody structure produced by B cells. The T-cell receptor must, however, recognize both foreign antigen and host cell histocompatibility proteins in close association. T cells will therefore not react to soluble antigen such as in the case of B cells. Class I major histocompatibility complex (MHC) proteins are present on almost all cells of the body and are recognized by CD8-bearing T-cells (cytotoxic and suppressor cells), whereas class II MHC proteins are found mainly on macrophages and other antigen-presenting cells and facilitate binding to T-helper cells via CD4.

Following the processing of soluble exogenous antigen by antigen-presenting cells, the antigen is presented to T-helper cells in association with class II cell proteins. The T-helper cells then release interleukin 2 which stimulates other T cells. T-helper cells are therefore able to augment specific innate immune responses by activating the myeloid cell lines and causing their division or multiplication. Cytotoxic T cells, in contrast, bind to endogenous antigen in association with host MHC I proteins on host cells. These cytotoxic T cells recognize MHC I molecules through interactions with CD8. They are therefore able to kill virus-infected cells that present components of endogenously synthesized virus proteins on their surfaces.

Many **lymphokines** have been characterized and these factors act as hormones between T cells and other immune cells. Lymphokines are neither antigen-binding nor antigen-specific. They are able to activate other T cells and B cells non-specifically. Lymphokines are either made by monocytes or by T cells and include interferons, tumor necrosis factors, interleukins 1 to 13 and colony-stimulating factors.

Antigen processing involves denaturation and/or fragmentation of complex antigens into smaller, simpler binding sites or epitopes. These epitopes determine the dominant direction and magnitude of immune responses. Presentation of antigen to antigen-sensitive lymphocytes evokes specific immune reactions against each distinct epitope. T lymphocytes and B lymphocytes represent two complementary and interactive arms of the immune response. These are thought to react with different non-cross-reactive repertoires of epitopes.

IMMUNOREGULATION

The primary regulator of the immune response is thought to be antigen, which may induce variable immune reactions depending on the host state of tolerance or reactivity. There are a number of other host-regulatory mechanisms which are intrinsic to the immune system.

Macrophages play a central role in cell-mediated immunity and initiate responses by acting as antigen-presenting cells. They may have effector functions as inflammatory, tumoricidal or microbiocidal cells in addition to their regulatory function. Macrophages are able to activate T and B cells by antigen processing and presentation. Macrophages are also able to produce pro-inflammatory molecules which activate lymphocytes (interleukins 1 and 6, tumor necrosis factor alpha).

Once T cells are activated by encountering antigens on the surface of macrophages they release lymphokines which are able to trigger and activate other T cells, B cells and non-specific phagocytes. The production of highly specific antibodies by B cells appears related to cooperation with T cells.

To summarize the important phenomena related to the induction and control of the immune response: macrophages process antigen and stimulate the induction of T-helper cells that secrete modulatory factors that influence lymphocytes. Helper T cells, helper B cells as well as other T cells are involved in delayed hypersensitivity and anti-microbial immunity. Suppressor T cells are also activated during immune responses. These eventually result in down-regulation of the immune response. T-suppressor cells are thought to inactivate T-helper cells and may also inhibit B-cell function. The elimination of antigen from macrophages results in down-regulation of responses. Specific antibodies bind available antigen and prevent subsequent cellular interactions with lymphocytes and monocyte-macrophages.

MECHANISMS OF HOST RESISTANCE

IMMUNITY TO BACTERIA

Host resistance to bacteria embraces all of the defense mechanisms the body can mobilize. These include non-immunological resistance and specific resistance mediated by the immune system. The predominant immune responses against bacteria include phagocytosis, humoral immunity and cell-mediated immunity. The mechanism or mechanisms operative for any specific bacterial infection depend on the nature of the organism in terms of antigens, as well as its ability to evade the host's immune responses and to enter phagocytes. The pathogenicity of the bacteria also governs the specific mode of resistance that the host is able to mobilize.

A protein found in most body secretions, called lysozyme, is primarily active against the cell walls of Gram-positive bacteria, including *Staphylococcus aureus*. Another innate immune barrier involves iron sequestration by the host. Bacteria are dependent on iron for their growth, therefore iron binding in tissues and body fluids by iron-binding proteins inhibits many bacteria.

Specific resistance is mediated by the immune system. The phagocytic cells are the first cells that respond to bacterial infections. These are present in the blood, in local lymph nodes, in the liver, spleen, and lungs. Humoral immunity provides additional anti-bacterial defenses by the ability of antibodies to neutralize toxins, to bind bacteria for phagocytosis, and to lyse bacteria in conjunction with complement. IgA, IgG, and IgM are the most important antibodies directed against bacteria.

Cell-mediated immunity is of major importance in bacterial infections that are resistant to antibody or phagocytic destruction. Bacteria of this type (e.g. *Mycobacteria* or *Listeria*) are able to survive for extended periods within macrophages. Activated T cells are required for the hyperstimulation of these macrophages, which in turn can kill the bacteria. This is usually associated with tissue damage. CD8-positive (class I MHC-restricted) cytolytic T cells play an important role in the resistance to intracellular bacteria by lysing infected cells and exposing the bacteria to activated immune cells. CD4 helper cells further augment this activity by the release of lymphokines, in addition to their role in activating macrophages.

The specific immune response pattern elicited during an infection depends on the type of causative agent. Humoral immunity restricts the harmful effects of extracellular microorganisms and soluble toxins, whereas a cell-mediated immune response controls the spread of intracellular pathogens. Generation of the appropriate immune effector mechanisms is regulated by the pattern of cytokines released by CD4+ helper T (TH) cells. They can be classified into two sub-sets: TH1 cells give rise to cell-mediated immunity (delayed hypersensitivity and stimulation of T cytotoxic cells) and are characterized by the production of interleukin 2 (IL-2) and gamma-interferon, whereas TH2 cells are more efficient in mediating antibody formation, and secrete IL-4, IL-5, IL-6 and IL-10. Many intracellular bacteria, protozoa, and viruses stimulate TH1 cells, whereas other bacterial and helminths induce TH2 cells. Recent evidence indicates that the molecular switch that initiates this polarized response in an infection is IL-12, which is produced by infected macrophages and promotes TH1 development. The production of IL-12 by infected macrophages is influenced by the type of pathogen and by host genetic factors; secretion of IL-12 may be inadequate or inappropriate resulting in failure to resolve the infection.

IMMUNITY TO VIRUSES

Immunity to viral infections depends on the induction of non-specific innate mechanisms and the development of an adaptive immune response to antigens present on the surface of viruses or of virus-infected cells. Certain viruses (retroviruses) are able to induce neoplastic disease by transforming the infected cells. The HIV and HTLV viruses are able to specifically infect and either kill or transform T lymphocytes and thereby subvert the immune response. The destruction of CD4-positive T cells by the HIV results in the clinical syndrome known as AIDS.

Within the first cycle of viral replication in cells interferons are released. Interferons inhibit viral replication and protect other cells from viral infection. Interferons activate natural killer cells that can specifically lyse virus-infected cells. Complement may inactivate free virus and limit viral replication in tissues. Macrophages inevitably become involved in virus infections and are important in the presentation of antigen in the generation of the specific immune response.

The adaptive immune mechanisms against viruses involve both soluble antibodies and cytotoxic T cells. Of the antibodies, secretory IgA is a major defense mechanism against viruses, which gain entry to the body via epithelial surfaces. IgA is likely to exert its effect by blocking viral receptors. IgG has an important role in neutralizing free viruses and, in combination with complement, may lyse viruses with lipid envelopes. Antibody coating of viruses may prevent them from uncoating and replicating inside phagocytic cells.

Infection of cells by viruses also leads to the induction of cytotoxic T cells which are able to bind to class I MHC proteins in association with viral proteins. Cytotoxic T cells appear early after infection and have an important role in promoting recovery from primary infection with viruses. The cytotoxic T cells are able to induce rapid and extensive disintegration of virus-infected cells but are not able to inactivate liberated virus, which must be cleared by antibody and complement. Therefore, persistent levels of antibodies are the main mechanism preventing reinfection of cells.

IMMUNITY TO PROTOZOA

Protozoa have developed a number of mechanisms to enable them to maintain their parasitic behavior by living both intra- and extracellularly. Antibodies in general may damage extracellular protozoa, whereas cell-mediated reactions governed by T cells and eosinophils are important mechanisms against intracellular parasites, such as *Plasmodia* and *Toxoplasma gondii*.

IMMUNITY TO HELMINTHS

Parasitic worms that infect man include trematodes (bilharzia), cestodes (tapeworms), and nematodes (roundworms). Helminths are complex multicellular organisms that occur in almost any locality in the host and evoke a wide variety of host reactions, both pathological and immunological. From an immunological point of view, the success of a parasite depends upon the degree to which it can disguise its presence and thus evade immune reactions.

The host immune responses to helminthic infections are both humoral and cell-mediated. Conventional antibodies of the IgE class are produced in response to helminths. These antibodies are elevated in parasitized humans. Eosinophils are able to interact with IgE bound on helminths and degranulate, with destruction of the helminth. Other antibodies are able to play a protective role by halting activity of the ova, larvae or adult helminths in human tissues.

Cell-mediated immune mechanisms against helminths are effective against helminths embedded in tissues or migrating through tissues. T cells may depress helminth activity by the inflammatory responses of delayed hypersensitivity and through cytotoxic T cells. The ability of T cells to react with helminths suggests that in certain instances, the helminth is able to mimic host antigen expression or wear shed host antigens like a coat.

HYPERSENSITIVITY AND GRAFT REJECTION

The above discussions have detailed the beneficial effects of the host response. At times, the host response may be exaggerated and lead to tissue damage and other reactions detrimental to the host. This is sometimes known as allergy. The major hypersensitivity reactions are those governed by antibody and cellular immunity. Type I hypersensitivity responses usually refer to anaphylaxis, such as in allergy to penicillin or other drugs, with a catastrophic reaction upon exposure to the allergen. This is governed by IgE and mast cells. Other types of hypersensitivity responses are usually related to antibody (IgG) production (type II), and to immune complex deposition (type III), such as in serum sickness. The delayed hypersensitivity response (type IV) is an accentuated cellular immune response. Type IV responses occur with organ transplantation or in the case of reactivation or secondary tuberculosis with tissue destruction and lung cavity formation. Interestingly, in organ transplantation less immunosuppression is required to maintain the graft after a certain period of adaptation, a process known as tolerance. The mechanisms may relate to clonal or functional depletion of effector cells or specific generation of T-suppressor cells.

AUTOIMMUNITY

Autoimmunity is a complex process in which there is loss of tolerance to self antigens. The major factors involved in autoimmunity are thought to be genetic, immunological defects, hormonal and environmental influences.

GENETIC FACTORS

Family studies have shown that genetic factors are important in triggering autoimmune diseases. Genetic impact is expressed chiefly on effectors of autoimmune damage, e.g. Gm allotypes of immunoglobulins and human leukocyte antigens (HLA) or MHC. The most common associations of MHC with autoimmune disease are those of the MHC sub-types B8, DR2, DR3 and DR4. Class II MHC proteins may be aberrantly expressed on cells normally lacking such proteins, allowing these cells to function in antigen presentation in local immunological reactions. However, cytokines are also known to induce MHC, so that some of these manifestations may be secondary or acquired paraphenomena.

IMMUNE DEFECTS

Cell reactivity is a physiological process and immunological control mechanisms permit this to take place without any harmful sequelae. However, impairments in immune regulation have been identified in precipitating autoimmunity. These include IgA deficiency, deficiencies of complement components (particularly C2 and C4), and associations between the immune response genes, predominantly DR3 and others.

Immune regulatory defects result in T- or B-cell effectors which may be activated by T-cell bypass or by polyclonal activation. Abnormalities in suppressor T cells no longer able to functionally suppress the effector T cell clones represent a further potential mechanism.

HORMONAL FACTORS

The hormonal impact on autoimmunity is well known and includes not only sex hormones but thymic hormones, corticosteroids and vitamin D3. These hormones have receptors on CD8 and CD4 cells. Altered sex hormone status has been reported in patients with autoimmune conditions. Auto-antibodies and suppressor T cell defects are more prevalent among healthy first-degree female relatives of patients with some autoimmune diseases.

ENVIRONMENTAL FACTORS

These are thought to act as inducing factors in individuals with an appropriate 'immuno-genetic/hormonal' background. Major environmental agents include sunlight, drugs, diet and infections. Pre-eminent among the drugs are penicillamine and hydrallazine.

Mechanisms by which drugs induce autoimmune disease include altered auto-antigens, immune complex formation and effects on T-cell function. Some drugs possess structures resembling auto-antigens and may result in what has been termed 'molecular mimicry'.

There are nutritional effects on autoimmunity. Low calorie, isocaloric low fat diets or diets supplemented by marine fish oils may delay autoimmune disease in animals. There are no human studies of note in this regard.

Infectious diseases have a major role in triggering autoimmune disease. These include hepatitis B virus infection linked to extrahepatic manifestations, and human immunodeficiency virus infection with autoimmune features. The mechanisms by which viruses, bacteria, and even parasites induce autoimmunity are as diverse as the agents themselves and include molecular mimicry, polyclonal B-cell activation, increased MHC expression, 'altered self', and idiotype cross-reaction. In the latter instance, auto-antibodies may be anti-idiotypes of anti-viral antibodies or anti-bacterial antibodies. The anti-mitochondrial antibodies seen in primary biliary cirrhosis may cross-react with gut bacterial enzymes. These bacterial enzymes show a close similarity to the E2 component of pyruvate dehydrogenase of humans.

Other factors which may have a significant role in autoimmunity include the modification of cell antigens (e.g. in diabetes or rheumatoid arthritis), or the effects of cancer or aging. Stress and even smoking may influence autoimmune disease.

ORGAN-SPECIFIC AND NON-ORGAN-SPECIFIC AUTOIMMUNE DISORDERS

There are different spectra of auto-antibodies which cross-react with cellular components that are widespread throughout the body, e.g. anti-nuclear factors, anti-DNA, or anti-ribonuclear proteins. These also include antibodies directed against microsomes (e.g. LKM antibodies) or mitochondria (e.g. anti-mitochondrial antibodies) (Chapter 9). The organ-specific antibodies include those directed at thyroglobulin, which may result in Hashimoto's thyroiditis. Organ-specific antibodies important in liver disease include antibodies directed at liver-specific proteins (LSP), liver membrane antigens (LMA) and the hepatic lectin, which is another term for the asialoglycoprotein receptor. These proteins are purported to be important targets for antibody-directed cellular toxicity in autoimmune chronic active hepatitis.

Viral proteins such as HBcAg may also be important in directing cytotoxic reactions in chronic active hepatitis associated with hepatitis B virus. In chronic autoimmune cholestatic diseases (e.g. primary biliary cirrhosis), biliary antigens seen in association with MHC appear to be recognized by effector T and B cells. One of these potential biliary antigens has shared, unique epitopes on human colonic mucosae, skin and biliary epithelium and this may explain several systemic manifestations of ulcerative colitis.

In the spectrum of autoimmunity from organ-specific to non-organ-specific systemic disease, Hashimoto's thyroiditis can be viewed as an organ-specific disorder, whereas systemic lupus erythematosus can be seen as a systemic disease involving skin, kidneys, tissues, joints, lungs, heart and bone marrow.

Chronic active hepatitis and primary biliary cirrhosis are somewhere in the middle of the spectrum. Although they are predominantly organ-specific, they are also associated with non-organ-specific manifestations. They also tend to overlap with other conditions in this spectrum, e.g. hemolytic anemia, thrombocytopenia, diabetes, etc.

IMMUNE DEFICIENCY SYNDROMES

This refers to either congenital or acquired deficiencies in the immune response. There may be deficiencies in antibody production, complement production, phagocytosis, T-and B-cell function and monocyte-macrophage abnormalities. The congenital immune deficiencies are rare, while the acquired immune deficiencies are common. Major acquired immune deficiencies occur in patients who are malnourished, who have chronic infections, such as tuberculosis or malaria, and in patients who have chronic kidney and liver failure. Other forms of immunodeficiency are associated with metabolic disorders such as diabetes, and with cancer.

Cytotoxic drugs used to treat leukemia and cancer have direct effects on the immune response by damaging lymphoid cells.

AIDS occurs as a result of infection with HIV, which specifically depletes the T-helper cells, resulting in impairment of immune responses in which the T cell responses are central. Patients with AIDS become much more susceptible to viral, protozoal and intracellular bacterial infections, such as tuberculosis. These patients are also prone to recurrent fungal infections, presenting as oral thrush, pneumonia or even fungemia.

IMMUNOSUPPRESSIVE DRUGS

Cytotoxic drugs are used as immunosuppressants in non-neoplastic disease and in cancer chemotherapy for their action on proliferating cells. Immunosuppressant drugs are usually given continuously, at low doses, whereas anti-cancer drug treatment often consists of intermittent, high-dose regimens.

The major drugs used to depress immune reactions are corticosteroids, antibiotics (such as cyclosporine and FK506), anti-metabolites (such as azathioprine) and alkylating agents (such as cyclophosphamide). Alkylating agents are able to damage the nucleic acid of proliferating cells and are particularly effective in certain autoimmune conditions. In transplantation, the usual drugs utilized are anti-metabolites, antibiotics and steroids.

CONCLUSIONS

This short review has aimed at achieving a broad understanding of immune responses in humans. We have attempted to show the clinical significance of the immune response in the control of bacterial, viral and other parasitic infections, and have alluded to the occasional tendency of the immune response to respond excessively and inappropriately, as in the case of hypersensitivity or autoimmune disease. Immunodeficiency has been described as an acquired disease often secondary to infection or drugs. Finally, immune reactions play an important role in transplant tolerance and rejection.

RECOMMENDED READING

Bach, F.H. and Sachs, D.H. (1987) Current concepts: immunology. Transplantation immunology. *N Engl J Med*, **317**, 489–92.

Barnett, E.V. (1986) Circulating immune complexes: their biologic and clinical significance. *J Allergy Clin Immunol*, **678**, 1089–96.

Brodsky, F.M. and Guagliardi, L.E. (1991) The cell biology of antigen processing and presentation. *Annu Rev Immunol*, **9**, 707–44.

Brostoff, J., Scadding, G.K., Male, D.K. and Roitt, I.M. (1991) *Clinical Immunology*, Gower Medical Publishing, London.

Buckley, R.H. (1987) Immunodeficiency disease. *JAMA*, **258**, 2841–50.

Condemi, J.J. (1987) The autoimmune diseases. *JAMA*, **258**, 2920–9.

Johnston, R. Jr. (1988) Current concepts: immunology, monocytes and macrophages. *N Engl J Med*, **318**, 747–52.

Kaufmann, S.H.E. (1993) Immunity to intracellular bacteria. *Annu Rev Immunol*, **11**, 129–63.

Kirkpatrick, C.H. (1987) Transplantation immunology. *JAMA*, **258**, 2992-3000.

Kishimoto, T., Toga, T. and Akira, S. (1994) Cytokine signal transduction. *Cell*, **76**, 253–62.

Life, death and the immune system (1993) *Scientific American* (special issue), September.

Mosmann, T.R. and Coffman, R.L. (1989) TH1 and TH2 cells: different patterns of lympokine secretion lead to different functional properties. *Annu Rev Immuol*, **7**, 145–73.

Nossal, G.J.V. (1987) Current concepts: immunology. The basic components of the immune system. *N Engl J Med*, **316**, 1320–5.

Roitt, I.M., Brostoff, J. and Male, D.K. (1989) *Immunology*, 2nd edn, Gower Medical Publishing, London.

29

Basic immunological and molecular biological techniques for medical practitioners

MARIO EHLERS, SIMON ROBSON and DAVID SHAFRITZ

INTRODUCTION

General medical journals are publishing an increasing number of studies that incorporate aspects of fundamental laboratory investigations, including cellular and molecular biology. Since these disciplines have become part of the modern undergraduate medical curriculum, most journals assume a certain background knowledge of the techniques and jargon used. Knowledge and awareness of basic methodology and scientific principles are therefore essential for the understanding and comprehension of the current medical literature. This chapter will cover techniques in immunology and molecular biology, two disciplines around which major advances in all areas of medicine, including hepatology, have evolved.

IMMUNOLOGY

Laboratory investigation of the immune system can be divided into two broad categories. First, tests which determine the number and the functions performed directly by cells of the immune system, and second, tests that determine the functions of soluble mediators released by these cells. Studies concerning both of these aspects may give information that can be used in the diagnosis, understanding and management of many diseases.

IMMUNE CELLS

These cells, produced in the bone marrow, undergo a process of maturation before their release. The predominant effector cells of immune responses are those of the myeloid cell line (granulocytes and monocytes) and the lymphoid cell series. Total cell numbers in peripheral blood and the phenotype of individual cells can be determined without prior separation and purification. However, to study individual functions and behavior, the cells need to be purified. This is generally achieved by exploiting known differences in the densities of these cells. The technique used relies on centrifuging whole, heparinized blood through a Ficoll–Hypaque density gradient. The centrifugal forces separate the different cell types into various iso-dense layers. Thus, mononuclear cells (PBMC) (monocytes, T and B lymphocytes) are found at the blood/density gradient interface, while neutrophils, which are more dense, are found with the clumped red blood cells at the bottom of the gradient. Lymphocytes and monocytes can be further separated by their adherence characteristics. Monocytes in the presence of serum stick to plastic *in vitro*, whereas lymphocytes do not. Neutrophils are separated from erythrocytes using differences in density following erythrocyte agglutination (6% dextran sedimentation) or by lysing the erythrocytes in hypotonic saline. Purified cells may then be utilized for both quantitative and qualitative functional assays.

PHENOTYPE DETERMINATION AND QUANTITATION

Cells are quantified either by simple counting using an electronic counter ('Coulter counter'), or by more complex methods using a fluorescence-activated cell sorter (FACS), which utilizes a laser. The latter method is used to determine numbers of cells displaying particular antigens or markers on their surfaces. The cells are incubated with a specific fluorescent-labeled antibody that binds to a particular surface antigen. The mixture of cells is then counted and is separated into fluorescent and non-fluorescent cells in the FACS. This technique is used frequently to determine the ratio of so-called T-helper cells (CD4-positive) to T-cytotoxic cells (CD8-positive).

FUNCTIONAL ASSAYS

Lymphocyte transformation

The response of T cells to antigen is reflected by a cycle of growth and division known as lymphocyte transformation or mitogenesis. Mitogens are agents that induce polyclonal proliferation and mitosis in mammalian cells. Plant lectins (meaning 'to bind') are among the most well-known mitogens and include concanavalin A (ConA) and phytohemagglutinin (PHA), which activate T cells. Pokeweed mitogen (PWM) stimulates both B and T cells. By using these compounds it is possible to study differential lymphocyte responsiveness in various diseases. In practical terms, purified peripheral blood mononuclear cells (PBMC) are incubated with varying concentrations of mitogens in the presence of ^{3}H-thymidine. As the cells are stimulated to divide, radioactive thymidine becomes incorporated into newly synthesized cellular DNA, which can be quantified by liquid scintillation counting after filtration of lysed cells and nuclei through glass-fiber filter paper.

Mixed lymphocyte reaction (MLR)

When mononuclear cells taken from two unrelated individuals are cultured together, a proliferative response is obtained (2-MLR). The majority of the responsive cells are T cells. As in the transformation assay, incorporation of radiolabeled thymidine into nucleic DNA is used as a measure of the mitotic response. Pretreatment of one population of mononuclear cells by irradiation or incubation with mitomycin to block cellular division enables the determination of unidirectional stimulation and proliferation *in vitro* (1-MLR). The MLR is often used clinically to select donor–recipient combinations for tissue transplantation. The method does not give information on the antigen composition of the donor and recipient, only on their compatibility.

CYTOTOXICITY ASSAYS

Cell-mediated cytotoxicity

CD8+T cells respond to foreign antigens, presented on the cell surface in the context of major histocompatability complex (MHC) class I molecules, by blastogenesis. Effector (cytotoxic) cells are then generated that will specifically lyse the relevant target cells. Cytotoxicity develops as a result of exposure to antigens which may include histocompatibility antigens and viral proteins. T cell-mediated cytotoxicity may be measured using ^{51}Cr-labeled target cells with the relevant antigen on their surfaces. After lysis of the target cells, the ^{51}Cr is released and can be counted in a gamma-counter. Other cells involved in target cell destruction are natural killer (NK) cells and null cells. NK cells need no previous exposure to the antigens of the target cell and are not target cell- or antigen-specific. Their recognition sites are undetermined.

Antibody-dependent cell-mediated cytotoxicity

In this phenomenon, target cells coated with very small amounts of antibody are killed by effector cells (K cells). K cells have receptors for the Fc region of the antibody and specifically recognize immune complexes bound to cells.

Complement-mediated cytotoxicity

This is often used for direct histocompatibility tests. Lymphocytes are incubated with various histocompatibility antisera from immunized individuals and test sera in the presence of complement to detect lymphocytotoxic (i.e. anti-lymphocyte) antibodies. If the lymphocytes have the specific antigens on their surfaces, these will combine with the antibodies and the cells will then be lysed by complement. The degree of cell killing is measured either by release of ^{51}Cr, or by manual counting.

SOLUBLE MEDIATORS OF THE IMMUNE RESPONSE

ANTIBODIES

Polyclonal and monoclonal antibody production

Antigens introduced into an animal generally stimulate a number of lymphocyte clones. This gives rise to a mixture of antibodies with a wide range of binding affinities, termed polyclonal antibodies. Non-specific or cross-reactive binding reactions by polyclonal antibodies may be a problem when antisera are used to identify or quantitate specific antigens on cell membranes. The need for homogeneous standardized antibodies as reproducible reagents was fulfilled by the advent of monoclonal antibodies (MoAbs) produced by hybrid cells or hybridomas.

MoAbs are made by fairly simple methodology. Mice are immunized with particular antigens and their immune spleen cells are fused with mouse plasmacytoma cells. This fusion between an antibody-producing and a malignant cell produces cells that grow like the tumor but retain the ability to synthesize and secrete antibody. These cells are aliquoted into culture wells and cultured in medium that selects for fusion hybrids. As the hybridomas grow, they secrete antibodies into the culture medium which can be assayed for antibodies to the specific antigen. Positive cultures are then diluted, so that each well contains a single cell ('cloning by limiting dilution'). Since each resulting colony has been derived from a single cell which multiplies rapidly, the entire population of cells in the colony represents a single clone. Clones producing antibody are again selected. Finally, the antibody is purified from other proteins in the culture medium.

MEASUREMENT OF ANTIGEN–ANTIBODY REACTIONS

The specific reaction of antibodies with antigens to form a complex can be used to detect and measure antibody or antigen in sera, culture fluids, or on cell membranes.

Immunodiffusion

This is one of the simplest detection methods, and is essentially qualitative. Antigens and antibodies are allowed to migrate towards each other in a gel; where the two reactants meet, insoluble complexes form which then precipitate. At the point of equivalence, when all the antibody and antigen is complexed, a sharp visible line is produced. A number of modifications of this technique, which render the method semi-quantitative are in use. Some of these modifications include the application of an electric field to the process of immunodiffusion, as in the technique known as rocket immunoelectrophoresis used for the measurement of serum proteins, complement and coagulation factors.

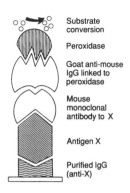

Figure 29.1 ELISA 'sandwich' technique.

Radio-immunoassay (RIA) and enzyme-linked immunosorbent assay (ELISA)

These are two quantitative methods for detecting antigen–antibody reaction that are used extensively in basic research and in clinical diagnostic services.

In RIA, the concentration of an unknown antigen is determined by measuring its ability to compete with a fixed amount of radiolabeled antigen for a limited quantity of antibody. Proteins are readily labeled with one of several radioactive isotopes by standard laboratory techniques. The antibody may be in solution, or may be immobilized on an insoluble support. The test sample, labeled protein, and antibody are mixed, allowed to react and the complexes formed are then separated from the remaining medium, and the amount of radioactivity in these complexes is determined. This 'bound' radioactivity is then compared to a standard curve of similar bound radioactivities obtained by running a range of known concentrations of pure antigen in the same assay.

In ELISA, either the antigen or the antibody is immobilized by attachment to a solid surface such as a plastic tube or microtiter plate (Fig. 29.1). The first reactant, i.e. the antigen or antibody to be assayed, is then added and incubated with the coated wells, followed by an enzyme-labeled antibody directed against the first reactant. The enzymes used are generally horseradish peroxidase or alkaline phosphatase. Enzyme substrate is then added, the colored reactants are read in a spectrophotometer and the absorbance values of the unknown samples compared with a standard curve. Advantages of the ELISA over the RIA include the absence of radioactivity and the stability of the enzymes and reagents.

Western blotting

A variant of the ELISA method that provides qualitative information about antigens is the Western blotting technique. In this method, proteins (antigens) are separated according to size by electrophoresis, transferred ('blotted') on to a membrane, and then identified by affinity binding of enzyme-linked antibodies (Fig. 29.2). The electrophoresis technique used is sodium dodecyl sulfate (detergent)–polyacrylamide gel electrophoresis (SDS–PAGE). The detergent, SDS, causes denaturation and all proteins become negatively charged, and thus separate only according to size. The samples are loaded at the cathode (negative) end of the gel, and when an electric current is applied, the proteins all move towards the anode (positive electrode). After separation, the proteins are electrically transferred out of the gel on to a nitrocellulose or nylon membrane, to which the proteins bind. This is then reacted with a series of specific antisera, in a similar fashion to an ELISA, culminating with an enzyme-linked antibody. Addition of substrate results in a band of colored product at the position of the antigen of interest. The molecular weight of this protein band can be determined by measuring the distance it migrated through the gel, compared with standard proteins of known molecular weights (Fig. 29.2).

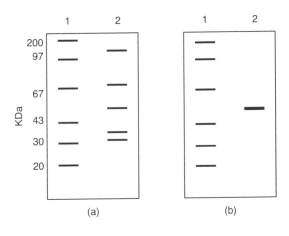

Figure 29.2 Electrophoresis and Western blotting of proteins. (a) Sodium dodecyl sulfate–polyacrylamide gel electrophoresis (SDS–PAGE) of proteins results in separation of proteins in a mixture according to their size. Lane 1 comprises standard proteins of known molecular weights (kDa); lane 2 comprises a sample mixture of five 'unknown' proteins. (b) Western blot of the sample proteins, achieved by transfer of the proteins from the gel on to a nitrocellulose membrane and detection of a particular protein by reaction with specific antibodies. Note that of the five proteins in lane 2, only one reacted with the antibody and was stained by the enzyme-linked reaction.

IMMUNE COMPLEXES

These complexes form whenever humoral immune responses to antigen are initiated, and antibody is synthesized. The complexes, which may or may not have incorporated complement, circulate for short periods (mainly in association with erythrocytes) and are then cleared by the immune system in several ways. The complexes may be solubilized by the complement component C1q, which interferes with Fc–Fc interactions of the immunoglobulin molecules, or they may bind to Fc receptors on cell surfaces, e.g. on macrophages, resulting in phagocytosis. The complexes can also bind the third component of complement, C3, which then binds specifically to the receptor CR1, found mainly on erythrocytes. The erythrocytes circulate via the liver and spleen where the immune complexes are removed.

Failure to clear immune complexes may result from properties of the antigen, inadequate specific antibody responses, impaired complement activation, abnormal or deficient complement receptors on erythrocytes, or dysfunction of the mononuclear phagocyte system ('blockade'). The circulating complexes are then deposited at target tissues, particularly in skin, blood vessels, renal glomeruli, choroid plexus and synovium. Tissue damage and inflammation may then result, particularly where complement is associated with the complex.

Techniques available to detect immune complexes deposited in or on tissues are simple and are superior to the procedures used to monitor them in body fluids. Frozen tissue sections are incubated with fluorescent-labeled antisera to human immunoglobulin or complement, and are then examined microscopically. Tests for circulating immune complexes are based on the distinct properties of complexed immunoglobulin molecules compared with free antibody, including physical characteristics (high molecular weight and changes in solubility) and biological properties (ability to react with complement components and cell receptors). However, all of these methods are subject to interference by substances other than immune complexes, and none can differentiate between true complexes and non-specifically aggregated immunoglobulins (caused, for example, by incorrect storage of sera or repeated freezing and thawing of samples). Erythrocyte binding of immune complexes is usually ignored. Despite this, a number of tests (C1q binding assays, precipitation of complexes with polyethylene glycol, and binding to Raji cell – a lymphocyte cell line – receptors), do distinguish pathological from normal sera.

ACUTE PHASE REACTANTS

The complex series of reactions that occurs in the body following local tissue injury or systemic infection are known as acute phase responses. An increase in the synthesis of acute phase proteins or reactants by the liver is a major feature of the systemic reaction. These proteins constitute a heterogeneous group. Their functional role is surmised on the basis of their normal functions, such as opsonization, anti-protease activity and the ability to scavenge free radicals.

In humans, the acute phase proteins can be divided into four broad groups, based on those proteins whose concentrations:

1. increase by about 50%, e.g. the third component of complement and ceruloplasmin;
2. increase by two to four-fold, e.g. alpha-1 acid glycoprotein, fibrinogen, alpha-1 antitrypsin;
3. increase by several hundred-fold, e.g. C-reactive protein (CRP) and serum amyloid A (SAA);
4. decrease, e.g. albumin and transferrin.

Determination of the concentrations of the acute phase proteins is important in the diagnosis and monitoring of disease processes, for example in rheumatoid arthritis, lupus erythematosus, and chronic infection. Methods of detection and quantitation of the individual reactants are all based on immunological reactions, such as ELISA, RIA, radial immunodiffusion and rocket immunoelectrophoresis.

COMPLEMENT

The complement system, consisting of 18 plasma proteins, mediates a variety of inflammatory effects, including bacteriolysis. The classic activation pathway of complement is triggered primarily by immune complexes formed between IgG or IgM antibodies and their antigens. The individual components of the system are synthesized mainly by the liver, and their synthesis appears to be linked to the acute phase response.

The most frequent complement abnormalities in patients are elevated levels in association with the acute phase response. However, other abnormalities include genetic conditions in which a component or regulatory factor is either not synthesized at all, or is produced at sub-normal levels; conditions in which hypercatabolism occurs; and conditions where structurally defective and therefore functionally inert proteins are synthesized. Sub-normal levels of complement components can also occur because of depletion by immune complexes *in vivo*.

Complement levels can be determined either by functional assays which measure the activity of groups of components, or by immunochemical assays which measure concentrations of individual components or fragments. The latter assays do not differentiate between active and inactive protein. Commonly used methods include the total hemolytic complement assay (which measures the ability of the test sample to lyse 50% of a standard suspension of sheep erythrocytes coated with rabbit antibody), nephelometric assays (which measure the increase in intensity of light scatter on formation of antigen–antibody complexes), and radial immunodiffusion techniques.

LYMPHOKINES

When mononuclear leukocytes are activated by mitogens or antigens, they produce a range of soluble mediators that affect or regulate the activities of other cells. These are collectively known as lymphokines, and their actions may be stimulatory or inhibitory. They act on diverse cell types, ranging from other cells of the immune system to hepatocytes, bone marrow cells and fibroblasts. These mediators include macrophage colony-stimulating factor (M-CSF or CSF-1), granulocyte colony-stimulating factor (G-CSF or CSF-β), tumor necrosis factor (cachectin), lymphotoxin, interferon and interleukins 1–13 (IL-1–13). This bewildering array of lymphokines can be simplified by classification into broad categories based on the putative cellular origin and distribution of specific receptors, e.g. IL-1 and IL-6 are predominantly synthesized by monocytes and have multiple effects on cells throughout the body, whereas IL-2, IL-3 and IL-4 are released predominantly by lymphocytes and affect mainly lymphocytes and other cells of the immune system. Further complexities may be developed with the sub-division of CD4+ helper T cells into TH_1(IL-2) and TH_2 (IL-4, IL-6, IL-10) (Chapter 28).

The systemic and local levels of lymphokines appear to be important. Abnormal concentrations have been associated with several diseases. IL-6 is raised in the serum of patients with malaria, in synovial fluids during active rheumatoid arthritis, in urine during rejection of renal allografts and in psoriatic skin. Serum interferon-gamma is decreased in lepromatous leprosy and AIDS. The measurement of lymphokines in patients may help explain underlying immunopathogenetic mechanisms. Lymphokines can be measured in biological fluids, such as serum, plasma and urine, which may reflect the levels (or spill-over effects) of the proteins *in vivo*. However, it is also possible to examine the ability of cells to synthesize the lymphokines *in vitro*. This may provide information on the regulation of lymphokine production, and on the functional integrity and state of 'activation' of the cells tested.

Bioassays measure the actual biological activity of the mediator. IL-1 assays measure the proliferation of thymocytes, or the production of IL-2 by a cell line, in response to IL-1. However, many natural inhibitors of lymphokines have been detected and, if present, would result in no active mediator being measured. In these cases, immunoassays, such as RIAs or ELISAs, are utilized, measuring immunologically active lymphokine irrespective of the presence of inhibitors.

GENETIC ENGINEERING AND MOLECULAR BIOLOGY

Over the past decade, a series of techniques evolving from basic molecular biology and variously referred to as genetic engineering, gene cloning or recombinant DNA technology have revolutionized the biological sciences, and biomedical research is no exception. Genetic engineering is 'the introduction of manipulated genetic material into a cell in such a way that it is replicated and passed on to progeny cells'.

The essential methods of recombinant DNA technology involve isolating nucleic acids, cutting these into variously sized pieces, amplifying sections of interest after recognition by specific probes, and then rejoining the pieces in new constructs, which are then inserted into mammalian cells, yeasts, bacteria or viruses.

The tools of this form of 'engineering' are bacterial enzymes. Polymerases use one strand of DNA as a template to synthesize DNA (replication) or RNA (transcription). Cellular mRNA may be used as a template to synthesize complementary DNA (cDNA) with the enzyme reverse transcriptase (RNA-dependent DNA polymerase). Restriction endonucleases are molecular scissors that cut DNA at specific 4–6-nucleotide recognition sequences, and ligases are enzymes that join (splice) severed fragments together again.

The basic steps involved in gene cloning include (Fig. 29.3):

1. Obtaining the specific piece of DNA (usually a gene or fragment thereof).
2. Insertion of this DNA into a suitable **vector** (a vehicle for replication and/or expression).
3. Return of the modified DNA to cells; so-called **transformation** if it is introduced into bacteria, or **transfection** if it is inserted into mammalian cells.
4. Selection of the appropriate **transformants** or **transfectants.**

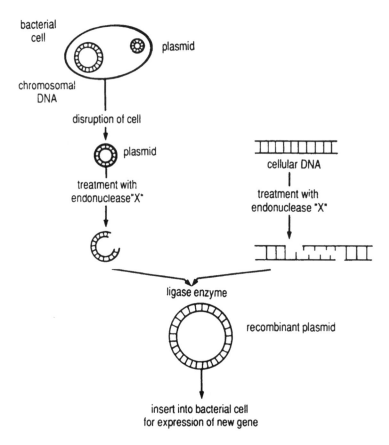

Figure 29.3 DNA Cloning. Cellular (chromosomal) DNA is cleaved with restriction endonucleases into various fragments, which can be recombined in various combinations and inserted into a plasmid (cut with the same restriction enzymes) by use of a ligase enzyme. The recombinant plasmid is then introduced into a bacterial cell (which becomes 'transformed'), which allows amplification of the recombinant DNA and/or expression of the DNA-encoded protein.

GENE CLONING

The first step is the most difficult, as the desired piece of DNA must be located within the cellular DNA and isolated. One approach to this problem involves searching for the desired DNA in a collection (or 'library') of genes or gene fragments. There are two types of libraries: **genomic** and **complementary DNA (cDNA)** libraries.

The first is constructed by cutting the entire genomic DNA of a suitable cell or tissue with a restriction enzyme (such as Eco R1 or Hind III), and inserting all the resulting fragments into bacterial **plasmids** (small, independently replicating, extrachromosomal, circular DNA molecules) or bacterial viruses **(phages)**, and then into bacterial cells (Fig. 29.3). This collection of DNA, cut into fragments and cloned into bacterial cells, is called a 'genomic library'. Each resulting bacterial colony then carries a different DNA insert (one of hundreds of thousands or millions), among which is the genomic sequence of interest.

The second type of library, or cDNA library, consists of DNA copies of all the mRNAs present in a particular cell, tissue, or organ. Unlike a genomic library, which consists of **all** the DNA making up the genome of an organism, cDNA libraries differ from tissue to tissue, because each tissue, or cell type, expresses a unique set of mRNAs that code for a specific set of proteins expressed in that cell type. Moreover, the DNA copies of these mRNAs (the cDNAs) represent the complete coding sequences for proteins (so-called exon sequences) without the often long and essentially non-coding intron sequences found in the genes (i.e. in the chromosomes).

Once a library has been constructed, it is 'screened' by using a suitable 'probe' that will identify the gene of interest. The probe is commonly either a nucleic acid or an antibody. **Nucleic acid probes** can be genes or fragments of genes homologous to the gene of interest, or short oligonucleotides synthesized on the basis of the codon usage for the amino acid sequence of the protein encoded by the gene of interest. In either event, the nucleic acid probe is radiolabeled and it then acts as a homing device or tracer by binding ('hybridizing') to the complementary (opposite) strand of the gene of interest.

Antibody probes can be used when a cDNA library is constructed in a vector (either phage or plasmid) that allows expression of the proteins encoded by the cDNA inserts, and therefore the cDNA of interest (i.e. the gene) can be isolated by detecting its protein product with an enzyme-linked antibody specific to that protein. Whichever type of probe is used, thousands of individual, unique clones within the library are screened, either in the form of bacterial colonies (plasmid vectors) or lysis plaques (phage vectors). Once identified, the desired DNA is isolated and transferred (sub-cloned) into a vector that facilitates subsequent manipulations, such as sequencing or expression of the encoded protein product.

GENE EXPRESSION

A variety of methods are available for introducing DNA into mammalian cells: calcium phosphate co-precipitation, DEAE–dextran electroporation, cell–cell fusion, and microinjection. If all the requirements are met (suitable promoters, enhancers and other regulatory regions), gene expression can occur. One step further than this is the introduction of a cloned piece of DNA into a fertilized egg, with subsequent growth of the embryo to birth, thereby creating a transgenic animal or plant. Successful incorporation of the DNA into the germ line can later be determined by analysis of genomic DNA in the offspring. Promoter constraints are the major limiting factor here and expression of proteins in the transgenic organism may be sporadic and unpredictable.

GENE DETECTION

A commonly used method in molecular biology is the **Southern blot**, named after the scientist, Ed Southern, who first described this technique. DNA is isolated, digested using sequence-specific restriction endonucleases, separated by electrophoresis, and transferred from the agarose gel to a nitrocellulose or nylon filter. It is then incubated with a specific radiolabeled DNA probe, which binds to target DNA of interest (Fig. 29.4). This allows detection of a gene in a genome and estimation of the number of copies present. A Northern blot is essentially a Southern blot except it involves the separation and detection of RNA, rather than DNA.

An application of Southern blotting is in the detection of **restriction fragment length polymorphisms (RFLPs)**. This refers to variations **(polymorphisms)** in the length of DNA fragments generated by cutting chromosomal DNA from numerous individuals with one or more restriction enzymes. These variations or polymorphisms exist because between homologous chromosomes there is a difference in sequence every 200 to 500 base pairs, which would equal about 1 million differences, on average, between each pair of homologous chromosomes. Variations in DNA sequence result in loss or gain of specific restriction enzyme cutting sites (so-called restriction sites) and also in insertions or deletions of short stretches of DNA. A consequence of these differences is the length of fragments generated by cleaving chromosomal DNA with a specific restriction enzyme, depending on whether a specific restriction site is present or absent. Of course, cutting total human DNA with one or more restriction enzymes results in millions of fragments, and therefore the specificity of RFLP analysis derives from the use of labeled probes in a Southern blotting procedure. The probe is a short stretch of DNA (up to a few hundred base pairs in length) that is complementary to, and therefore hybridizes to (recognizes), a stretch of human DNA on a chromosome (the probe may be part of a previously isolated gene). If, in the vicinity of the probe, there is a variation in DNA sequence resulting in a change of a restriction site or loss or gain or an inserted sequence, then cutting the DNA with an appropriate restriction enzyme, separating the fragments by size by agarose gel electrophoresis, and probing the fragments with the radiolabeled probe (by Southern blotting) will show different restriction fragment lengths for different individuals (Fig. 29.4). Hence the term restriction fragment length polymorphisms (polymorphism means 'many forms'). These sequence variations can occur within genes or between genes. In fact, in most cases they are between genes because only about 5% of the DNA in the total human genome is comprised of genes (sequences coding for specific proteins or RNA molecules). The positions of these variations on chromosomes are referred to as genetic loci, and the variations are also called alleles. The greater the number of alleles at a locus, the greater the usefulness of this locus as a genetic marker.

Using hundreds of different combinations of probes and restriction enzymes, thousands of RFLPs have been identified, many of them useful genetic markers. These markers are enormously useful in diagnosing genetic diseases and indeed have contributed substantially to the isolation of unknown disease genes in conditions such as cystic fibrosis, muscular dystrophy and Huntington's disease, and more recently cancer states.

POLYMERASE CHAIN REACTION (PCR)

PCR is the most recent and spectacular addition to the arsenal of recombinant DNA methods. It is an ingenious procedure that enables greater than a million-fold amplification of vanishingly small amounts of DNA.

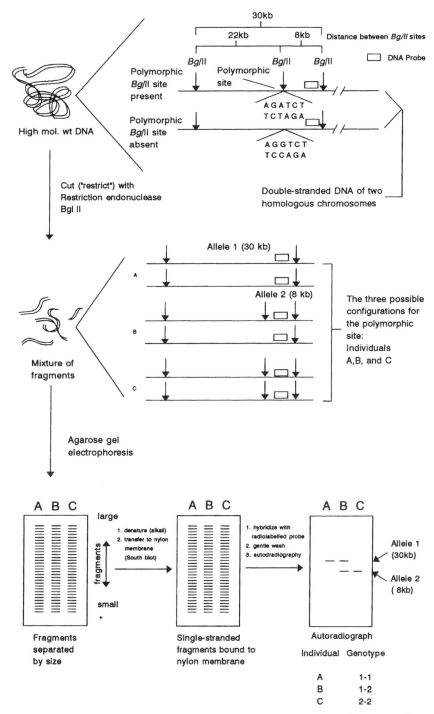

Figure 29.4 The technique of Southern blotting and its use in the detection of restriction fragment length polymorphisms (RFLPs). See text for details.

307

PCR rests on a few simple principles. DNA is a double-stranded molecule. Each strand can serve as a template for synthesis of the complementary strand by the enzyme DNA polymerase. Before DNA polymerase can initiate DNA synthesis it requires a primer, i.e. a short sequence of DNA complementary to the template strand, such that initiation of DNA synthesis begins at a stretch of double-stranded DNA. Based on these principles, the PCR method works as follows (Fig. 29.5).

(a) The starting material is double-stranded DNA.

(b) The strands are separated by heating (typically to 94°C) to generate single-stranded DNA templates (step 1). The DNA is then cooled to between 50 and 60°C to allow short, single-stranded oligonucleotides (typically about 20 nucleotides in length) called primers to bind to sites at the end of the target sequence, one on each strand (step 2). Note that the primers bind because they are complementary in sequence to the target sequence, such that the primer that binds to the -ve (antisense) strand (primer 1) has a sequence identical to that of the stretch of complementary DNA on the +ve (sense) strand, and vice versa for the primer that binds to the +ve strand (primer 2).

(c) DNA polymerase synthesizes new strands of DNA starting from the primers, complementary to the template, extending a variable distance beyond the position of the primer binding site on the other template (step 3).

(d) The mixture is heated again to separate the strands; after cooling, primers once again bind to both the original strands and to the two new strands (repeat of steps 1 and 2).

(e) DNA polymerase again synthesizes new strands (repeat of step 3); extension of the strands complementary to the newly synthesized strands produced in (c) is limited precisely to the target sequence. Thus in this step, two of the four newly synthesized strands span exactly the region specified by the primers.

(f) Steps 1 to 3 are repeated for 25 to 40 cycles until the target sequence has been amplified over a million-fold.

Note that with every cycle the number of newly synthesized strands increases exponentially such that the original template strands become vanishingly rare, and the overwhelming proportion of PCR-generated DNA molecules are precisely bounded by the region specified by the primers.

Note also that there is no requirement for addition of fresh DNA polymerase after every cycle. Although the reaction mixture is heated to 94°C during every cycle, a special thermostable DNA polymerase has been identified, called Taq polymerase, from the bacterium *Thermus aquaticus* that grows in hot springs; this polymerase is not denatured by temperatures up to 100°C.

If the introduction of molecular biology and recombinant DNA methods into biomedical science and medicine is regarded as a revolution, then PCR is a revolution within a revolution. It has accelerated enormously the pace of molecular and genetic research by enabling the retrieval and analysis of DNA that is present in such small amounts that previously it could not even be detected. The method has already spilled over into clinical application, such as in detecting mutant genes in genetic diseases, and in detecting pathogen-specific DNA from bacteria such as *M. tuberculosis*, and viruses such as HBV, HCV and HIV which are frequently difficult to detect by conventional means.

CONTRIBUTION OF MOLECULAR BIOLOGY TO MEDICINE

The introduction of molecular biology and the

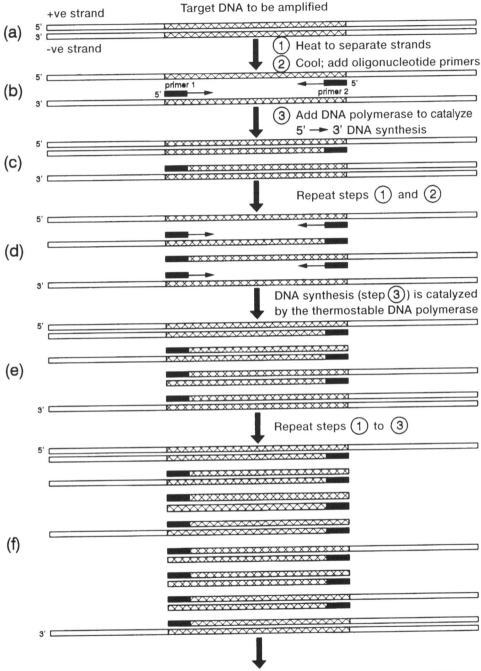

(a) +ve strand / Target DNA to be amplified
-ve strand

① Heat to separate strands
② Cool; add oligonucleotide primers

(b) primer 1 / primer 2

③ Add DNA polymerase to catalyze 5' → 3' DNA synthesis

(c)

Repeat steps ① and ②

(d)

DNA synthesis (step ③) is catalyzed by the thermostable DNA polymerase

(e)

Repeat steps ① to ③

(f)

After 25 cycles, the target DNA has been amplified about 1 million-fold

Figure 29.5 The polymerase chain reaction (PCR). See text for explanatory notes. The circled numbers represent the 'steps' referred to in the text.

application of recombinant DNA methods in biomedical research has resulted in an exponential growth of knowledge in the past two decades which has led us to an unprecedented depth and precision of understanding of human physiology and disease. We are finally in a position where many of the previously inscrutable processes in medicine can be cracked open and exposed, and now as never before rational treatments can be devised for human diseases. Not only are more and more diseases being unraveled in molecular and genetic terms, but already trials are underway in the USA and Europe to correct serious diseases by gene therapy, that is, by correcting the underlying gene defect. For many of the most serious diseases plaguing mankind, including diabetes, heart disease, cancer and mental illnesses, the prospects are at hand for a real and lasting cure as opposed to only partial and symptomatic treatments. The significance of this cannot be overstated. Indeed these developments will bring us to the next great era in medicine, namely the era of molecular medicine. The impact of molecular biology on the practice of medicine in the early 21st century will be as great as, if not greater than, the impact of anesthetics and modern surgical techniques in the late 19th century and antibiotics in the mid 20th century.

CONCLUSION

It is hoped that this review has provided a basis for understanding these principles and techniques and a desire to learn more about them. Readers are referred to the list of recommended reading for further, more detailed information.

RECOMMENDED READING

Barnett, E. (1986) Circulating immune complexes: their biologic and clinical significance. *J Allergy Clin Immunol*, **78**, 1089–96.

Caskey, C.T. and Cournoyer, D. (1993) Gene therapy of the immune system. *Annu Rev Immunol*, **11**, 297–329.

Catty, D. (ed.) (1989) Antibodies. *A practical approach*, IRL Press, Oxford.

Davis, L., Dibner, M. and Battey, J. (1986) *Basic Methods in Molecular Biology*, Elsevier, New York.

Gardner, E.J., Simmons, M.J. and Snustad, D.P. (1991) *Principles of Genetics*, 8th edn, John Wiley, New York.

Hamblin, A. (1988) *Lymphokines*, IRL Press, Oxford.

Hudson, L. and Hay, F. (1989) *Practical Immunology*, 3rd edn, Blackwell Scientific Publications, London.

McMichael, A. and Fabre, J. (eds) (1982) *Monoclonal Antibodies in Clinical Medicine*, Academic Press, London.

Van der Valk, P. and Herman, C.J. (1987) Biology of disease: leucocyte function. *Lab Invest*, **56**, 127–37.

Walker, J.M. and Gingold, E.B. (1988) *Molecular Biology and Biotechnology*, 2nd edn, Royal Society of Chemistry, London.

Watson, J.D., Gilman, M., Witkowski, J. and Soller, M. (1992) *Recombinant DNA*, 2nd edn, Scientific American Books, New York.

Index

Page numbers in **bold** type refer to figures; those in *italic* type refer to tables